Eat
Right
Your For 4
Baby

Titles by Dr. Peter J. D'Adamo with Catherine Whitney

Eat Right 4 Your Type: The Individualized Diet Solution to
Staying Healthy, Living Longer, and Achieving Your Ideal Weight

Cook Right 4 Your Type: The Practical Kitchen Companion
to Eat Right 4 Your Type

Live Right 4 Your Type: The Individualized Prescription for
Maximizing Health, Metabolism, and Vitality
in Every Stage of Your Life

Eat Right 4 Your Type Complete Blood Type Encyclopedia

Eat Right for Your Baby: The Individualized Guide to Fertility and Maximum Health
During Pregnancy, Nursing, and Your Baby's First Year

Blood Type O: Food, Beverage and Supplement Lists

Blood Type A: Food, Beverage and Supplement Lists

Blood Type B: Food, Beverage and Supplement Lists

Blood Type AB: Food, Beverage and Supplement Lists

Cancer: Fight It with the Blood Type Diet

Diabetes: Fight It with the Blood Type Diet

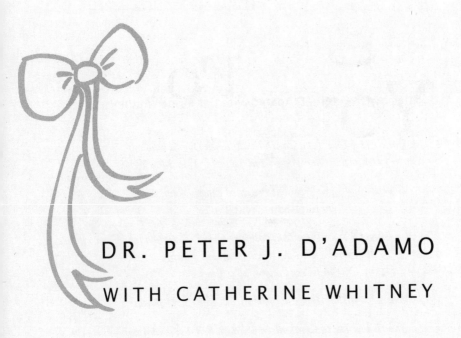

DR. PETER J. D'ADAMO

WITH CATHERINE WHITNEY

BERKLEY BOOKS
NEW YORK

Eat Right For Your Baby

THE INDIVIDUALIZED GUIDE TO FERTILITY AND MAXIMUM HEALTH DURING PREGNANCY, NURSING, AND YOUR BABY'S FIRST YEAR

A Berkley Book
Published by The Berkley Publishing Group
A division of Penguin Group (USA) Inc.
375 Hudson Street
New York, New York 10014

PRINTING HISTORY
G. P. Putnam's Sons hardcover edition / March 2003
Berkley trade paperback edition / July 2004

Berkley trade paperback ISBN: 0-425-19614-3

The Library of Congress has catalogued the G. P. Putnam's Sons
hardcover as follows:

D'Adamo, Peter J.
    Eat right 4 your baby : the individualized guide to fertility and
maximum health during pregnancy, nursing, and your baby's first
year / by Peter J. D'Adamo with Catherine Whitney.
        p.   cm.
    Includes index.
    ISBN 0-399-14996-1
    1. Pregnancy—Nutritional aspects.   2. Prenatal care.   3. Moth-
ers—Nutrition.   I. Title: Eat right for your baby.   II. Whitney,
Catherine (Catherine A.).   III. Title.
RG559.D334   2003   2002031714
618.2'4—dc21

PRINTED IN THE UNITED STATES OF AMERICA

10   9   8   7   6   5   4   3   2   1

ACKNOWLEDGMENTS

I AM PARTICULARLY DELIGHTED to introduce *Eat Right 4 (for) Your Baby*, a book I have wanted to write since Martha and I gave birth to our first child almost twelve years ago. Today, Martha and I are the parents of two healthy daughters. I have discovered such a deep wellspring of joy in my spirited, happy children that I feel tremendous compassion for the couples who come to me with their myriad problems—couples who are striving to attain the same experiences that have become the cornerstones of my life. With this book I am able to offer the best that naturopathic and blood type science have to offer, to guide parents-to-be through the most significant journey of their lives.

This effort has been a collaborative process, and I want to express my deep thanks to the people who have been involved in its creation.

I am most grateful to Martha Mosko D'Adamo, not only my partner in life and in parenting but also my partner in bringing the valuable wisdom about blood type to the world. Martha daily provides love, support, insight, and inspiration to all of my endeavors.

Catherine Whitney, my writer, and her partner, Paul Krafin, are invaluable word masters, who have once again captured exactly the right tone in tackling this sensitive topic. Their agent, Jane Dystel, continues to provide advice and encouragement.

I would also like to acknowledge others who have made significant contributions to this book: my colleague Bronner Handwerger, N.D., whose research and clinical abilities helped make this book comprehensive and practical; my friend Cathy Rogers, N.D., a naturopath/midwife whose compassion and understanding of the emotional and medical concerns of pregnant women has added a wonderful element to this book; and my associate Heidi Merritt, who continues to make an important contribution to the work.

My literary agent and friend, Janis Vallely, always takes time to listen and advise. Her quiet guidance and personal support make the work possible.

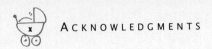

Amy Hertz, my editor at Riverhead/Putnam, has been the force behind the success of all the blood type books, and she continues to guide my work with dedication and skill.

As always, I am extremely grateful to the wonderful staffs at Riverhead Books and Putnam. They have been tireless and enthusiastic, and their efforts have made it possible to continue bringing this important work to the market.

PETER J. D'ADAMO, N.D.

CONTENTS

Introduction: A Personal Word from Martha D'Adamo   1

1 Blood Type and Fertility: A Vital Connection   5
A Question of Compatibility   5
Not for Women Only   8
Why Diet Matters   9
The Genetic Power of Blood Type   10
The Rh Factor   11
Eat Right for Your Baby   12

2 Your Pregnancy: A Naturopathic Primer   15
Get Started *Before* You're Pregnant   15
    Pre-pregnancy Checklist   16
    Detoxification Guidelines   17
    A Word to Dad   18
Your Pregnancy: The Three Trimesters   20
    First Trimester Basics   20
       Common First Trimester Conditions   20
          Morning sickness and nausea   20
          Mood swings   21
          Constipation   21
          Fatigue   22
          Food aversions and cravings   22
       Prenatal Supplements   23
          Medications to avoid during pregnancy   24
          Herbs to avoid during pregnancy   24
       Exercise Guidelines   25
          Exercise caution   26
    Second Trimester Basics   26
       Common Second Trimester Conditions   26
          Allergies   26

          Bleeding gums/nosebleeds 26

          Blood sugar imbalance 27

          Hemorrhoids and varicose veins 27

      Exercise Guidelines 27

   Third Trimester Basics 28

      Common Third Trimester Conditions 30

          Lack of appetite 30

          Constipation 30

          Edema 30

          Shortness of breath/fatigue 30

          Indigestion and heartburn 30

          High blood pressure 30

          Urinary tract infections 31

      Exercise Guidelines 31

      Dads Take Note: Stress and Weight Gain 31

Labor and Delivery Basics 32

3 The Type O Pregnancy   37

The Type O Diet 37

Before You Get Pregnant 52

   Pre-pregnancy Diet Strategies 53

   Pre-pregnancy Supplement Guidelines 56

   Improve Your Emotional Health 57

   Pre-pregnancy Exercise Guidelines 58

Your Pregnancy: Type O Three-Trimester Plan 59

   Diet Strategies 59

      First Trimester 59

      Second Trimester 69

      Third Trimester 77

   Exercise Guidelines 85

   Supplement Guidelines 89

Labor and Delivery 93

4 The Type A Pregnancy   95

The Type A Diet 95

Before You Get Pregnant 110

   Pre-pregnancy Diet Strategies 111

   Pre-pregnancy Supplement Guidelines 112

   Improve Your Emotional Health 114

   Pre-pregnancy Exercise Guidelines 115

Your Pregnancy: Type A Three-Trimester Plan   116
    Diet Strategies   116
        First Trimester   116
        Second Trimester   126
        Third Trimester   135
    Exercise Guidelines   143
    Supplement Guidelines   148
Labor and Delivery   151

5 The Type B Pregnancy   153
The Type B Diet   153
Before You Get Pregnant   168
    Pre-pregnancy Diet Strategies   168
    Pre-pregnancy Supplement Guidelines   172
    Improve Your Emotional Health   173
    Pre-pregnancy Exercise Guidelines   173
Your Pregnancy: Type B Three-Trimester Plan   174
    Diet Strategies   174
        First Trimester   174
        Second Trimester   184
        Third Trimester   194
    Exercise Guidelines   203
    Supplement Guidelines   207
Labor and Delivery   211

6 The Type AB Pregnancy   213
The Type AB Diet   213
Before You Get Pregnant   228
    Pre-pregnancy Diet Strategies   228
    Pre-pregnancy Supplement Guidelines   231
    Improve Your Emotional Health   232
    Pre-pregnancy Exercise Guidelines   232
Your Pregnancy: Type AB Three-Trimester Plan   233
    Diet Strategies   233
        First Trimester   233
        Second Trimester   243
        Third Trimester   253
    Exercise Guidelines   261
    Supplement Guidelines   264
Labor and Delivery   268

7 The "Fourth" Trimester (After the Birth)   269
   Easing Postpartum Discomfort   269
   Handling Postpartum "Blues" and Depression   270
   Getting Back into Shape   271
   The Type O Mother   271
   The Type A Mother   275
   The Type B Mother   279
   The Type AB Mother   282

8 A Healthy Start for Baby   287
   Breast-feeding Diet Strategies   287
       All Blood Types   288
       Type O Mother—Breast-feeding Power Foods   292
       Type A Mother—Breast-feeding Power Foods   292
       Type B Mother—Breast-feeding Power Foods   293
       Type AB Mother—Breast-feeding Power Foods   293
   Starting Solids—All Blood Types   294

9 The Type O Baby   297
   Type O Baby Health Issues   297
   Type O Remedies for Common Conditions   297
       Food Allergies   297
       Gastric Distress   297
       Diarrhea   298
       Ear Infections   299
       Diaper Rash   299
       Restlessness/Hyperactivity   299
   The Type O Baby Diet   299
       Type O Beneficial Baby Foods—First Year   300
       Type O Avoid Baby Foods—First Year   301

10 The Type A Baby   303
   Type A Baby Health Issues   303
   Type A Remedies for Common Conditions   303
       Ear Infections/Overproduction of Mucus   303
       Colds and Congestion   303
       Eczema-like Skin Rashes   304
       Colic   304
       Diarrhea   304
       Diaper Rash   304

Restlessness/Sleep Problems 305
The Type A Baby Diet 305
Type A Beneficial Baby Foods—First Year 305
Type A Avoid Baby Foods—First Year 307

11 The Type B Baby   309

Type B Baby Health Issues 309
Type B Remedies for Common Conditions 309
Respiratory/Ear Infections 309
Food Allergies 310
Diarrhea 310
Diaper Rash 310
Restlessness/Hyperactivity 310
The Type B Baby Diet 310
Type B Beneficial Baby Foods—First Year 311
Type B Avoid Baby Foods—First Year 312

12 The Type AB Baby   315

Type AB Baby Health Issues 315
Type AB Remedies for Common Conditions 315
Ear Infections/Overproduction of Mucus 315
Colds and Congestion 315
Diarrhea 316
Diaper Rash 316
The Type AB Baby Diet 316
Type AB Beneficial Baby Foods—First Year 316
Type AB Avoid Baby Foods—First Year 318

Appendix A

Blood Type Friendly Recipes for Mom and Baby   321
For Mom 321
For Baby 411

Appendix B

Resources and Products   417

Index   423
A Final Note   431

INTRODUCTION

A Personal Word from Martha D'Adamo

BLOOD TYPE AND BABIES are two realities that have forever changed my life. Blood type came first, in 1985, when I met Peter D'Adamo. He transformed the way I viewed food and, in the process, transformed who I was as an individual. Babies arrived later—Claudia in 1991 and Emily in 1994.

When we decided to start our family, Peter and I had the same concerns every other young couple has—could we conceive, would our child be healthy, would we be good parents? As we looked forward to the future, we also looked back into our family histories for information that would be helpful.

Although our backgrounds were very different, neither of us had family histories of troubled pregnancies, births, or miscarriages. Further, we knew our blood types—I am Type O and Peter is Type A. This gave us important information about our genetic profiles, as well as a basis for establishing nutritional needs. What we didn't know was what we would actually experience. Every couple is unique, every pregnancy is different, and every baby is unlike any other baby that came before.

I was lucky that my mother was still alive during both my pregnancies. I pestered her with questions about her pregnancies unmercifully, until one day she said, "When I was having all my children, I went to the doctor, he told me to drink lots of fluids—it didn't matter what, just that it was fluid. He said when I started to have contractions, get to the hospital. I went to the hospital, they knocked me out, and when I woke up, I had a baby."

This was a stunning example of how things have changed so dramatically in the world of obstetrics. In the fifties, most obstetricians were men, and the system seemed to be set up to accommodate them rather than their pregnant patients. Women were rarely encouraged to ask questions about their pregnancies and about all the changes they were experiencing. Little or no nutritional guidance was provided. Nor was there much attention given to toxic behaviors like smoking or alcohol consumption—issues that are well understood today. Breast-feeding had become déclassé, as the development of formula was heralded as "better than mother can provide" and more convenient.

Today we live in a vastly different environment. Pregnancy, birth, and women's health in general are getting more attention than ever before. Maternity centers in major hospitals are "patient-centered" with birthing rooms, labor tubs, midwife consultants, doula referrals, childbirth educators, and in-house lactation consultants. Nutritional support, stress reduction techniques, exercise programs, and a host of natural remedies for pregnancy-related conditions are widely available.

I was very fortunate with both my pregnancies, since Peter was there to serve as my loving and supportive husband as well as my in-house medical consultant. My midwives were open to incorporating naturopathic and blood type–related practices into my pregnancy and birth plans. For my first pregnancy, Peter helped me work out a nutritional plan to support each trimester, and he recommended an exercise and supplement program that enhanced the diet. We made refinements for the second pregnancy based on what we'd learned.

We didn't realize it at the time but Peter was actually creating the template for *Eat Right 4 (for) Your Baby*. What you will find as you read through the book are the dietary, exercise, and supplement guidelines that we used for both my pregnancies, adapted for the four blood types. refined to include the wisdom that came from our experiences.

I was also fortunate during my two pregnancies to have our good friend, Dr. Cathy Rogers, as my long-distance midwifery consultant. Cathy is a naturopath/midwife who organized the Seattle Midwifery School and has been a leader in the field of naturopathy for twenty-four years. Cathy was invaluable in guiding me through the physical preparation for birth, postpartum issues, and nursing. Every year as I celebrate Claudia's and Emily's birthdays, I recall the phone calls with Cathy, tracking the contractions, making suggestions to ease the discomfort of labor, her nursing suggestions, and her calm and gentle guidance as I made the shift into new motherhood. She was such a wonderful support for both of us that Peter and I decided to incorporate her wisdom into *Eat Right 4 (for) Your Baby*.

The journey to conception, pregnancy, birth, and motherhood is wondrous and mysterious. For some women it occurs without complications, and for others it is a challenging, frustrating, and a sometimes deeply disappointing experience. By utilizing the key concepts of blood type diet, we are able to strengthen our overall health and optimize our genetic individuality. Although this won't guarantee a trouble-free pregnancy, it will assist in the best of all possible outcomes— increased energy levels, appropriate weight gain during pregnancy and loss of the weight afterward, and an overall enhanced sense of well-being. As Peter often says, the blood type information is a way of zeroing in on the exact health and nutrition information that corresponds to your biological profile. Armed with this new information, you can make choices about your diet, exercise regimen, and general health that are based on the dynamic natural forces within your own body.

In *Eat Right 4 (for) Your Baby,* he custom-tailors this concept to address all the health and physical issues that are present during pregnancy, birth, postpartum, and the first months of your baby's life. By supporting these dietary recommendations with the most current naturopathic and midwifery advice, he has created a primer for women who are in all the various stages of the childbearing years and who are committed to having the best of all possible pregnancies and raising strong, healthy children.

Our children are the greatest gifts in our lives, and there's no better gift we can give them than a healthy start in life that celebrates and supports their individuality. The blood type diet is an invaluable tool in bringing them into the world, and it provides the legacy of optimum health and well-being as they grow and develop.

Peter and I have grown tremendously because of our children. They have brought joy, love, and an expansive quality into our lives that touches everything we do. *Eat Right 4 (for) Your Baby* represents not only good science and the evolution of the blood type diet, but also the "on the job" training we received as we became new parents. I hope as you read this book you will find the guidance, support, and wisdom that will assist you on your journey to becoming a parent.

MARTHA MOSKO D'ADAMO

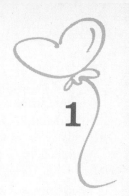

Blood Type and Fertility:
A Vital Connection

EARLY IN MY PRACTICE AS A NATUROPATH, I discovered, almost by co-incidence, that when my female patients followed the correct diet for their blood type, fertility increased dramatically. Even women with long-standing fertility problems, including repeated miscarriages, were able to conceive and carry their babies to term.

It wasn't immediately apparent why this was so. Just a couple of decades ago, our overall understanding of genetics was still fairly limited. Like so many discoveries, observation predated the explanation. Today, we have the knowledge to explain what once appeared to be simply a happy phenomenon. I am now able to predict with some degree of accuracy which of my patients will have problems conceiving, and am able to offer blood type–specific guidelines that effectively overcome those problems. It has been one of the more gratifying aspects of my work.

A Question of Compatibility

Rachel and Eric were typical of many couples who come to my clinic. I first met with them in July 1993, after they had tried for almost ten years to have a child. During that time, Rachel had become pregnant twelve times. But each hopeful beginning had ended in a devastating miscarriage within the first two months. For the last couple of years, Rachel and Eric had been treated by a physician who specialized in reproductive health, and Rachel had become pregnant twice more. But again, both pregnancies had ended in miscarriage. At thirty-seven, Rachel was running out of time—and hope.

Rachel initially heard about me from a woman she'd met in her fertility specialist's waiting room. Even though she decided to go ahead and see me, she was clearly skeptical of the concept that making changes in her diet according to her blood type could enhance her fertility. "I don't even know my blood type," she admitted. "But I guess I have nothing to lose."

I began by blood typing Rachel and Eric and found that Rachel was Type O and Eric was Type A. The result wasn't surprising. Research has shown that many of the problems associated with fertility result from some form of blood type incompatibility, either between the mother and her fetus, or between the mother and the father.

Why would this occur? Each blood type is a chemical marker called an antigen. These blood type antigens can act like barriers against foreign intruders, such as bacteria, viruses, and parasites. When our immune system encounters a harmful foreign intruder, it creates antibodies against it. These antibodies serve as an early warning system. The next time the foreign intruder is encountered, it will be attacked and destroyed. The antibodies we make against other blood types are actually induced early in life by bacteria and sometimes by the first foods we eat.

Blood Type O carries anti-A and anti-B antibodies and rejects anything with an A-like or B-like antigen. Type A carries anti-B antibodies, and Type B carries anti-A antibodies. Only Type AB carries no anti-blood type antibodies, which is why Type AB individuals can receive blood transfusions from anybody.

The Antigen-Antibody Dynamic

IF YOU ARE . . .	YOU PRODUCE ANTIBODIES TO . . .
Type O	A and B
Type A	B
Type B	A
Type AB	None

Several studies conducted over the past forty years have concluded that infertility and habitual miscarriage may be the result of antibodies in the woman's vaginal secretions reacting with blood type antigens in the man's sperm. In one of these studies, it was determined that the majority of miscarriages were of Type A or Type B fetuses, caused as the result of incompatibility with Type O mothers who produced anti-A and anti-B antibodies. What seems to be missing in many physicians' understanding of miscarriage is that these anti-blood type antibodies are often the result of provocations produced by eating the wrong foods for one's blood type. These foods act in many ways as a "bad blood transfusion," sensitizing the person against future exposure to foreign blood type antigens—including that of a spouse.

Since Rachel was Type O and Eric was Type A, there was a heightened chance that Eric's sperm could be rejected, although that didn't seem to be the case here, as Rachel was able to repeatedly conceive. More likely, the incompatibility was between Rachel and her fetus, which would occur if the fetus were Type A.

A Type O mother and a Type A father can produce either Type O or Type A offspring—although A is dominant over O. If Rachel's fetus was Type A, blood type incompatibility could not be ruled out as the cause of miscarriage.

The good news is that mixed–blood type parents can have healthy babies, even if they produce antibodies against each other's blood type antigens. How? By creating the properly balanced immune system and minimizing provocations that might compromise it.

Rachel began following the Type O diet, being especially careful to avoid foods that triggered an antigen-antibody reaction. Eric began following the Type A diet, which contributed not only to his overall health, but to the health of his semen. I suggested to Rachel that she follow the protocol for at least six months before trying to conceive.

Ten months after her first visit, Rachel became pregnant again. In her sixth month, she came to see me for a checkup. She looked wonderful. Her mood matched her looks.

"Everything seems to be going well, Doctor," Rachel beamed at me. "I feel good, Eric is ecstatic, and we're both taking it step by step. We've never gotten this far before, so we're just trying to relax and enjoy every second." It was clear that Rachel was thrilled, but she was also very nervous. Now, in addition to her previous miscarriages, she was worried about her age and the possibility of her fetus having Down's syndrome or some other developmental disorder. Her obstetrician recommended amniocentesis, which is common for women over age thirty-five. I advised against it, because the procedure carries a risk of miscarriage, there was not a family history of Down's syndrome, and their religious beliefs had convinced them that any child is a gift from God, so abortion was out of the question. After talking with Eric, Rachel decided to forgo the amniocentesis. In January 1995, Rachel and Eric gave birth to a perfectly healthy baby girl they named Rebecca.

Even though Rebecca was blood Type A, Rachel had been able to create a welcome environment in her womb. Rachel and Eric assured me that they would continue to make the blood type diet a part of their lives—and a part of their daughter's life when she began eating solid food.

Not for Women Only

Naftali is a Blood Type O patient I "inherited" from my dad, who had been his physician since he was a boy in the years following World War II. Naftali had contracted a very high fever either from a viral or bacterial infection when he was young, which had apparently damaged the cells in the testicles responsible for manufacturing sperm. Naftali and his parents are Hasidic Jews originally from Eastern Europe, and the family had very limited medical care immediately after the Holocaust.

Fertility is a big issue in Naftali's community, and as the son of a renowned rabbi, he was expected to produce an heir. Consequently, this caused a lot of stress for him and his wife.

Pious Jews do not easily consent to semen analysis, since semen is viewed as a precious seed. However, when it comes to health, Judaism is a remarkably flexible religion, and after much consultation Naftali was allowed to have his semen analyzed.

Result: Naftali's semen had no sperm in it.

When I began working with him I could only promise to do my best. Naftali's wife had no fertility problems, but would be following the diet for her blood type, which was AB. I began Naftali on the basic Type O diet, plus a few herbal supplements, and he followed it assiduously. Six months later we again tested his semen.

Result: Semen showed one sperm cell, nonmotile (not able to move).

Well, anyone else might have been discouraged, but this man was relentless. If any individual could do the program perfectly, it was Naftali. "One cell!" he exclaimed. "It's working!"

Four months later Naftali came in with the good news that his wife was pregnant, and they have since had another child. I cannot tell you the final results of his sperm count; the rabbis have now decided that since his "seed" is viable, it cannot be tested anymore. Why tell you this story? Because you might think that following the blood type diet is only for females.

But this is not true. Fertility is a joint endeavor.

I'm not trying to give infertile couples unrealistic hopes. Obviously, blood type incompatibility is not the only cause of infertility. Nor does the blood type diet magically resolve all fertility problems. But it's just common sense to approach pregnancy in the optimum state of health. Following a dietary regimen that is geared precisely for your blood type seems an excellent choice for enhancing your system's response to the many stresses involved in bringing a child to full term. And there is no question in my mind that you can minimize the risk of incompatibility with the right diet.

Why Diet Matters

So, what does diet have to do with fertility?

Simply put, there is a chemical reaction between your blood type antigen and the food you eat. That's because the proteins in foods have antigens as well, and these antigens are similar to the blood type antigens. If you eat food that contains a foreign antigen, your immune system will create anti–blood type antibodies to it, and it will be rejected by your system.

These antibody reactions can dramatically affect your health—weakening your immune system, increasing inflammation, disturbing your digestive processes, and upsetting your metabolic balance. They can also be a factor in infertility or miscarriage when a mother and father have opposing blood types or when a mother is carrying a fetus of an opposing blood type.

It stands to reason that the best way to minimize the chances of blood type incompatibility is to eat foods that are right for your blood type and avoid foods that trigger an antibody or antigen reaction. To this day my wife, Martha, credits her easy pregnancies and the delivery of two healthy daughters to the fact that she "lived in the land of the beneficials." That is, she ate the foods that were most beneficial for her blood type.

Ramona, Type B, is a case in point. Ramona was in her early thirties and about 50 pounds overweight. She had been unable to conceive after nearly six years of trying, and I was her last stop on the way to a fertility clinic. In addition to her weight problem, Ramona had problems with recurrent urinary tract infections and persistent allergies. Ramona's husband, Franklin, was Type A, and it appeared that an antibody reaction to his sperm was being exacerbated by Ramona's infections and allergies.

I have found that most of the problems Type Bs have with infections and allergies can be resolved with a change in diet. There is a direct connection between our digestive activity and our immune system. In fact, more than 50 percent of all immune function occurs in our digestive tracts.

Ramona's weight was an impediment to fertility as well. Obesity can disrupt a woman's menstrual cycle, change her hormonal balance, and interfere with fertility. Most of the overweight women I've treated in my practice have histories of menstrual irregularity.

In addition to her excess weight, Ramona's dieting history was a factor. She admitted that during the past ten years she had frequently tried to lose weight by going on extremely low-calorie diets. That was a significant piece of information.

When you go on a very low-calorie diet, you are telling your body not to get pregnant. Nature is very smart. It has endowed us with automatic signals designed to guarantee the survival of our species. One of these is related to nutrition. In times of famine, women's reproductive abilities shut down—nature's way of preventing the growth of a population during a period when mothers do not have the fat stores to nurture more children. Modern women who follow starvation diets are inadvertently triggering that protective signal.

Ramona's challenge was to lose weight in a gradual, healthy way, while also improving her immune function by avoiding foods that made her more vulnerable to allergies and infections. Numerous studies of blood Type B cells have conclusively demonstrated that specific foods caused hemolytic (blood cell–destroying) and allergic reactions—among them chicken, corn, lentils, peanuts, and buckwheat. Not surprisingly, chicken was a staple of Ramona's diet. I created a diet plan for her that would substitute beneficial foods for problem foods—for example, turkey and lean venison instead of chicken, rice instead of wheat, and abundant green vegetables instead of problematic beans. I also encouraged Ramona to begin including daily servings of low-fat dairy foods. Most Type Bs thrive on dairy, and cultured dairy foods such as yogurt and kefir are instrumental in the health of the intestines and the prevention of infections.

I also put Ramona on an exercise program specifically designed for Type B— a combination of moderate aerobic activity and calming exercises such as yoga. This combination has been shown to dramatically reduce stress and promote fitness for Type Bs. Chronic stress itself is a factor in obesity and also interferes with ovulation and fertility.

In my experience, when people follow the blood type diet, they lose weight naturally, without having to significantly lower their calorie levels, and this happened with Ramona. Within six months on the diet she had lost 35 pounds, her allergic symptoms had disappeared, and she had had no further problems with urinary tract infections. She continued on the program, and on the first-year anniversary she and her husband decided she was ready to try conceiving. This time Ramona got pregnant with relative ease. During her pregnancy we continued to adapt the Type B diet to her special needs, and she delivered a healthy baby boy.

Ramona likes to talk about her "miracle baby." I agree that life is a miracle, but I also believe that we have the power to help miracles happen by listening to the wisdom of our bodies.

The Genetic Power of Blood Type

Blood type is the most powerful genetic connection you have with your ancestors and therefore plays a vital role in reproduction. Your blood type is the key to your body's entire immune system. Blood type determines and controls the influence of viruses, bacteria, infections, chemicals, stress, and any other invaders and conditions that might compromise your immune system.

Like the color of your eyes or hair, your blood type is determined by two sets of genes—the inheritance you receive from your mother and father. It is from those genes commingling that your blood type is selected at the moment of your conception. Like genes, some blood types are dominant over others. In the cellular creation of a new human being, the A gene and B gene are dominant over O. If at conception the embryo is given an A gene from the mother and an O gene from the father, the infant's blood will be Type A, although it will continue to carry the father's O gene unexpressed in its DNA. When the infant grows up and passes these genes on to its offspring, half of the genes will be for Type A blood and half will be for Type O blood. Because A and B genes are equally strong, you are Type AB if you received an A gene from one parent, and a B gene from the other. Finally, because the O gene is recessive to all the others, you are Type O only if you receive an O gene from each parent.

It is quite possible for two Type A parents to conceive a child who is Type O. This occurs when the parents each have one A gene and one O gene, and both pass the O gene on to their offspring. In the same way, two brown-eyed parents can conceive a blue-eyed offspring if each carries within them the dormant recessive gene for blue eyes.

Both of my parents are Type A. I presume that I received an A from each parent (making me genotype AA) because my two daughters are both Type A. My wife Martha is Type O and can only have two Os, so it is certain that our daughters are genotypically *AO*.

Blood Type Inheritance

PARENTS' BLOOD TYPES	POSSIBLE BLOOD TYPES OF CHILDREN
Both A	A or O
Both B	B or O
Both AB	A, B, or AB
Both O	O
One A and one B	A, B, AB, or O
One A and one O	A or O
One A and one AB	A, B, or AB
One B and one O	B or O
One B and one AB	A, B, or AB
One AB and one O	A or B

The Rh Factor

When your blood is typed, you also learn whether you are "negative" or "positive." Many people don't realize that this is an additional blood type called the Rhesus or Rh system, and it really has nothing to do with your ABO blood type. However, it has everything to do with reproduction. The Rh system is named for the rhesus monkey, a commonly employed laboratory animal in whose blood it was first discovered. For many years, it remained a mystery to doctors why some women who had normal first pregnancies developed complications in their second and subsequent pregnancies, which often resulted in miscarriage and even the death of the mother. In 1940, the mystery was solved by Dr. Karl Landsteiner, an Austrian-American scientist. Landsteiner discovered that these women were carrying different blood types than their babies, who took their blood types from their fathers. The babies were Rh-positive, which meant that they carried the Rh antigen on their blood cells. Their mothers were Rh-negative, which meant that this antigen was missing from their blood.

Unlike the ABO system, where the antibodies to other blood types develop from birth, Rh-negative women do not make an antibody to the Rh antigen unless they are first sensitized. This sensitization usually occurs when blood is exchanged between the mother and infant during birth, so the mother's immune system does not have enough time to react to the first baby. However, should a later conception result in yet another Rh-positive baby, the mother, now sensitized, will produce antibodies to the baby's blood type. The result is an attack on the baby's blood cells that can be devastating and potentially fatal. Complications include severe anemia, hemorrhage, decline in the number of blood cells, and heart failure. Reactions to the Rh factor can only occur in Rh-negative women who conceive the children of Rh-positive fathers. If the mother and father are both Rh-negative, there is no problem. Rh-positive women, who comprise 85 percent of the population, have nothing to worry about.

Today we have a simple immunization given to Rh-negative women after the birth of their first child, which protects against the effects of this incompatibility. Rh immune globulin (Rho-GAM, GammulinRH) is routinely given to Rh-negative women after delivery—although if you are delivering in an underdeveloped country you'll want to make certain it is available.

Rh sensitization is not just an issue in full-term deliveries. Even if you have a miscarriage, ectopic pregnancy, or abortion, you will need to receive Rh immune globulin. Since there's a small chance that fetal blood can enter a woman's bloodstream during amniocentesis, it is recommended that Rh-negative women receive Rh immune globulin after this procedure.

Eat Right for Your Baby

A successful pregnancy is a miraculous holistic event. The atmosphere that you create for this extraordinary happening is one that is formed long before you conceive. Pregnancy is an excellent example of body/mind integration, involving every physical and neurological function.

How can you use your knowledge about your blood type's role in nutrition and health to maximize your well-being before pregnancy, improve your condition during pregnancy, and give your baby the best start in life—from the moment he or she is conceived?

I have said many times that blood type science is about individuality, and perhaps no experience is as completely individual as pregnancy and childbirth. Chances are you will hear many stories from others during your pregnancy and receive more advice than you care to. Some of it will be contradictory. Some of it will not conform to your experience. Your blood type advisory is a touchstone that can offer you reliable individualized recommendations. All of these recommendations are safely within our current scientific and medical understanding of reproduction and childbirth. This book is not designed to replace that knowledge, but to enhance and personalize it.

In the following sections you will learn how to maximize your chances of enjoying a healthy, successful pregnancy by employing strategies that have been individually crafted for your blood type. Obviously, blood type is not the sole factor involved in a healthy pregnancy. So your plan is really a combination of the best naturopathic advice and the best blood type–factored advice.

Every so often I'll see a pregnant woman in my practice who is so obsessed with doing everything perfectly that she's a nervous wreck. She's convinced that if she makes one bad choice or eats one food that isn't right for her blood type, she'll jeopardize her baby's health.

Although it's wonderful to live in an era when we have so much knowledge about how to keep both mother and baby healthy during pregnancy, I always advise mothers-to-be (and dads-to-be, too) not to go overboard in monitoring their compliance with every detail of the blood type diet and other recommendations. Such rigidity is a big stress-inducer, and right now you need to be eliminating stress, not adding to it. For the most part, your body will let you know if you've gone astray.

Pregnancy can be a uniquely rich and satisfying period. Don't miss the opportunity to savor the totality of this experience.

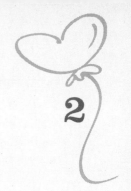

2

Your Pregnancy:
A Naturopathic Primer

THE FOLLOWING ADVICE APPLIES TO ALL BLOOD TYPES. In combination with your specific blood type guidelines, it constitutes the best of naturopathic wisdom.

Get Started *Before* You're Pregnant

Your level of fitness at conception is a critical factor in the long course that will finally lead to birth. Consider: A microscopic fetus's heart, lungs, liver, kidneys, limbs, and nervous system are being formed before many women have even missed their period. This is the best reason to consider your state of health before you become pregnant.

If infertility is an issue, you and your partner should both evaluate the factors in your lifestyle and health history that may be contributory. For example:

Impediments to female fertility include:

- Pelvic inflammatory disease (PID), chlamydia, or any other sexually transmitted diseases
- History of menstrual irregularities
- Taking medications for allergies
- Use of tobacco or recreational drugs
- Excessive alcohol consumption
- Thyroid disease

Impediments to male fertility—especially sperm production—include:

- Use of tobacco, recreational drugs, and steroids
- Excessive consumption of alcohol
- Treatment of cancer with radiation or chemotherapy
- Exposure to radiation, chemicals, and toxins in the workplace
- Sexually transmitted diseases
- Use of saunas or hot tubs
- Wearing tight underwear

In your pre-pregnancy blood type advisory, you will find strategies for achieving the best condition possible. These strategies, which you should employ at least six months prior to pregnancy, emphasize individualized dietary guidelines for losing weight if you need to, controlling chronic conditions that may interfere with conception and pregnancy, and ridding your body of toxins. In addition, there are supplementary protocols, using vitamins, minerals, and herbs; and a blood type–specific exercise and stress-reduction plan.

All blood types should use the following pre-pregnancy checklist:

Pre-pregnancy Checklist

In the months before you become pregnant, take care of these crucial matters.

LAB TESTS
- Blood test to determine blood type and Rh status (both partners)
- Blood test to screen for thyroid activity, anemia, and sexually transmitted diseases (both partners)
- Diabetes screening—especially if you've previously gained excessive weight in pregnancy or have given birth to a baby weighing more than 9 pounds
- Test for urinary indican levels and levels of serum albumin; high levels are indicators of toxicity.

EXAMS
- Full physical exam
- Pap smear and gynecological exam
- Dental checkup and the performance of any necessary dental work

INFORMATION GATHERING
- Family and personal health history, including any genetic factors (both partners)

- Evaluation of weight and body composition
- Evaluation of all current medications and natural supplements you're using

Detoxification Guidelines

Resolve to rid your body of any toxins that diminish your health, sap your strength, and heighten the risks for you and your baby. What exactly do I mean by toxins? These are the by-products of bacterial activity on unabsorbed foods that grow in your intestinal tract. In my conservative estimate, at least 50 percent of all the illnesses I treat involve some sort of toxicity. Hippocrates, the father of modern medicine, knew the elemental importance of what he advised physicians in the treatment of their patients: "First, cleanse the bowels."

Follow these guidelines to detoxify:

- *Eat only those foods that are recommended for your blood type.* When you eat foods on the "avoid" list, they are poorly digested and leave toxic by-products in your digestive tract.
- *Eat organic.* Chemicals, pollutants, and improper storage make foods harder to digest and leave toxins lingering in your digestive tract.
- *Eat natural.* Avoid artificial sweeteners, colors, and flavorings.
- *Eat fresh.* Limit your consumption of packaged, frozen, and canned foods.
- *Eat safe.* Avoid nitrates and nitrites—found in smoked, cured, and pickled foods. Avoid fish high in mercury—swordfish, tuna, shark (canned tuna is okay). Avoid fish that contain potentially harmful PCBs—bluefish, striped bass, fresh-water fish. Avoid shellfish—shrimp, crab, lobster, clams, oysters. Forgo raw fish and sushi during your pregnancy.
- *Avoid excessive use of fermented foods (cheese, beer, and yeast extracts) and canned and frozen foods.* These foods are particularly high in proteins that are destructive to the intestinal tract.
- *Stop smoking, drinking alcohol, and taking recreational drugs.* If you smoke, it's important to stop well before you become pregnant. You may already be aware that smoking during pregnancy can result in low birth weight and even birth defects. But smoking *before* pregnancy can have a lingering ill effect. Smoking impedes circulation and reduces your oxygen supply—making it much harder to deliver the necessary nutrients to your fetus. Studies show that smoking during pregnancy has been associated with low birth weight and even the development of ADD. Similarly, excessive alcohol consumption and the use of recreational drugs place you in a nutrient-deprived state—hardly a welcoming

environment for fetal growth. Lead and other heavy-metal exposures have also been linked to ADD.

• *Follow safe food preparation guidelines.*

  • Meat and fish: Take this added measure before cooking. Bring a pot of water to a boil. Turn off water and let meat or fish soak for 3 to 5 minutes. This will help remove any chemicals and kill bacteria. Then, be sure to cook the meat and fish thoroughly.
  • Use a vegetable/fruit wash to clean the skin and outer surface of fruits and vegetables before you slice into them.
  • Don't cook in copper, aluminum, or pewter pots. These metals can get into the food.

A Word to Dad

During the vital pregnancy preparation stage, don't consider yourself a bystander. You're able to command a leading role in determining the health of your offspring. You, too, need to rigorously comply with your own blood type diet and work toward a maximum state of health and fitness. In particular, eliminate bad habits that can interfere with the quality of your sperm. There are extensive studies clearly indicating that smoking, inhaling secondhand smoke, and exposure to toxic chemicals can have a negative influence on your sperm count. Studies also show that infants born to alcohol-free fathers are healthier and have higher birth weights. Never underestimate the influence you have over the well-being of your future son or daughter. This is truly a combined effort in which you play a crucial role.

TIPS FOR DAD
1. Follow the diet appropriate for your blood type. Clinical experience has shown that following the blood type diet as a couple increases your overall chances for a healthy conception.
2. Drink a cup of green tea once or twice daily.
3. Take 250 milligrams of vitamin C daily, preferably from food sources, such as acerola cherry or rose hip.
4. Take a daily multivitamin (preferably blood type–specific) to assure adequate levels of certain nutrients necessary for sperm count and motility.
5. Consult your physician if you take prescription medications. Some can interfere with fertility.

MALE FERTILITY-ENHANCING SUPPLEMENTS

VITAMIN C protects sperm from oxidative damage. Supplementing vitamin C improves the quality of sperm in smokers. When sperm stick together (a condition called agglutination), fertility is reduced. Vitamin C reduces sperm agglutination, increasing the fertility of men with this condition. Many doctors of natural medicine recommend 250 to 500 milligrams of vitamin C per day (preferably from acerola cherries or rose hips) for infertile men, particularly those diagnosed with sperm agglutination.

ZINC supplementation can raise testosterone levels and increase fertility if you have low semen zinc levels. The standard recommendation is 25 milligrams daily.

ARGININE is an amino acid found in many foods. It is needed to produce sperm. Most research shows that several months of arginine supplementation (1 to 2 grams daily) increases sperm count and quality and, therefore, fertility.

COENZYME Q_{10} is a nutrient used by the body in the production of energy. While its exact role in the formation of sperm is unknown, there is evidence that as little as 10 milligrams per day (over a two-week period) will increase sperm count and motility.

VITAMIN E deficiency in animals leads to infertility. In a preliminary human trial, 100 to 200 international units of vitamin E given to each man and woman of infertile couples led to a significant increase in fertility. (Type Os may want to limit vitamin E intake, except from foods.)

VITAMIN B_{12} is needed to maintain fertility. Vitamin B_{12} injections have increased sperm counts in men with low numbers. These results have been duplicated in double-blind research. Men seeking B_{12} injections should consult a nutritionally oriented physician.

CARNITINE is a substance made in the body and also found in supplements. It appears to be necessary for normal functioning of sperm cells. Supplementing with 250 milligrams to 1 gram per day for four months has helped normalize sperm in men with low sperm quality in several studies.

If you plan to implement any of these recommendations, be sure to talk them over with your physician.

Your Pregnancy: The Three Trimesters

It is helpful to understand what you can basically expect from each trimester of your pregnancy, as a context for the recommendations made in your individual blood type section. Your nutrient and exercise needs change as your fetus grows. In addition, each trimester brings with it a number of common conditions. Through blood type recommendations, you will be able to control the severity of your symptoms.

First Trimester Basics

The first trimester is the most critical time in your pregnancy. Although the fetus at the end of three months is only about 4 inches long and weighs less than 1 ounce, all of its functions have begun to form—major organs and nervous system, heartbeat, arms, fingers, legs, toes, hair, and buds for future teeth.

This is not a time to skimp on food or count calories. You're not quite eating for two people, but you do need extra nutrients for your growing fetus. The general recommendation is to eat about 300 extra calories a day. You'll need to gain 25 to 35 pounds during your pregnancy. This will allow you to nourish your fetus and store nutrients for breast-feeding. Expect to gain at least 3 to 4 pounds during the first trimester.

For many women, the first trimester is also the period when you experience the most profound changes. Although you may not appear pregnant, you'll certainly feel all of the differences.

COMMON FIRST TRIMESTER CONDITIONS

MORNING SICKNESS AND NAUSEA. The nausea—"morning sickness"—that many women experience during the first trimester of pregnancy is the result of hormonal changes. Morning sickness (which isn't necessarily limited to mornings) may actually be a positive thing—though you may not feel particularly grateful. Some scientists believe that morning sickness evolved as a natural way of protecting women against foods that might contain dangerous microorganisms or parasites, or foods whose chemical compositions might prove harmful to a developing fetus, by expelling those foods. Also, increasing levels of the hormone beta-hcg have been linked to nausea. Since high levels of beta-hcg tend to protect against miscarriage, look on the bright side: Your morning sickness may well be an early sign that your pregnancy is off to a good start. Morning sickness usually disappears after the first trimester.

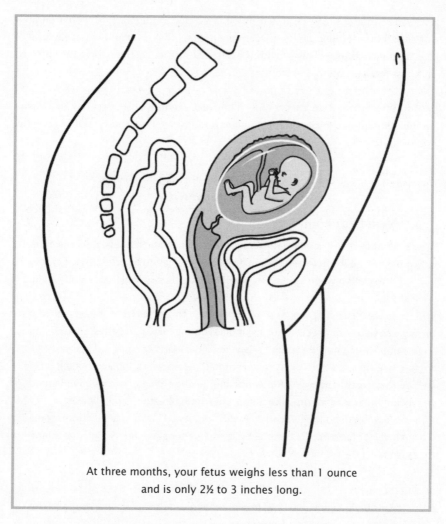

At three months, your fetus weighs less than 1 ounce
and is only 2½ to 3 inches long.

MOOD SWINGS. Women are often surprised that they don't feel more buoyant at the start of pregnancy—especially when it is a long-awaited result. The stresses of the first trimester can produce many emotional ups and downs. Although you may be delighted that you're pregnant, the hormonal adjustments you're experiencing can make you feel anything but joyous. You may experience mood swings, fatigue and insomnia, anxiety about your ability to experience a successful pregnancy, and fear about what will happen.

CONSTIPATION. Constipation is a fact of life for most pregnant women. Hormonal changes are largely responsible, signaling food to move more slowly through your system as it nourishes your fetus.

FATIGUE. Your entire system is fully engaged in creating a healthy environment for your fetus—producing the placenta, a process that is completed at the end of the third month, as well as providing sufficient nutrients. Every organ is engaged in a vast reorganization. No wonder you're tired.

FOOD AVERSIONS AND CRAVINGS. The food cravings and aversions that many women experience during pregnancy are something of a mystery. While you may

Advice from the Naturopath Midwife
Cathy Rogers, N.D.

RELIEVING YOUR ANXIETY

It's normal to feel some ambivalence early in your pregnancy. In a way, it would be odd if you *weren't* ambivalent. You're inviting a perfect stranger into your body! Even when a pregnancy is planned, the physical reality of it can be a shock.

If you're feeling anxious, it's important to address the issues beneath your anxiety. Get specific. For example, you may have anxieties about being a mom. Or you may be feeling exposed to the world (pregnancy is a very visible "out there" state). If you have compulsivity about eating and body image, you may worry about what is happening to the shape of your body. Remind yourself that you are growing a new life within. Breathe—and allow it.

This is a good time to connect with your mate—who may be having some anxieties of his own. Talk about what you want as parents. Solidify as a family unit.

Anti-Anxiety Soak

This bath, taken at neutral (tepid) temperature calms the nervous system. Neutral means body temperature, not hot.

1 ounce rose
1 ounce lavender

Mix the herbs together and tie them into a cotton scarf.

Place the scarf over the tub nozzle. Run hot water through the herbs until the tub is half full, then add cold water to bring it to the right temperature. As the water cools while you're soaking, add more warm water.

An alternative method is to mix a few drops of rose and lavender essential oils with a teaspoon of olive oil and pour it into the tub once the water has reached the right temperature.

crave what's good for you and be repelled by foods that are harmful, it doesn't always work that way. Your best strategy is to eat what's right for you and try to find replacements within your diet for the harmful foods you may crave.

PRENATAL SUPPLEMENTS

Vitamins are very important to the developing fetus. However, you should be aware that overdoing supplements can cause grave problems in the baby, so consult your physician before taking *any* vitamins or supplements.

Virtually any of the commercial prenatal multivitamins will be effective. But many are made with synthetic components rather than the preferred whole food ingredients. Choose a blend of the B vitamins, along with antioxidants. Look for quality, not quantity. Not all formulations release the specified amount of nutrients on the label. When researchers at the University of Maryland tested nine prescription prenatal vitamin tablets to see whether the folate contained would dissolve, only three passed the muster. Two failed so miserably that they released less than 25 percent of the folate specified on the label. That means that if swallowed by someone, more than 75 percent of the folate in those pills could possibly travel right through the body with very little chance of being absorbed by the blood and transported to various tissues, including tissues belonging to the fetus. If possible, use powder-in-capsule versus compacted pills: Evidence suggests that dissolvability is a big problem with many prenatals. Encapsulated ingredients do not need to dissolve.

Your daily prenatal vitamin/mineral supplement probably doesn't give you enough calcium. Most of the daily prenatal formulas only contain about 200 to 300 milligrams of calcium—about 1,000 milligrams less than you and your baby need every day. So check the label on your bottle or talk to your doctor. You'll want to make sure that you are getting at least 1,200 milligrams of calcium every day from natural food sources and supplements.

If you wish to take a prenatal supplement specifically formulated for your blood type, see appendix B for information about Healthy Start ABO Prenatal.

SPECIAL NOTE: DHA SUPPLEMENTATION: A natural nutrient for humans of all ages, DHA, an omega-3 long-chain polyunsaturated fatty acid, is one of the essential building blocks of human brain tissue. Found naturally in breast milk, DHA is also present in egg yolk and oily fish, such as salmon and sardines. What does having enough DHA mean for you and your baby? Whether you're a baby or an adult, DHA is important for signal transmission in the brain, eye, and nervous system. Your developing baby receives the DHA through the blood, via the placenta and umbilical cord. Seventy percent of the brain cells are formed before birth. These cells are mainly composed of essential fatty acids, with DHA being the most important because it gives great flexibility to the cell membranes. Flexibility is essential for fast and accurate message transfer in the brain. During pregnancy, the recommended intake of DHA is 300 milligrams per day, in food and supplements. Studies have shown that mothers' diets deficient in DHA are often linked with low head circumference, low placental weight, and low birth weight in their babies.

Medications to Avoid During Pregnancy

Certain prescription and over-the-counter medications can potentially harm a growing fetus. Avoid these during your pregnancy.

OTC PAINKILLERS	ACNE MEDICATIONS	ANTICONVULSANTS
Aspirin	Accutane	Diazepam
Acetaminophen (Tylenol)	Retin-A	Clonazepam
Ibuprofen (Advil, Nuprin)	And similar medications	Lorazepam
And similar medications		And similar medications
ANTIBIOTICS	**TRANQUILIZERS**	**MAO INHIBITORS**
Tetracycline	Librium	Isocarboazid
Streptomycin	Miltown	Phenelzine
And similar medications	Valium	And similar medications
	And similar medications	

Herbs to Avoid During Pregnancy

Herbs are medicine just like drugs and should be respected during pregnancy. Just as you would not take an unnecessary drug, avoid unnecessary herbs.

Aloe vera	Fenugreek	Poke root
Angelica	Feverfew	Rosemary
Arnica	Ginger	Rue
Black cohosh	Ginseng	Sage
Bladderwrack	Goldenseal	Senna
Bloodroot	Gugul	St. John's wort
Blue cohosh	Horsetail	Thuja
Celery seed	Indian tobacco	Turmeric root
Chaste berry	Iris	Uva ursi
Chichona	Licorice	Vervain
Cinnamon	Male fern	Wormwood
Coltsfoot	Motherwort	Wild carrot
Comfrey	Nutmeg	Wild indigo
Curcumin	Parsley	Yarrow
Ephedra	Pennyroyal	

EXERCISE GUIDELINES

There are tremendous benefits to maintaining your exercise program throughout your pregnancy. Regular exercise improves your condition and reduces the risk factors associated with pregnancy. It can also alleviate many of the uncomfortable side effects of early pregnancy, such as fatigue and morning sickness.

One of the most important functions of exercise is its ability to reduce stress and improve your mental condition. Pregnancy itself can be stressful. Throughout your pregnancy, you are also grappling with the effects this new reality will have on your relationship to the world. Your feelings, fears, and expectations about yourself, your family, and the impending arrival of your baby are important, too. To make matters a bit more complicated, your emotions can be affected by the dramatic hormonal changes you're experiencing. This is especially true during the first trimester.

Exercising three to four times a week, according to the blood type recommendations contained in chapters 3 to 6, will help you reduce stress, fight fatigue, and stabilize your emotions.

Exercise is good for your baby, too. Studies show that babies born to moms who exercise during pregnancy may benefit from better stress tolerance and advanced neurobehavioral maturity. These children are leaner at five years of age and have better early neurodevelopment. The new findings are added to the already-known benefits of exercise during pregnancy, including improved cardiovascular function, improved attitude and mood, easier and less complicated labor, quicker recovery, and improved fitness.

In addition to individual blood type guidelines, all blood types should bear in mind the following:

- All aerobic exercise is not of equal value. If your regular workout involves contact sports or in-line skating, I'd suggest you forgo them during pregnancy, to avoid any potential injury to the abdominal area.
- Make your aerobic exercises the low-impact variety. If you are taking dance or movement classes, keep your feet on the floor. No jumping or bouncing. Or choose exercises such as cycling, swimming, or brisk walking that have little or no impact risks.
- Take extra time to warm up and properly stretch your muscles before exercising.
- Wear a good support bra to protect your breasts and limit discomfort, especially if they are feeling tender.
- Drink plenty of water throughout the workout.
- Don't exercise on an empty stomach. Eat a snack 30 minutes before exercising.

EXERCISE CAUTION. Though exercise in pregnancy is generally safe, moms-to-be embarking on an exercise program should be aware of warning signs. If any of these symptoms occur, stop exercising and contact your practitioner: sudden and severe abdominal pain; uterine contractions lasting 30 minutes once exercising stops; dizziness; and vaginal bleeding. Other signs to watch for are decreased fetal activity, visual disturbances, or numbness in any part of the body.

For some women, such as those with heart disease, blood clots, recent pulmonary embolism, or for those who have a "high-risk" pregnancy, exercise may not be recommended. In taking the complete medical history, your practitioner will determine if maternal conditions limit, or exclude, an exercise program.

Second Trimester Basics

As you enter your second trimester, your pregnancy begins to show. The chance of miscarriage is substantially lessened, and you may begin to relax as some of the more uncomfortable symptoms—morning sickness, constipation, fatigue—begin to disappear.

During the second trimester you should gain about 1 pound a week—for a total of 12 to 14 pounds. You may experience a greater appetite, especially if you no longer suffer from nausea. Monitor your weight, and, if needed, increase your calorie intake by 100 to 300 calories a day.

Fetal growth is rapid during the second trimester, and you'll experience a number of physiological changes related to that growth. As your blood volume increases to pump more nutrients to your fetus, you may find yourself more susceptible to nosebleeds and bleeding gums due to extra pressure on these sensitive membranes. You'll also be more vulnerable to conditions that can be dangerous to the health of your fetus if they are not kept in check.

COMMON SECOND TRIMESTER CONDITIONS

ALLERGIES. If you are susceptible to allergies, they may be exacerbated during this time by hyperimmunity—the increased vigilance of your immune system designed to protect your fetus.

BLEEDING GUMS/NOSEBLEEDS. High levels of reproductive hormones circulating in your body increase blood flow to the delicate mucus membranes of the nose and mouth. This can bring easy bleeding when you stress these areas—by brushing your teeth too vigorously or by blowing your nose too hard. If you have allergies, a runny nose can make the problem worse.

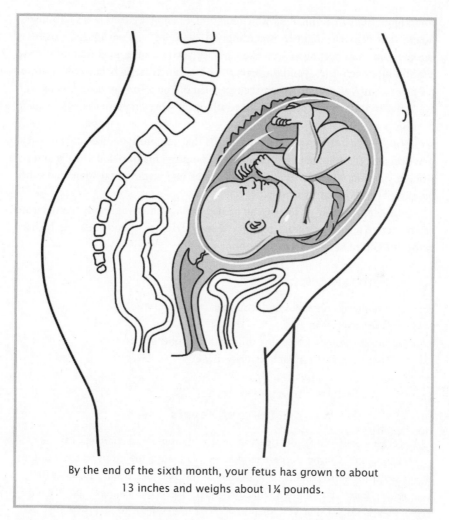

By the end of the sixth month, your fetus has grown to about
13 inches and weighs about 1¼ pounds.

BLOOD SUGAR IMBALANCE. Most pregnant women have more sugar (glucose) in their blood during the second trimester. This is normal, since your fetus requires more nourishment. However, elevated blood sugar can lead to a dangerous condition called gestational diabetes, which can cause premature birth and even birth defects.

HEMORRHOIDS AND VARICOSE VEINS. These are inflammatory conditions. Hemorrhoids are actually varicose veins of the anus.

EXERCISE GUIDELINES

As your pregnancy progresses, the extra weight and its unwieldy distribution place stress on your joints and muscles, especially in the lower back and pelvis.

You might also have problems with circulation, causing leg cramps and dizziness. Adapt your exercise regimen accordingly. If you are still engaging in rigorous workouts, such as cycling or step exercises, this would be a good time to shift to less strenuous activities—and those that don't require careful balance. As your fetus has grown, your center of gravity has shifted. You also may have less oxygen available, so reduce the pace of your routines, or stop altogether if you become breathless.

After the first trimester, avoid exercises that require lying flat on your back. The weight of your expanding uterus can compress major blood vessels and restrict circulation. Do your abdominal exercises in a standing position, and other floor exercises lying on your side.

Overheating during exercise can be dangerous. Keep your body temperature at a moderate level. An increase of more than one degree of body heat can be dangerous. If you're not sure, wear a monitor.

WHEN *not* TO EXERCISE

> You have pregnancy-induced high blood pressure
> You have asthma
> You experience bleeding during the second trimester
> You have a history of late miscarriage

Do Your Kegels

Kegel exercises should be a part of your daily routine, beginning in the second trimester. During the last months of pregnancy the growing fetus puts pressure on your bladder, which makes you feel the need to urinate frequently. Sometimes women limit their fluids when this happens, but it's absolutely essential that you keep your fluid intake high to stay hydrated. A better solution: Kegel exercises to strengthen the muscles around your urethra. Here's how: Contract the muscles in your vagina, urethra, and anus—as if you were trying to hold back urine. Hold for 5 to 7 seconds, then release. Repeat 10 to 20 times a day.

Third Trimester Basics

The third trimester is dedicated to intensive fetal growth. Your fetus will gain fully half its weight during this period. In the final months there will be further essential lung and brain development. The food you eat during the final three months is directly utilized in increasing your baby's birth weight. The quality of the food you eat continues to be of primary importance.

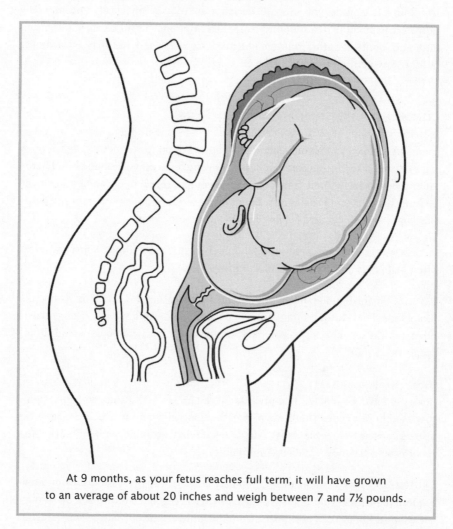

At 9 months, as your fetus reaches full term, it will have grown to an average of about 20 inches and weigh between 7 and 7½ pounds.

As you approach the birth of your baby, typically after some forty weeks, it's normal to feel equal measures of excitement and apprehension. If this is your first pregnancy, you're entering the great unknown. You may find your thoughts filled with worries about whether your baby is all right, and dread about what you'll experience during labor.

If you've participated in childbirth classes and have a strong partnership with your doctor or midwife, some of that anxiety will be alleviated. And if you've adhered to your blood type plan, you can have some degree of confidence that you've done the best you can to assure a healthy baby.

The key now, as you prepare for labor, is to be as physically and mentally prepared as possible. Continue to gain about 1 pound per week during the seventh and eighth months. Your weight may stabilize—and you may even drop a pound or two during the ninth month.

COMMON THIRD TRIMESTER CONDITIONS

LACK OF APPETITE. Many women find they have far less appetite later in pregnancy. One reason is the pressure of the growing fetus on your abdomen. There's simply less room for food. The best way to combat this is to eat something, even a small snack, every 3 to 4 hours. Don't drink water or juice with a meal. Liquid fills your stomach quickly, leaving less room for solid food.

CONSTIPATION. Constipation, which afflicts many women in the first trimester, often reappears in the final months of pregnancy.

EDEMA. Sluggish metabolism, often triggered by eating the wrong foods for your blood type, leads to an accumulation of extracellular water, which, in turn, causes edema. Mild swelling, especially in your legs and feet, is to be expected during pregnancy.

SHORTNESS OF BREATH/FATIGUE. By the third trimester, you'll be carrying a heavy and awkward load. The pressure of the expanding uterus on your respiratory system can cause shortness of breath even with mild exertion. Fatigue can also be caused by sleeplessness. Many women have trouble sleeping in the final months because they can't get comfortable.

INDIGESTION AND HEARTBURN. You may find that the pressure from your growing fetus constricts your digestive tract, forcing stomach contents back up through the esophagus. You can minimize acid reflux or heartburn by eating small, regular meals, chewing food thoroughly, and eating slowly. Don't lie down for at least an hour after eating.

HIGH BLOOD PRESSURE. If your edema is more serious, it could be a sign of preeclampsia. Eclampsia is a severe condition associated with elevated blood pressure. Even women who are not normally at risk for high blood pressure sometimes develop a pregnancy-induced hypertension. High blood pressure can restrict blood flow to the placenta and rob your fetus of oxygen and vital nutrients. If you have hypertension, you'll need to get more rest and even stay off your feet.

URINARY TRACT INFECTIONS. UTIs are very common during pregnancy. In the third trimester they are more serious because of the potential for developing a kidney infection. Kidney infections can provoke preterm labor.

EXERCISE GUIDELINES

Keep in mind that exercise is not only tolerated, it can prevent potentially serious complications, such as high blood pressure that can lead to preeclampsia. Exercise during pregnancy may also prevent some of the aches and pains associated with carrying extra weight and the changes in gait. However, pregnancy is such a different experience for each individual that, according to your own level of fitness and your needs at this time, it is best to approach your exercise program with great care and scrupulous attention to both form and function. Don't hesitate to adapt your daily workout according to your needs. It is common for women in the final months to feel short of breath, especially when exercising. Awkwardness, leg cramps, and pelvic aching can all hinder your ability to exercise as fully as you once did. Care should be taken to rise gradually from the floor to avoid dizziness.

Advice from the Naturopath Midwife
Cathy Rogers, N.D.

PERINEAL MASSAGE

Your body is making lots of new hormones that enhance the relaxation and elasticity of your muscles. This elasticity allows your abdomen and pelvis to accommodate the rapidly growing fetus. You can use this to your benefit by beginning to stretch the vaginal opening to ease the delivery of your infant's head and minimize the need for an episiotomy.

Recline comfortably, either on your bed or the floor. Place a small amount of warm almond or olive oil on your thumb. Insert your thumb into the vaginal tract, and gradually apply light pressure downward toward your feet. Do this for a count of 10, then allow another count of 10 for relaxation. Repeat five to six times. Practice this stretching routine daily in the third trimester—and invite your partner to participate.

DADS TAKE NOTE: STRESS AND WEIGHT GAIN

As your wife's pregnancy progresses, be aware of your own stress triggers. A recent study showed that men gained an average of 3 to 4 pounds during their wives' pregnancies. First-time fathers tended to eat and drink too much in response to stress.

Labor and Delivery Basics

I can assure you of one thing. No matter what your individual circumstances, good nutrition and regular exercise throughout your pregnancy will make your delivery far easier. Prepare for delivery the same way you would prepare for a strenuous athletic event.

- Pack more protein into your meals.
- Don't skimp on healthful complex carbohydrates, especially those found in vegetables and fruits, and blood type–friendly selections of grains and beans. These will increase your energy and balance your metabolism.
- Increase your consumption of vitamin C– and vitamin A–rich foods. These vitamins are essential for wound healing and tissue repair—especially for the genital and eliminative tissues, which will be so severely stressed during labor and delivery.
- Eat vitamin K–rich foods every day to improve circulation and blood-clotting factors.

Prepare Yourself: Prelabor Guidelines

As you approach the birth of your baby, typically around forty weeks, it's normal to feel equal measures of excitement and apprehension. If this is your first pregnancy, you're entering the great unknown. You may find your thoughts filled with worries about whether your baby is alright and dread about what you'll experience during labor.

If you've participated in childbirth classes and have a strong partnership with your doctor or midwife, some of that anxiety will be alleviated. And if you've adhered to your blood type plan, you can have some degree of confidence that you've done the best you can to assure a healthy baby.

The key now, as you prepare for labor, is to be as physically and mentally prepared as possible.

Consider enlisting the services of a doula. *Doula* (pronounced DOO-la) is a Greek word that, roughly translated, means "an experienced woman who helps other women." Doulas are specially trained women who provide pregnant women with nonmedical emotional and physical assistance from late pregnancy through labor and delivery, and into the first weeks of a newborn's life. In the past, it was common for female friends and family members of a woman in labor to gather at the birth and offer assistance. Today, doulas offer a way for women to gain this support before, during, and after labor. Studies have shown that in hospitals with high cesarean rates, a doula's presence lowers the chances of a cesarean. Women have shorter labors and need less chemical intervention to speed birth or reduce pain.

Women's satisfaction with their birth experiences, postpartum psychological state, success in breast-feeding, and interactions with their newborns are improved.

Doulas don't replace Dad. In fact, they make Dad's role more effective. With a doula present to relieve some of the stress and burden, dads take fewer breaks, remain closer to the mother, touch her more, and give her more support.

There are several thousand doulas working in the United States, and their number and use are increasing. Most have undergone special doula training. See appendix B for information on finding a doula in your area.

Advice from the Naturopath Midwife Cathy Rogers, N.D.

HOSPITAL OR HOME DELIVERY?

The setting of the birth is an important decision. Many hospitals today are labor-friendly, so you'll want to check out the hospitals in your area and visit their maternity floors.

When you're deciding between home or hospital birth, the important factors are: a practitioner you can communicate with and whom you trust, and a setting that offers a sense of safety. Some women need the medical environment to feel safe—and it *will* be necessary if you have a high-risk pregnancy. Other women feel safest in their own homes. They equate hospitals with being sick. Talk it over with your mate and your doctor/midwife, and do your research.

Whatever you decide, remember that a meaningful birth experience is less about *where* and more about how completely you involve yourself in the birth.

THE STAGES OF LABOR: WHAT TO EXPECT

The first stage of labor is called cervical dilation. It is the longest period, normally lasting several hours to a day. During this stage the cervix will fully dilate to 10 centimeters.

In the second stage of labor, you will begin to voluntarily push the baby down the birth canal with contractions, which become very strong and can be painful. Each contraction lasts about 60 seconds. The contractions do, however, space out to about 2 to 3 minutes apart. The usual length of the second stage of labor for a first-time mother is about 2 hours. The second stage culminates in the birth of your baby.

The third stage comes after the birth and continues through the delivery of the placenta.

There is a fourth stage of labor, which is often ignored. The fourth stage begins after the birth of the baby and the delivery of the placenta, and lasts for about an hour. The fourth stage is a healing and mending time for the mother, and a time for her and her new child to begin to get acquainted. During this stage, the midwife or doctor will examine the placenta and the umbilical cord, look for episiotomy tears, and suture them and the episiotomy, if one was performed. The uterus will be firm or hard to the touch. This is the adjustment period to the stresses of labor. Many of the physiological changes that occurred in labor will stabilize within the first hour following the birth.

EASING YOUR LABOR

The exertion of labor has sometimes been compared to running a marathon race. Your state of fitness and the steps you take to keep your energy levels high will play a major role in how well you do during labor. Realistically, you can probably expect to have a longer labor if it is your first child. Some women begin experiencing mild contractions one to two days before the birth. If you have followed your blood type diet and lifestyle guidelines throughout your pregnancy, you should be at a peak level of fitness. Here are some tips:

- In the weeks and especially days before delivery, get plenty of rest. If you experience sleep disturbances, institute a relaxing routine before bedtime, such as a warm bath and a light snack to raise your blood sugar.
- Keep your nutrition levels high. You'll need those extra nutrients for the job ahead.
- During the first stage of labor, when contractions begin and the dilation of your cervix occurs, stay as active as possible. Distract yourself by engaging in regular activities. Delay the time you have to give your full attention to the contractions. (Cathy Rogers suggests that you not consider yourself in "active" labor until you can't talk through a contraction.) Walk around as much as possible, as walking helps the cervix dilate.
- If you're using breathing exercises, such as the Lamaze technique, start them when the contractions become intense enough that you have difficulty speaking.
- The first stage of labor can last many hours. Drink plenty of liquids and keep a light snack nearby. A strengthening broth of miso, vegetables, or chicken can be helpful in the early stages of labor. Ginger tea (okay now that you're in labor) can also help you avoid exhaustion.
- Be sure to discuss in advance with your doctor or midwife what the policy is about eating light foods or drinking liquids during labor.
- During the second stage of labor, when contractions are more intense and

closer together, you'll be working harder to push the baby into the birth canal. Try to change positions frequently—at least every 30 minutes. This will reduce the pressure and keep you more flexible.

SAFE PAIN CONTROL

In my experience, most of the anxiety women experience prior to and during labor is related to fears that the pain will be too great to handle, or they won't be able to stay focused or in control. There are many artificial painkillers available in hospitals today. Some are analgesics, which carry some risk since they affect your baby as well. Others, such as the epidural, are regional blocks. Before you hand yourself over to a medicalized childbirth, I urge you to investigate the many nonmedical pain-relief strategies that are available. Not only are they safe, they also allow you to be totally present for the birth experience.

EIGHT NATURAL PAINKILLERS

1. *Relaxation techniques.* Visualization, meditation, and mild hypnosis can take the focus off your pain, relieve your anxiety, and make labor go a lot easier. See appendix B for resources.
2. *Movement.* Changing position frequently enables the force of gravity to work with you, not against you. This decreases the feeling of pressure.
3. *Massage.* Prior to delivery, practice massage with your partner. In labor, light massage to your shoulders, scalp, legs, thighs, brow, face—wherever tension needs easing—can make you feel much better. Deeper massage can also be used at specific points. Counterpressure can be effective. This is pressure applied to areas of the body that are causing pain during labor. See appendix B for more information on massage techniques.
4. *Hydrotherapy.* Water labor and birth can significantly increase your comfort and help you relax during labor. See box on page 36.
5. *Acupressure.* Acupressure is the stimulation of specific pressure points on the body to relieve pain. Refer to appendix B for additional resources.
6. *Acupuncture.* The insertion of tiny needles into nerve centers to block pain.
7. *Doula.* Studies show that doulas reduce a woman's need for pain medication by alleviating stress and the negative impact of high levels of stress hormones.
8. *Homeopathy.* The homeopathic remedy Gelsemium (in either the 6x or 30cc dilution or potency) can help to dilate the cervical opening. Homeopathic remedies are very gentle dilutions of a variety of plants, animals, and minerals. You can take two to three pellets of homeopathic Gelsemium under your tongue every 10 to 20 minutes.

Advice from the Naturopath Midwife
Cathy Rogers, N.D.

LABOR BATHS AND SHOWERS

Water labor is gaining in popularity, for good reason. Contractions are less painful if you are in water. Water equalizes the pressure, relieving pain. It also allows you to change positions easily, which reduces the discomfort. Water puts you in a state of physiological relaxation.

Whether you are delivering at a hospital or at home, you can order a labor tub. There are a number of companies across the country that specialize in providing labor tubs (see appendix B). You can order the tub in advance, call their service when you are in labor, and the tub will be delivered. It has a hard plastic shell wrapped around a soft foam interior. A sturdy reusable liner wraps the whole tub and a disposable liner wraps it a second time. A circular foam pad is used as a base. Most services include setup, support, cleaning, takedown, and removal of the tub.

You can also use your own tub or ask for a hospital room with a private tub. If it's not deep enough to cover your belly, cover your belly with a washcloth and continuously pour water over it.

If you only have access to a shower, sit on a towel-covered stool in the shower stall and direct the spray where it will help the most.

You can also use moist hot or cold compresses throughout labor— whichever is most comfortable. Use a washcloth and wring it well, then apply it to the brow, abdomen, lower back, or perineum. If you cover the hot washcloth with plastic, it will retain the heat longer.

In the next four chapters you will find individualized advice according to your blood type. Combined with this basic naturopathic wisdom, it will provide a complete plan for your healthy pregnancy.

The Type O Pregnancy

THE HEALTHY TYPE O WOMAN IS LEAN, strong, metabolically efficient, and perfectly suited for childbearing. The fact that Type O remains the dominant blood type is a testament to its genetic hardiness. However, if you don't follow the diet and lifestyle guidelines for your blood type, conditions can develop that may compromise your health and your ability to pursue a successful pregnancy. There is good evidence that Type Os who consume too much wheat, simple carbohydrates, and sugar have problems regulating their blood sugar, which can be especially dangerous during pregnancy, potentially leading to gestational diabetes and preventing vital nutrients from reaching the fetus. Type O also has a tendency to suffer from hormonal and metabolic disorders, which are a major impediment to fertility. The Type O's hyperactive immune defenses can lead to allergies, inflammation, chronic fatigue, and a number of other autoimmune disorders that can interfere with the ability to conceive. These disorders can also create problems during pregnancy.

Following the blood type diet provides an essential foundation, enabling you to optimize your health and prepare for an energetic and enjoyable pregnancy.

The Type O Diet

The following food lists comprise the Type O Diet. Note that the values for certain foods change in preparation for pregnancy, during pregnancy, and/or while you are breast-feeding. I call these Chameleon Foods, and they are contained in the following table. Use this table for quick reference. Chameleon Foods are also marked with an asterisk (*) in the specific food lists.

Values are calculated for secretors. If you are a non-secretor and want a higher level of compliance, refer to *Live Right 4 Your Type*.

TYPE O CHAMELEON FOODS

Chameleons are foods whose values change before pregnancy, during pregnancy, and/or while breastfeeding.

FOOD	PRE/POST PREGNANCY	PREGNANCY	FACTORS
SEAFOOD			
Bass	Beneficial	Avoid	Heightened risk of contamination
Bluefish	Neutral	Avoid	Heightened risk of contamination
Carp	Neutral	Avoid	Heightened risk of contamination
Flounder	Neutral	Avoid	Heightened risk of contamination
Grouper	Neutral	Avoid	Heightened risk of contamination
Halibut	Beneficial	Avoid	High mercury content
Mahimahi	Neutral	Avoid	Heightened risk of contamination
Shark	Neutral	Avoid	High mercury content
Swordfish	Beneficial	Avoid	High mercury content
Tilapia	Neutral	Avoid	Heightened risk of contamination
Tuna	Neutral	Avoid	High mercury content
Whitefish	Neutral	Avoid	Heightened risk of contamination
DAIRY/EGGS			
Egg/chicken	Neutral	Beneficial	Good source of DHA
OIL			
Borage	Neutral	Avoid	Uterine stimulant
Linseed (flaxseed)	Beneficial	Neutral	Limit intake; can be a uterine stimulant in large amounts.*
NUTS/SEEDS			
Flaxseed	Beneficial	Neutral	Limit intake; can be a uterine stimulant in large amounts.
VEGETABLES			
Parsley	Beneficial	Neutral	Limit intake; can be a uterine stimulant in large amounts.
SPICES			
Bladderwrack	Beneficial	Avoid	Potentially harmful to fetus
Cayenne Pepper	Beneficial	Neutral	May cause digestive difficulties
Chocolate	Neutral	Avoid	Contains caffeine
Fenugreek	Beneficial	Avoid	Uterine stimulant

FOOD	PRE/POST PREGNANCY	PREGNANCY	FACTORS
Ginger	Beneficial	Avoid	May cause miscarriage in large amounts.
Licorice	Neutral	Avoid	Can influence estrogen levels
Parsley	Beneficial	Neutral	Limit intake; can be a uterine stimulant in large amounts.
Turmeric	Beneficial	Avoid	Uterine stimulant
HERBAL TEAS			
Catnip	Neutral	Avoid	Uterine stimulant
Chamomile	Neutral	Beneficial	A calmative and sleep aid
Dong quai	Neutral	Avoid	Can start uterine bleeding
Fenugreek	Beneficial	Avoid	Uterine stimulant
Ginger	Beneficial	Avoid	May cause miscarriage in large amounts.
Licorice	Neutral	Avoid	Can influence estrogen levels
Raspberry leaf	Neutral	Beneficial	Supports the pregnancy
Vervain	Neutral	Avoid	Uterine stimulant
Yarrow	Neutral	Avoid	Uterine stimulant
BEVERAGES			
Tea, green	Neutral	Avoid	Contains caffeine; start weaning yourself before pregnancy, and avoid during pregnancy.
Wine, red	Neutral	Avoid	Alcohol should be completely avoided during pregnancy.

Meats and poultry

Eat only lean, organic meat and poultry of the highest grade available. If you are of African descent, emphasize lean red meats and game over fattier, more domestic choices like lamb or chicken. Avoid all pork and processed meat products, such as ham and bacon. They contain nitrites, which can be toxic for you and your fetus.

HIGHLY BENEFICIAL

Beef

Buffalo

Heart/Sweetbreads

Lamb

Liver (calf)

Mutton

Veal

Venison

NEUTRAL

Chicken

Cornish hen

Duck

Goat

Goose

Grouse

Guinea hen

Horse

Ostrich

Partridge

Pheasant

Rabbit

Squab

Squirrel

Turkey

AVOID

All commercially
processed meats

Bacon

Ham

Pork

Quail

Turtle

Seafood

Seafood, the second most concentrated animal protein, is well suited for Type O, but pregnant women must use special caution to avoid fish that may contain PCBs or that are otherwise potentially toxic. Check with your local health department about the safety of fish caught in local waters. In addition, avoid certain fish that are especially vulnerable to contamination by environmental pollutants, such as pesticides and PCBs. These include bass, bluefish, grouper, mahimahi, fresh salmon, tilapia, and whitefish. Also avoid fish that may contain a high level of mercury—halibut, swordfish, shark, and fresh tuna.

HIGHLY BENEFICIAL

Bass*

Cod

Halibut*

Perch (all)

Pike

Rainbow trout

Red snapper

Shad

Sole (except gray sole)

Sturgeon

Swordfish*

Tilefish

Yellowtail

Foods with different values than the standard Type O diet are indicated with an asterisk (*).

NEUTRAL

Anchovy
Beluga
Bluefish*
Brook trout
Bullhead
Butterfish
Carp*
Caviar (sturgeon)
Chub
Clam
Crab
Croaker
Cusk
Drum
Eel
Flounder*
Gray sole
Grouper*
Haddock
Hake
Halfmoon fish
Harvest fish
Herring (fresh)
Lobster
Mackerel
Mahimahi*
Monkfish
Mullet

Mussels
Opaleye fish
Orange roughy
Oysters
Parrot fish
Pickerel
Pompano
Porgy
Rosefish
Sailfish
Salmon
Sardine
Scallop
Scrod
Sea trout
Shark*
Shrimp
Smelt
Snail (*Helix pomatia*/
    escargot)
Sucker
Sunfish
Tilapia*
Tuna*
Weakfish
Whitefish*
Whiting

AVOID

Abalone
Barracuda
Catfish
Conch
Frog
Herring (pickled)

Muskellunge
Octopus
Pollack
Smoked salmon
Squid (calamari)

Foods with different values than the standard Type O diet are indicated with an asterisk (*).

Eggs and Dairy

Type Os should severely restrict the use of dairy products. Your system is not designed for their proper metabolism, and there are no highly beneficial foods in this group. Eggs are a good source of DHA, which is a beneficial nutrient for your health and the health of your developing fetus. Choose organic eggs only.

Since pregnant women need at least 1,200 milligrams of calcium daily, Type Os need to be sure to get plenty of calcium from nondairy sources. Calcium-enriched rice milk, almond milk, soy milk, and soy cheese are good alternatives, in addition to a calcium supplement.

HIGHLY BENEFICIAL
None

NEUTRAL

Butter	Feta
Egg (chicken)*	Ghee (clarified butter)
Egg (duck)	Goat cheese
Farmer cheese	Mozzarella

AVOID

American cheese	Jarlsberg
Blue cheese	Kefir
Brie	Milk (cow, goat)
Buttermilk	Monterey jack
Camembert	Muenster
Casein	Neufchatel
Cheddar	Paneer
Colby	Parmesan
Cottage cheese	Provolone
Cream cheese	Quark cheese
Edam	Ricotta
Egg (goose)	Sherbet
Egg (quail)	Sour cream
Emmenthal	String cheese
Gouda	Swiss cheese
Gruyère	Whey
Half & half	Yogurt (all varieties)
Ice cream	

Foods with different values than the standard Type O diet are indicated with an asterisk (*).

Oils and Fats

When cooking, give preference to the healthful monounsaturated olive oil. Linseed (flaxseed) oil, normally beneficial for Type O, should be limited during pregnancy; in large amounts it may be a uterine stimulant. Borage oil should be avoided.

HIGHLY BENEFICIAL

Linseed (flaxseed)*	Olive

NEUTRAL

Almond	Cod liver oil
Black currant seed	Sesame
Borage*	Walnut
Canola	

AVOID

Castor	Peanut
Coconut	Safflower
Corn	Soy
Cottonseed	Sunflower
Evening primrose	Wheat germ

Nuts and Seeds

Nuts and seeds are normally a good source of supplemental vegetable protein for Type O. However, you may find them difficult to digest during pregnancy, especially if you have a very sensitive stomach. Occasional use of nut butters or purees may be more palatable. Again, limit your consumption of flaxseeds during pregnancy.

HIGHLY BENEFICIAL

Flaxseed*	Walnut (black/English)
Pumpkin seed	

NEUTRAL

Almond	Macadamia
Almond butter	Pecan/butter
Almond cheese	Pignolia (pine nut)
Almond milk	Safflower seed
Butternut	Sesame butter (tahini)
Filbert (hazelnut)	Sesame seed
Hickory	

Food with different values than the standard Type O diet are indicated with an asterisk (*).

AVOID

Beechnut	Peanut butter
Brazil nut	Pistachio
Cashew/butter	Poppy seed
Chestnut	Sunflower butter
Litchi	Sunflower seed
Peanut	

Beans and Legumes

Type Os of Asian ancestry utilize beans well because they are culturally accustomed to them. Even so, beans and legumes are not an important part of *any* Type O diet. They contain proteins that can interfere with other nutrients in your diet. Try to get most of your protein from animal foods instead. One exception is soy-based products, such as soy milk and soy cheese, which are a good source of calcium—extremely important during pregnancy, especially for dairy-free Type Os.

HIGHLY BENEFICIAL

Adzuki bean	Black-eyed pea

NEUTRAL

Black bean	Pea pod
Cannellini bean	Snap bean
Fava (broad) bean	Soy bean
Garbanzo bean (chickpea)	Soy cheese
Green bean	Soy milk
Green pea	Soy, miso
Jicama bean	Soy, tempeh
Lima bean	Soy, tofu
Mung bean, sprouts	String bean
Northern bean	White bean

AVOID

Copper bean	Navy bean
Kidney bean	Pinto bean
Lentil bean	Tamarind bean

Grains, Breads, and Pasta

Type Os do not tolerate whole wheat products at all, and you should eliminate them completely from your diet. They contain lectins or glutens that react both with your blood and your digestive tract and interfere with the proper absorption of beneficial foods.

Overall, Type O should limit the amount of grains in your diet.

HIGHLY BENEFICIAL

Essene bread (manna bread)

NEUTRAL

Amaranth
Artichoke pasta (pure)
Buckwheat/kasha
Ezekiel 4:9 bread
   (100% sprouted)
Gluten-free bread
Kamut
Millet
Oat bran
Oat flour
Oatmeal
Quinoa
Rice bran
Rice bread
Rice cake
Rice (cream of)
Rice milk
Rice (puffed)
Rice (white, brown, basmati)
Rye bread (100%)
Soba noodles (100%
   buckwheat)
Soy flour bread
Spelt
Spelt flour products
Tapioca
Teff

AVOID

Barley
Corn flour (white/yellow/
   blue)
Cornflakes
Cornmeal
Couscous (cracked wheat)
Cream of Wheat
English muffin
Familia
Farina
Gluten flour
Grape-Nuts
Grits
Matzo
Popcorn
Pumpernickel
Seven-grain bread/cereal
Shredded wheat
Sorghum
Spinach pasta
Wheat (bran)
Wheat bread (sprouted
   commercial—not Essene/
   Ezekiel)
Wheat (germ)
Wheat (gluten flour products)
Wheat (refined unbleached)
Wheat (semolina flour
   products)
Wheat (white flour products)
Wheat (whole-wheat
   products)

Vegetables

There are a tremendous number of vegetables available to Type Os, and they form a critical component of your diet. You cannot, however, simply eat all vegetables indiscriminately. Several classes of vegetables cause big problems for Type Os. For example, certain members of the Brassica family—cauliflower and mustard greens—can inhibit thyroid function, which is already somewhat temperamental in Type Os. Thyroid irregularity can interfere with ovulation and fertility and also present problems during pregnancy. Leafy green vegetables rich in vitamin K, like kale and collards, are very good for Type Os. This vitamin is critical for blood clotting. Type Os have lower levels of certain clotting factors and need vitamin K to help blood clot properly. This is particularly important as your delivery date approaches.

Alfalfa sprouts contain components that, by irritating the digestive tract, can aggravate Type O hypersensitivity problems. The molds in domestic and shiitake mushrooms, as well as fermented olives, tend to trigger allergic reactions in Type Os. The nightshade vegetables, like eggplant and potatoes, cause arthritic conditions in Type Os, because their lectins cause immune reactions against the tissues. Corn lectins may affect the sensitivity of your body to insulin and can cause blood sugar imbalances—potentially dangerous during pregnancy.

Fennel and parsley should be minimized during pregnancy, as these are potential uterine stimulants. Also note that although onions and garlic are beneficial for Type O, you may want to avoid or limit them while you're breast-feeding. Some babies experience colic when moms eat these foods.

Values for whole vegetables apply to their juices, unless otherwise noted.

HIGHLY BENEFICIAL

Artichoke (globe, Jerusalem)	Okra
Beet greens	Onion (all)
Broccoli	Parsley*
Chicory	Parsnip
Collard greens	Potato (sweet)
Dandelion	Pumpkin
Escarole	Seaweeds
Horseradish	Spinach
Kale	Swiss chard
Kohlrabi	Turnip
Lettuce (Romaine)	

Foods with different values than the standard Type O diet are indicated with an asterisk (*).

NEUTRAL

Arugula
Asparagus
Asparagus pea
Bamboo shoot
Beet
Bok choy
Brussels sprouts
Cabbage (Chinese, green,
   red, white)
Carrot
Celeriac
Celery
Chili pepper
Daikon
Eggplant
Endive
Fennel*
Fiddlehead fern
Garlic
Lettuce (bibb, Boston,
   butter, iceberg, mesclun)
Mushroom (abalone, enoki,
   maitake, oyster,
   portabello, straw)

Olive (Greek, green,
   Spanish)
Oyster plant
Parsley*
Pea (green, pod, snow)
Pepper (all)
Radicchio
Radish, sprouts
Rappini (broccoli rabe)
Rutabaga
Sauerkraut
Scallion
Shallot
Squash, (all types except
   pumpkin)
String bean
Tomato
Water chestnut
Watercress
Yam
Zucchini

AVOID

Alfalfa sprouts
Aloe
Cauliflower
Corn
Cucumber
Leek

Mushroom (shiitake, silver
   dollar)
Mustard greens
Olive (black)
Potato (purple, red, white,
   yellow)

Fruits

Many wonderful fruits are available on the Type O diet. Fruits are not only an important source of fiber, vitamins, and minerals, but they can be an excellent alternative to breads and pasta. If you eat a piece of fruit rather than a slice of bread, your system will be better served. Oranges and tangerines should be avoided due

Foods with different values than the standard Type O diet are indicated with an asterisk (*).

to their high acid content and tendency to increase intestinal toxicity. Most berries are okay, but stay away from blackberries, which contain a lectin that aggravates Type O digestion. Unless noted separately, all values of the whole fruits apply to their juices as well.

HIGHLY BENEFICIAL

Banana	Mango
Blueberry	Pineapple juice
Cherry (all)	Plum (all types)
Fig (fresh, dried)	Prune
Guava	

NEUTRAL

Apple	Mulberry
Apricot	Musk melon
Boysenberry	Nectarine
Breadfruit	Papaya
Canang melon	Peach
Casaba melon	Pear
Christmas melon	Persian melon
Cranberry	Persimmon
Crenshaw melon	Pineapple
Currants (black, red)	Pomegranate
Date	Prickly pear
Dewberry	Quince
Elderberry (dark blue, purple)	Raisin
Gooseberry	Raspberry
Grape (all types)	Sago palm
Grapefruit	Spanish melon
Kumquat	Star fruit (carambola)
Lemon	Strawberry
Lime	Watermelon
Loganberry	Youngberry

AVOID

Asian pear	Honeydew melon
Avocado	Kiwi
Bitter melon	Orange
Blackberry	Plantain
Cantaloupe	Tangerine
Coconut	

Spices and Sweeteners

Spices can be either helpful or dangerous, and this is especially true during pregnancy. A number of spices are uterine stimulants and should be avoided during pregnancy, especially if you have a high-risk pregnancy or a history of miscarriage. Ginger can be an excellent remedy for digestive ailments. However, it can cause miscarriage in high amounts, so limit its use to pre- and post-pregnancy. Bladderwrack, normally beneficial for Type O, should also be avoided during pregnancy. However, you may consume seaweed in food form. Chocolate contains caffeine and should be avoided. Type Os should also limit the consumption of sugars.

Certain spices, normally used in tiny amounts for cooking, should be minimized during pregnancy, including cinnamon, marjoram, nutmeg, oregano, parsley, rosemary, sage, and thyme.

If you have problems with heartburn, nausea, or morning sickness, which occur mostly in the first trimester, you may find it helpful to eliminate strong spices such as curry and horseradish. However, if you don't have digestive problems, go ahead and use these spices.

HIGHLY BENEFICIAL

Bladderwrack*	Ginger*
Carob	Horseradish
Cayenne pepper*	Parsley*
Curry	Turmeric*
Fenugreek*	

NEUTRAL

Agar	Chili powder
Allspice	Chive
Almond extract	Chocolate*
Anise	Cilantro (coriander leaf)
Apple pectin	Cinnamon
Arrowroot	Clove
Barley malt	Coriander
Basil	Cream of tartar
Bay leaf	Cumin
Bergamot	Dill
Blackstrap molasses	Garlic
Caraway	Gelatin, plain
Cardamon	Honey
Chervil	Licorice*

Foods with different values than the standard Type O diet are indicated with an asterisk (*).

Maple syrup

Marjoram

Molasses

Mustard (dry)

Nutmeg

Oregano

Paprika

Peppermint

Rice syrup

Rosemary

Saffron

Sage

Savory

Sea salt

Soy sauce

Spearmint

Stevia

Sucanat

Sugar (brown, white)

Tamari (wheat-free)

Tamarind

Tapioca

Tarragon

Thyme

Vanilla

Vinegar (apple cider)

Wintergreen

Yeast (baker's, brewer's)

AVOID

Acacia (gum Arabic)

Aspartame

Capers

Carrageenan

Cornstarch

Corn syrup

Dextrose

Fructose

Guar gum

Guarana

Juniper

Mace

Maltodextrin

MSG

Pepper (black ground,
     white ground)

Vinegar (except apple cider)

Condiments

There are no highly beneficial condiments for Type Os. If you must have mustard, mayonnaise, or salad dressing on your foods, use them in moderation and stick to the low-fat, low-sugar varieties. Another option is to make your own from acceptable ingredients. Although Type Os can have tomatoes occasionally, avoid ketchup, as it also contains ingredients like vinegar and corn syrup. All pickled foods are indigestible for Type Os. Replace these condiments with healthier seasonings like olive oil, lemon juice, and garlic. There are a number of recipes in appendix A for healthy, delicious dressings.

HIGHLY BENEFICIAL

None

NEUTRAL

Apple butter

Jam (from acceptable
fruits)

Jelly (from acceptable fruits)

Mustard (prepared,
vinegar-free)

Salad dressing (low-fat, from
acceptable ingredients)

AVOID

Ketchup

Mayonnaise

Pickle relish

Pickles (all types)

Worcestershire sauce

Herbal Teas

Herbal teas can deliver strong doses of herbs, and for this reason many are not advised for pregnant women. However, certain teas are particularly beneficial, especially late in pregnancy. Raspberry leaf is rich in vitamins and nourishes the uterus. Chamomile is excellent as a calming tea and sleep aid. Dandelion tea aids digestion. Rose hip tea is a good source of vitamin C. Slippery elm tea is an excellent remedy for intestinal problems.

HIGHLY BENEFICIAL

Chickweed

Dandelion

Fenugreek*

Ginger*

Hops

Linden

Mulberry

Peppermint

Rose hip

Sarsaparilla

Slippery elm

NEUTRAL

Catnip*

Chamomile*

Dong quai*

Elder

Ginseng

Hawthorn

Horehound

Licorice root*

Mullein

Raspberry leaf*

Skullcap

Spearmint

Valerian

Vervain*

White birch

White oak bark

Yarrow*

Foods with different values than the standard Type O diet are indicated with an asterisk (*).

AVOID

Alfalfa	Red clover
Aloe	Rhubarb
Burdock	Senna
Coltsfoot	Shepherd's purse
Corn silk	St. John's wort
Echinacea	Strawberry leaf
Gentian	Yellow dock
Goldenseal	

Miscellaneous Beverages

Start eliminating caffeine and alcohol three to six months before pregnancy and continue until you are no longer breast-feeding. The common caffeine withdrawal symptoms—headache, fatigue, and irritability—won't occur if you wean yourself gradually.

HIGHLY BENEFICIAL

Seltzer water
Tea, green*

NEUTRAL

Wine, red*

AVOID

Beer	Tea (black regular and
Coffee (regular and decaf)	decaf)
Liquor	Wine, white
Soda (all types)	

Before You Get Pregnant

The best guarantee for a healthy pregnancy is to be in top condition before you get pregnant. Start getting ready at least six months before you conceive.

Foods with different values than the standard Type O diet are indicated with an asterisk (*).

Pre-pregnancy Diet Strategies

Get Serious About the Type O Diet

Check the Type O Chameleon Foods in the table on page 38. Some of these show different values for the pre-pregnancy period.

Begin to increase your compliance to the Type O diet at least six months prior to attempting to conceive. The most efficient approach is to add to the number of Type O beneficial foods you consume. These beneficial foods exert a powerful medicinal influence on your system, creating the optimal atmosphere for conception. At the same time, make an effort to eliminate foods in the avoid category.

Control Your Weight

If you are overweight, take steps to reduce to a healthy weight before you get pregnant. Type Os utilize animal protein quite efficiently, but gain weight when too many grains, breads, legumes, and beans are eaten. The worst offenders are the lectins, glutens, and gliandins found in wheat germ and whole wheat products. It is unfortunate that wheat is ubiquitous in almost all cereal and grain products. The vast majority of Type Os report weight loss and a gradual decrease in water retention solely by eliminating wheat from their diets.

Type Os have a special susceptibility to metabolic disorders which can be a factor in both obesity and infertility.

TYPE O HEALTHY WEIGHT-LOSS GUIDELINES

1. Eat a high-protein diet, emphasizing organic, chemical-free meats.
2. Minimize carbohydrates found in grains, beans, and legumes, except those allowed for Type O.
3. Include sources of essential fatty acids, especially omega-3 oils found in fish.
4. Eat plenty of fresh vegetables and fruit to provide proper natural fiber. This will aid in the eliminative process.
5. Avoid stimulants found in alcohol, caffeine, and refined sugars.
6. Eliminate carbonated flavored sodas, even diet sodas.
7. Engage in rigorous aerobic exercise several times a week.

Type O

THESE FOODS PROMOTE WEIGHT LOSS	THESE FOODS PROMOTE WEIGHT GAIN
Lean, organic red meat	Wheat gluten
Seafood	Dairy foods
Kelp (seaweed)	Corn
Kale, spinach, broccoli	Kidney beans
Pineapple	Navy beans
	Lentils
	Cabbage
	Potatoes

Regulate Thyroid Activity

In my clinical experience, Type Os tend to have "tippy" thyroids. That is, they have problems with both overactive and underactive thyroids. Both hyperthyroidism and hypothyroidism can interfere with fertility and upset your metabolic balance. If you have the following symptoms, have your thyroid levels tested.

HYPOTHYROIDISM	HYPERTHYROIDISM
Hair loss	Unexplained weight loss
Dry skin	Heavy sweating
Fluid retention	Palpitations
Cold intolerance	Frequent bowel movements
Constipation	Bulging eyeballs
Fatigue	Goiter
Unexplained weight gain	

To regulate your thyroid activity, follow the Type O diet and adhere to the following protocol for a period of four weeks.

TYPE O METABOLIC ENHANCEMENT PROTOCOL
(Use *before* pregnancy only.)

- Dandelion (*Taraxacum officinale*). 250 mg, 1 capsule, twice daily.
- Gum Guggul (guggulsterones of types E and Z). 1 capsule, once or twice daily.
- Selenium. 50–75 mcg daily.

- Lectin-blocking formula ("Deflect") specific for Type O. 2 capsules with meals. See appendix B.
- Green tea. 1 to 3 cups daily.
- Diet. Increase consumption of sea vegetables, such as seaweed.

Incorporate Detoxifiers into Your Diet

Toxins are the by-products of bacterial activity on unabsorbed foods that grow in your intestinal tract. Most often these toxins are the result of eating foods that are poorly digested by your blood type—including foods that are overly processed and chemically treated.

SIGNS OF TOXICITY IN TYPE O
- Water retention
- Difficulty losing weight
- Inflammation and joint pain
- Bad breath
- Bowel problems—cramping, flatulence, and constipation
- Fatigue; mental hyperactivity

To aid in detoxification before pregnancy, follow this protocol for one week.

TYPE O DETOXIFICATION PROTOCOL
(Do not use during pregnancy.)

- Standardized Chinese garlic extract (*Allium sativum*). 400 mg, 1 capsule, twice daily.
- Prune powder or boiled prunes. 1 tablespoon before bed with a large glass of water.
- Saunas and steam treatments as appropriate for your physical health and constitution.
- Probiotic supplement (friendly bacteria). Twice daily, preferably blood type specific (see appendix B).
- Larch arabinogalactan (soluble fiber supplement). 1 tablespoon mixed with water or juice, twice daily.

Detoxifying foods that are especially effective for Type O include soy products, such as miso, natto, okara, soy sauce, and tempeh. These do not replace meat for Type O. You still need plenty of lean, organic meat protein. However, the cultured soy foods are excellent supplements for intestinal health. Be sure to choose wheat-free varieties.

Pre-pregnancy Supplement Guidelines

VITAMINS	MINERALS	HERBS
Vitamin B complex— daily, with: 400–600 mcg folic acid, 500 mcg vitamin B$_{12}$	Calcium citrate— 1,000 mg daily	Horsetail (equisetum)— 250 mg daily as a source of trace minerals and the mineral silica.
Vitamin C from rose hip or acerola cherry—250 mg daily		Dandelion—250-mg capsule daily; also use fresh in salads or as tea
Vitamin K—food sources only		Green tea—1 to 3 cups daily *before* pregnancy
		Licorice (DGL) 150-mg. capsule or chewable tablet as needed

The Type O diet offers abundant quantities of important nutrients, such as protein and iron. It's important to get as many nutrients as possible from fresh foods, and only use supplements to fill in the minor blanks in your diet. In addition to vitamins, minerals, protein, carbohydrates, and fats, many grains, beans, vegetables, and fruits are excellent sources of fiber, which is necessary for proper digestion. In addition, fresh vegetables are an important source of phytochemicals, the substances in foods that strengthen the immune system and help prevent cancer and heart disease.

VITAMINS

VITAMIN B. I have found that Type Os often benefit from a high-potency vitamin B complex, which seems to have an energizing effect on metabolism. If you take a B supplement, be sure to choose one that is free of fillers or binders. Avoid any formula that contains yeast or wheat germ. Make sure that your supplement provides at least 400 to 600 micrograms of folic acid and 500 micrograms of vitamin B$_{12}$ (methylcobalamin form is best) at the standard dose.

VITAMIN K. Type Os have lower levels of several blood-clotting factors, which make you "thin-blooded" and can cause bleeding problems. You definitely want to boost your clotting factors as much as possible before pregnancy. However, vitamin K is generally not advisable in supplement form. Instead, take supplemental vitamin C (250 milligrams daily, preferably from food sources, such as acerola cherry or rose hips), and incorporate vitamin K–rich foods into your diet. These include liver, egg yolks, and green leafy vegetables, such as spinach, kale, and Swiss chard.

MINERALS

CALCIUM. Type Os should always include a calcium supplement, since your diet does not include dairy foods, which are the best sources of this mineral. It is especially important now, since pregnancy is a very calcium-intensive condition. A mother's calcium stores are constantly being depleted to furnish the fetus with nourishment for the growth of bone and tissue.

SILICA. The most commonly known benefit of silica is its role in preventing osteoporosis and restoring bone density by assisting the utilization of calcium within the bones. It also improves the strength of hair and nails by stimulating the production of keratin and collagen. Horsetail (Equisetum) grass is one of the best sources of natural silica, with high bio-availability. Silica is available in most health-food stores. A typical dose is 250 to 500 milligrams daily.

HERBS

DANDELION (*Taraxacum officinale*). Very effective for mild water retention. It can be used in salads, as a tea, or in capsule form. Take one 250-milligram capsule daily.

GREEN TEA (*Camellia sinensis*). Regular consumption of green tea appears to enhance chances of conception. Drink one to three cups daily, before pregnancy only.

LICORICE (DGL). DGL licorice can be used to control heartburn. Do not use "whole-herb" forms of licorice: They can encourage water retention. Use DGL licorice before pregnancy only—a 150-milligram capsule or chewable tablet as needed.

Improve Your Emotional Health

Your emotional well-being—especially your ability to adapt to stress—is every bit as important to your overall health as the physical. Indeed, the two are inextricably linked.

Studies show that Type Os are susceptible to an imbalance of the stress hormones called catecholamines. One effect of this imbalance is a marked tendency toward so-called "type A behavior," which is known to be much more common in Type Os than in the other blood types. People who exhibit type A behavior have an intense, competitive desire for achievement; an exaggerated sense of urgency;

are afraid of the passage of time; are always in a hurry; and display frequent aggression or hostility toward others. These people often try to do two or more things at once and believe that the only way to get something done right is to do it themselves. They're often fast talking, fast thinking, and abrupt. They are typically too busy to notice the things around them, like the color of the wallpaper in the dining room, or to be interested in things of beauty such as art, music, or sunsets.

Not surprisingly, I've found that Type Os who exhibit these characteristics have an especially difficult time getting pregnant. When they do get pregnant, they are likely to be plagued with sleep disturbances, digestive problems, and severe mood swings.

It is crucial that you take steps to regulate your stress levels before you become pregnant. The key to Type O stress regulation is the Type O diet combined with intense aerobic exercise. In addition, you can benefit from adaptogens, which help regulate your stress response. The most effective is *Rhodiola rosea*, which literally helps your body stay in the adaptive stage of stress—a relatively safe place that prevents stress from causing a physiological breakdown.

In addition, Type Os generally need an ample supply of B vitamins to balance stress hormones. Of particular importance are B_1 (50 milligrams once daily), pantethine (500 milligrams once daily), and B_6 (50-milligram capsules once daily). (Dosages suitable *before* pregnancy only.)

A SPECIAL NOTE FOR TYPE OS WHO ARE PREPARING FOR PREGNANCY. There is a powerful, synergistic relationship between the release of the neurochemical dopamine and feelings of satisfaction. Type Os are more prone to dopamine imbalances than are the other blood types. In conditions of stress, when dopamine levels plummet, you may feel drawn to substitute "rewards" to boost that sensation. Cigarette smoking, alcohol, caffeine, and recreational drug use can all result from that compulsion. These substances must be avoided during your pregnancy, so if you have a tendency to turn to any of them when you're anxious, bored, or fatigued, now is the time to begin finding effective alternatives to stress reduction.

Pre-pregnancy Exercise Guidelines

For Type O, stress regulation and overall fitness depend on engaging in brisk regular exercise that taxes the cardiovascular and muscular/skeletal systems. More than any other blood type, Type O relies on physical exercise to maintain health and emotional balance. Below is a list of exercises that are recommended for Type O. Choose from among these exercises for a minimum regimen of 45 minutes, three to four times a week. Later, I'll give you the appropriate adjustments for each trimester of pregnancy.

EXERCISE	DURATION	FREQUENCY
Aerobics	40–50 minutes	3–4 × week
Weight training	25–35 minutes	3–4 × week
Running	40–45 minutes	3–4 × week
Calesthenics	30–45 minutes	3 × week
Treadmill	30 minutes	3 × week
Kick boxing	30–45 minutes	3 × week
Cycling	30 minutes	3 × week
Contact sports	60 minutes	2–3 × week
In-line/roller skating	30 minutes	2–3 × week

Your Pregnancy: Type O Three-Trimester Plan

Diet Strategies

First Trimester

Choose Type O Beneficial Foods

Continue your compliance with the Type O diet, paying special attention to the Type O Chameleon Foods in the table on page 38. These are foods whose normal values are different during pregnancy. If you are new to the Type O diet, your most important first steps are inclusion of high-quality protein found in lean, organic meat and the avoidance of wheat and dairy foods.

The first trimester is such a critical time that you should emphasize your highly beneficial foods whenever possible. These foods act as medicine for Type O. While many foods are good choices of important nutrients, your power foods offer an extra benefit. For example:

- Choose lean, organic beef over chicken.
- Choose greens—collard, dandelion, kale, Swiss chard, or spinach—over asparagus, mushrooms, or squash.
- Choose olive oil over canola oil.
- Choose blueberries, plums, and pineapple over apples and grapefruit.

Emphasize Pregnancy Power Foods

There are some nutrients that have special importance. These include protein, calcium, folic acid, and iron.

Blood Type O Pregnancy Power Foods

PROTEIN	CALCIUM	IRON	FOLIC ACID
Lean, organic beef	Sardines (unboned)	Lean, organic beef	Liver, kidney, muscle meats
Beef liver	Canned salmon (unboned)	Heart	Fish
Lean, organic venison	Calcium-enriched rice or almond milk	Sweetbreads	Dark green leafy vegetables
	Soy milk*		
	Seaweed		
	Broccoli		
	Spinach		

Minimize Digestive Discomfort

Type O has naturally high levels of stomach acid, which can add to the digestive discomfort common in the first trimester of pregnancy. If you keep your stomach acid levels in check, you'll experience far less heartburn, nausea, and "morning sickness."

HEARTBURN

- Eat frequent, small meals.
- Eat slowly and chew thoroughly.
- Bend at the knees, not at the waist.
- Avoid acid-stimulating foods, such as oranges, tangerines, and strawberries.
- Avoid coffee, chocolate, mints, and black tea, all of which can provoke heartburn.
- Avoid sugars and sweets.
- Avoid wheat and dairy.
- Don't lie down directly after meals.
- Supplement with slippery elm bark or drink slippery elm tea. Slippery elm promotes the health of the membranes of the stomach, intestine, and urinary tract. Slippery elm bark is also soothing to intestinal tissue and encourages the growth of good bacteria. (See Supplement Guidelines, page 89.)
- Keep your head and upper body elevated while sleeping.
- Avoid eating while lying down.

- Use this simple reflexology technique for heartburn and nausea: Place your fingers above the navel in the midline. Press at 10-second intervals. Stimulating this point should bring substantial relief.

> **NOTE:** Before taking any medications, such as antacids, talk with your doctor. Not all medications, no matter how benign they may appear to be, are safe during pregnancy.

CONSTIPATION

- Get plenty of exercise.
- Drink lots of water.
- Include dietary sources of inulin, a form of soluble fiber found in over 30,000 plants such as cabbage, chicory, onion, and asparagus. Inulin helps increase stool volume and intestinal motility.
- Take a daily probiotic supplement to keep your intestines healthy. (See Supplement Guidelines, page 89).
- Get plenty of fiber from fresh fruits and vegetables.

MORNING SICKNESS

- Adhere to the blood type diet.
- Drink plenty of water and nonacidic juices (no caffeine—it dehydrates).
- Eat frequent, small meals throughout the day.
- Do not mix fluids with meals.
- Dry carbohydrates are usually well tolerated. Eat a rice cracker with almond or walnut butter before bed.
- Exercise to reduce stress, which can promote nausea.
- Avoid the sight and smell of offensive foods.
- Avoid being around smokers.
- Wear an acupressure wrist band, used by travelers to prevent motion sickness.
- There is some evidence that vitamin B_6 minimizes nausea. Foods rich in vitamin B_6 include fish and bananas.

> **SPECIAL NOTE:** Two herbal remedies for high stomach acid normally recommended for Type O should not be used during pregnancy. They can increase the risk of miscarriage. They are: ginger rhizome and DGL licorice.

Balance Your Moods

Mood swings are common in the first months of pregnancy, triggered by the many hormonal changes that are occurring, as well as the extra stress that comes with a major life change. The hyperintensity characteristic of many Type Os won't serve you well during this time. Here are some suggestions for maintaining your emotional balance:

• Find a support group or friend you can share your anxieties with. The typically extroverted Type O releases stress by engaging in a supportive conversation.
• Keep a journal detailing what you are experiencing.
• Break up your workday with physical activity, especially if your job is sedentary. You'll feel more energized, and exercise serves as a natural mood elevator.
• Plan ahead to have foods on hand for a quick energy snack when you're feeling tired or moody. Mood changes can be triggered by a decrease in blood sugar.
• Type Os who suffer from mood swings should always supplement with extra folic acid, along with other B-complex vitamins. Folic acid has the additional benefit of being essential for fetal development. (See Supplement Guidelines, page 89).

Handle Your Cravings and Aversions

I've seen many Type O pregnant women who've developed a strong aversion to red meat during the first trimester. Since red meat is the best source of high-quality protein for Type O, this aversion isn't necessarily based on healthy instincts. I encourage these women to incorporate very small amounts of red meat into vegetable and rice dishes, and make sure to trim all visible fat—similar to Chinese-style cooking. Sometimes the real aversion is to the fat, rather than to the meat itself.

If you crave foods that are not beneficial for your blood type, find healthy blood type–friendly substitutes. For example:

WHEN YOU CRAVE . . .	EAT . . .
Sugar	Raisins or a plum; any suitable fruit
Salty foods	Nori (seaweed) snack; miso soup
Ice cream	Frozen fruit ice or sorbet; soy- or rice-based ice cream

| Fatty foods | A banana or walnuts |
| Creamy foods | Vegetable puree—sweet potato, onion, pumpkin, or turnip; fruit smoothie |

First Trimester Menu Plans

The following menus offer a guide to healthy eating during the first trimester of your pregnancy. They are designed to offer well-balanced, delicious meals that include the primary values critical for Type O:

- They emphasize lean meats, fish, and fresh fruits and vegetables.
- They provide an extra boost of calcium and protein with Type O–specific smoothies.
- They provide many foods to help overcome first trimester problems, such as constipation, fatigue, and morning sickness.
- They break the daily diet into six meals/snacks a day—aiding digestion and reducing fatigue by avoiding an empty stomach.

The menus are flexible and can be mixed and reorganized according to your personal needs. I have purposely not included portion sizes for most dishes, since caloric needs vary depending on your height and weight. However, try to eat about 300 calories a day more than normal during the first trimester.

Although beverages are listed with some meals, I suggest you drink them half an hour before or after eating. Liquids consumed with solid foods dilute the digestive juices. Don't forget to keep drinking water throughout the day.

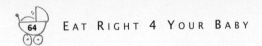

Menus

DAY 1

BREAKFAST
One-Egg Omelet with Fresh Spinach
  and Feta*
Glass of Calcium-enriched rice milk
Pineapple slices
Red raspberry tea

MID-MORNING SNACK
Sassy Smoothie*

LUNCH
Mozzarella, tomato, and basil on
  spelt bread
Mixed green salad

MID-AFTERNOON SNACK
Beneficial fruit or protein

DINNER
Pan-Fried Liver and Onions*
Baked sweet potato
Steamed broccoli

EVENING SNACK
Super Baby Smoothie*

DAY 2

BREAKFAST
Spelt flakes with raisins and soy milk
Mixed berries
Slippery elm tea

MID-MORNING SNACK
Beneficial fruit or protein

LUNCH
Farmer's Vegetable Soup*
Mesclun Salad*

MID-AFTERNOON SNACK
Type O Trail Mix-1*
Almond milk

DINNER
Broiled Lamb Chops*
Wild rice
Braised leeks

EVENING SNACK
Super Baby Smoothie*

DAY 3

BREAKFAST
Spinach Frittata*
Fruit Salad
Slippery elm tea

MID-MORNING SNACK
Apricot Silken Tofu Shake*

LUNCH
"Watch Dog Salad"*
Essence bread with almond butter

MID-AFTERNOON SNACK
Toasted Tamari Pumpkin Seeds*
Glass of calcium-enriched rice milk

DINNER
Sesame Chicken*
Green Bean Salad with Walnuts and
  Goat Cheese*
Beneficial vegetable

EVENING SNACK
Sliced banana with soy milk
Chamomile tea

DAY 4

BREAKFAST
Fruit Silken Tofu Scramble*
Pineapple juice
Spelt toast

MID-MORNING SNACK
Beneficial fruit or protein

LUNCH
Salmon with Wakame Seaweed*
Cuban Black Bean Soup*

MID-AFTERNOON SNACK
Type O Trail Mix-2*

DINNER
Great Meatloaf*
Pureed sweet potato
Braised Collards*

EVENING SNACK
Super Baby Smoothie*

DAY 5

BREAKFAST
Date-Prune Smoothie*
Poached eggs
Rose hip tea

MID-MORNING SNACK
Beneficial fruit or protein

LUNCH
Leftover meatloaf sandwich on spelt
  bread, with Romaine lettuce and
  tomato

MID-AFTERNOON SNACK
Sliced apple with walnuts and raisins

DINNER
Broiled filet of beef
Steamed spinach
Faro Pilaf*

EVENING SNACK
Tofu Banana Pudding*
Chamomile tea

DAY 6

BREAKFAST
2 scrambled eggs
½ grapefruit
Spelt toast
Slippery elm tea

MID-MORNING SNACK
Banana-Papaya Smoothie*

LUNCH
Mushroom Barley Soup with Spinach*
Mesclun Salad*

MID-AFTERNOON SNACK
Beneficial fruit or protein
Pineapple Seltzer*

DINNER
Baked red snapper
Steamed Artichoke*
Wild Rice Salad*

EVENING SNACK
Super Baby Smoothie*

DAY 7

BREAKFAST
Wheat-free Waffles*
Mixed berries
Rose hip tea

MID-MORNING SNACK
High-Energy Protein Shake*

LUNCH
Sardine Salad*
Rye vita crackers
Apple slices

MID-AFTERNOON SNACK
Rice cakes with prune butter

DINNER
Pasta with Rappini*
Glazed Turnips and Onions*
Beneficial vegetable

EVENING SNACK
Super Baby Smoothie*

DAY 8

BREAKFAST
Vegetable Frittata*
Ezekiel toast with almond butter

MID-MORNING SNACK
Banana Yogurt Drink*

LUNCH
Adzuki Bean and Pumpkin Soup*
Spinach Salad*

MID-AFTERNOON SNACK
Beneficial fruit

DINNER
Grilled filet of beef
Grilled Portabello Mushrooms*
2 Beneficial vegetables

EVENING SNACK
Super Baby Smoothie*

DAY 9

BREAKFAST
Poached egg on toasted Ezekiel bread
Pineapple juice
Rose hip tea

MID-MORNING SNACK
Beneficial fruit or protein

LUNCH
Leftover sliced beef on bed of Romaine
Vegetable Crudite
Apple slices

MID-AFTERNOON SNACK
Type O Trail Mix-1*

DINNER
Sesame Chicken*
Brown Rice Pilaf* with carrots and
onions

EVENING SNACK
Super Baby Smoothie*

DAY 10

BREAKFAST
Heidi's Early Morning Shake*
Essene toast with almond butter

MID-MORNING SNACK
Beneficial fruit or protein

LUNCH
Grilled Chicken Salad* on a bed of
Romaine
Plums
Rice crackers

MID-AFTERNOON SNACK
Raisins and chopped walnuts
Glass of soy-rice milk

DINNER
Shrimp Kabobs*
Stir-fried leeks
Artichoke and Vidalia Onion Tart*

EVENING SNACK
Super Baby Smoothie*

DAY 11

BREAKFAST
Spelt flakes with fresh berries and soy
milk
Soft-boiled egg
Slippery elm tea

MID-MORNING SNACK
Pineapple-Apricot Silken Smoothie*

LUNCH
Carrot-Tofu Soup with Dill*
Mesclun Salad*

MID-AFTERNOON SNACK
Beneficial fruit

DINNER
Pan-Fried Liver and Onions*
Braised Swiss chard*
Wild rice

EVENING SNACK
Super Baby Smoothie*

DAY 12

BREAKFAST
Tropical Salad*
Ezekiel toast with cherry preserves
Vegetable juice
Slippery elm tea

MID-MORNING SNACK
Beneficial fruit or protein

LUNCH
Black-Eyed Peas with Leeks*
Carrot-Raisin Salad*

MID-AFTERNOON SNACK
Type O Trail Mix-2*

DINNER
Cellophane Noodles with Grilled
    Sirloin and Green Vegetables*
Beneficial vegetable

EVENING SNACK
Super Baby Smoothie*

DAY 13

BREAKFAST
Leftover sirloin and eggs
Spelt toast
Red raspberry tea

MID-MORNING SNACK
Super Baby Smoothie*

LUNCH
Super Broccoli Salad*
Sliced chicken on a bed of Romaine

MID-AFTERNOON SNACK
Beneficial fruit or protein

DINNER
Baked red snapper
Glazed Turnips and Onions*
Steamed asparagus

EVENING SNACK
Sliced banana with soy milk
Chamomile tea

DAY 14

BREAKFAST
Banana Spelt Muffin*
Poached egg
Mixed fruit
Slippery elm tea

MID-MORNING SNACK
Rice cakes with apple butter

LUNCH
Speltberry and Basmati Rice Pilaf*
Green salad

MID-AFTERNOON SNACK
Type O Trail Mix-1*

DINNER
Grilled Loin of Lamb Chops*
Sautéed greens
Romaine-feta salad

EVENING SNACK
Super Baby Smoothie*

* You can find recipes for asterisk-marked items in appendix A.

Second Trimester

Adjust to an Increased Appetite

Fetal growth is rapid during the second trimester, and you may experience a greater appetite, especially if you no longer suffer from the nausea that may have plagued you during the first three months. Use your extra calories to maximum benefit.

EMPHASIS FOR EXTRA CALORIES
- High-quality protein—lean red meat, fish
- Calcium-rich foods—sardines, unboned canned salmon, calcium-enriched rice milk, almond milk, soy milk
- Vitamin C–rich foods—dark green leafy vegetables, plums, pineapple, bananas

Keep Your Blood Sugar in Check

For Type O, blood sugar irregularities are usually the result of carbohydrate intolerance—especially if you're eating too many grains, beans, and potatoes. While some increase in blood sugar is normal during pregnancy, be aware that severely elevated blood sugar leads to a dangerous condition called gestational diabetes, which can cause premature birth and even birth defects. The following symptoms should alert you to blood sugar imbalances:

Sweating
Palpitations
Extreme hunger
Restlessness
Anxiety
Dizziness and light-headedness

To restore a proper balance:

- Increase the protein and decrease the carbohydrates in your diet.
- Eliminate refined sugars and starches.
- Eat fiber-rich foods every day.
- Never skip meals. Preferably, eat six small meals a day.

Reduce Allergic Reactions

Type Os have a greater susceptibility to respiratory and food allergies than the other blood types—and pregnancy can make your allergies worse. Follow the Type O diet to rid your intestinal tract of lectins, which can exacerbate allergic tendencies. In addition:

- *Drink stinging nettle leaf as a tea.* This herb tends to promote a more balanced immune system and can be helpful to allergy sufferers. Drink one to two cups per day.
- *At the first sign of allergies, take a teaspoon of rose hip concentrate,* and continue every 30 minutes as needed. Or drink a strong tea made from rose hips one to three times a day.
- *Eliminate the allergen.* Reduce your exposure to allergens by removing dust-collecting furniture, carpets, and draperies; using plastic covers over mattresses and pillows; wet-mopping and dusting frequently; reducing the humidity level; and installing a high-efficiency air filter.
- *Avoid black pepper.* Specifically, commercially ground black pepper can provoke allergies. When the protective outer covering of the peppercorn is broken, several species of molds can settle on the soft inner pepper parts. All Type Os should avoid black pepper, but it's especially crucial if you have a history of allergies, especially to mold.

Minimize Problems with Varicose Veins and Hemorrhoids

Varicose veins and hemorrhoids are inflammatory conditions very common to pregnant women. (Hemorrhoids are basically varicose veins on the anus.) Type Os are particularly inclined toward inflammatory conditions.

- Avoid wheat and dairy foods, which trigger inflammatory conditions in Type Os.
- Avoid nightshade plants, which exacerbate inflammatory conditions. These include tomatoes, white potatoes, peppers, and eggplant.
- Increase your intake of safe deep-ocean fish to add helpful fish oils.

NATURAL REMEDY FOR HEMORRHOIDS: This cold compress can be quite soothing. Pour witch hazel on an absorbant minipad and freeze. Apply to the area.

Prevent Candida Infections

In general, Type Os are more inclined to Candida hypersensitivity than other blood types. During pregnancy, many women find that they have more problems with vaginal Candida, commonly called yeast infections. The best way to prevent these infections is to improve your overall bowel health. Here are some recommendations in addition to the Type O diet:

- Increase your consumption of olive oil by using it whenever possible in cooking and making dressings.

- Cut back on sugary foods.
- Take a probiotic supplement every day—preferably blood type–specific.

Improve Your Blood-Clotting Ability

Studies show that Type Os have lower levels of certain blood-clotting factors, giving you "thin" blood. This can be a problem during the second trimester. The effort of pumping extra blood to the placenta can strain the blood vessels, causing nosebleeds and bleeding gums. Incorporate plenty of vitamin K– and vitamin C–rich foods into your diet to minimize this tendency.

One side effect of the extra blood volume experienced during pregnancy is inflammation of the mucous membranes. For Type Os, this can increase the tendency for gum problems.

NATURAL REMEDY FOR SORE OR BLEEDING GUMS: Dissolve two 400-microgram tablets of folic acid in 1 to 2 ounces of water and swish around in your mouth, coating the gums, then swallow. Do this once a day.

Second Trimester Menu Plans

The following menus offer a guide to healthy eating during the second trimester of your pregnancy. They include some adjustments from the first trimester, taking into account the special emphasis on this period in your pregnancy.

- The menu suggestions place an even greater emphasis on lean meats, fish, and fresh fruits and vegetables—all foods that help regulate blood sugar.
- They include more calories than the first trimester menus, to accommodate the growing nutritional needs of your fetus.
- They provide an extra boost of calcium and protein with Type O–specific smoothies.
- They provide additional foods that will help to overcome second trimester problems, such as hemorrhoids, varicose veins, bleeding gums, and allergic sensitivities.

The menus are flexible and can be mixed and reorganized according to your personal needs. I have purposely not included portion sizes for most dishes, since caloric needs vary depending upon your height and weight. However, these menus do offer more foods than the first trimester—and you should try to increase your intake by 100 to 300 calories per day.

NOTE: Although beverages are listed with some meals, I suggest you drink them half an hour before or after eating. Liquids consumed with solid foods dilute the digestive juices. Don't forget to keep drinking water throughout the day.

Menus

DAY 1

BREAKFAST
Silken Scramble* with fruit
Ezekiel toast
Fresh vegetable juice
Stinging nettle leaf tea

MID-MORNING SNACK
2 plums
Glass of soy-rice milk

LUNCH
Salmon with Wakame Seaweed*
Rice crackers
Mixed fruit

MID-AFTERNOON SNACK
Beneficial fruit or protein

DINNER
Roast Chicken with Garlic and Herbs*
Glazed Turnips and Onions*
Brown Rice Pilaf*

EVENING SNACK
Super Baby Smoothie*

DAY 2

BREAKFAST
Spinach and Feta Omelet*
Poached fruit
Grapefruit juice
Rose hip tea

MID-MORNING SNACK
Pineapple-Apricot Silken Smoothie*

LUNCH
Mushroom Barley Soup with Spinach*
Caesar Salad*

MID-AFTERNOON SNACK
Beneficial fruit

DINNER
Fried Monkfish*
Grilled Pepper Medley*
Wild and Basmati Rice Pilaf*

EVENING SNACK
Baked Apple*
Glass of calcium-enriched almond
   milk

DAY 3

BREAKFAST
Wheat-Free Waffles*
Cherry preserves
Banana
Grape juice
Rose hip tea

MID-MORNING SNACK
Beneficial fruit or protein

LUNCH
Grilled Chicken Salad*
Rye crisps
Mixed greens

MID-AFTERNOON SNACK
Type O Trail Mix-2*

DINNER
Pan-Fried Liver and Onions*
Steamed broccoli
Pureed sweet potato*

EVENING SNACK
Super Baby Smoothie*

DAY 4

BREAKFAST
Scrambled eggs
Poached Fruit*
Ezekiel toast
Raspberry leaf tea

MID-MORNING SNACK
Sassy Smoothie*

LUNCH
Broiled lean ground beef patty with
    melted goat cheese, lettuce,
    tomato, and onion
Mixed green salad

MID-AFTERNOON SNACK
Beneficial fruit or protein

DINNER
Broiled Salmon with Lemongrass*
Black-Eyed Peas with Leeks*
Steamed spinach

EVENING SNACK
Super Baby Smoothie*

DAY 5

BREAKFAST
Heidi's Early Morning Shake*
Spelt toast with almond butter

MID-MORNING SNACK
Beneficial fruit or protein

LUNCH
Jerusalem Artichoke Soup*
Super Broccoli Salad*
Rice crackers

MID-AFTERNOON SNACK
Super Baby Smoothie*

DINNER
Broiled beef filet
Brown rice
Carrots and Parsnips with Garlic
    and Cilantro*

EVENING SNACK
Tofu Banana Pudding*
Glass of calcium-enriched rice milk

DAY 6

BREAKFAST
Poached eggs on toasted spelt bread
Fresh pineapple slices
Slippery elm tea

MID-MORNING SNACK
Date-Prune Smoothie*

LUNCH
Spicy Stir-fried Tofu with Apricots and
    Almonds*
Miso Soup*

MID-AFTERNOON SNACK
Beneficial fruit or protein

DINNER
Beef Stew with Green Beans and
    Carrots*
Romaine salad with Olive Oil and
    Lemon Dressing*

EVENING SNACK
Baked Apple*
Glass of calcium-enriched rice milk

DAY 7

BREAKFAST
Silken Scramble with Sautéed Pears*
Ezekiel toast
Raspberry leaf tea

MID-MORNING SNACK
Beneficial fruit or protein

LUNCH
Farmer's Vegetable Soup*
Mesclun Salad*

MID-AFTERNOON SNACK
Sassy Smoothie*

DINNER
Grilled Loin of Lamb Chop*
Steamed Artichoke*
Pureed root vegetables*

EVENING SNACK
Super Baby Smoothie*

DAY 8

BREAKFAST
Pumpkin Spelt Muffin*
Stewed plums
Soft-boiled egg
Pineapple juice

MID-MORNING SNACK
Beneficial fruit or protein

LUNCH
Sardine Salad*
Rice crackers
Apple slices

MID-AFTERNOON SNACK
Super Baby Smoothie*

DINNER
Steamed Whole Red Snapper*
Grilled Sweet Potato Salad*
Steamed broccoli

EVENING SNACK
Tofu Banana Pudding*
Chamomile tea

DAY 9

BREAKFAST
Tofu Carob Protein Drink*
Mixed berries
Raspberry leaf tea

MID-MORNING SNACK
Beneficial fruit or protein

LUNCH
Spinach Salad*
Spelt pita
Apple

MID-AFTERNOON SNACK
Super Baby Smoothie*

DINNER
Pan-Fried Liver and Onions*
Vegetable Fritters*
2 Beneficial vegetables

EVENING SNACK
Fresh Fig Salad*
Glass of calcium-enriched
    almond milk

DAY 10

BREAKFAST
Steak and eggs
Vegetable juice
Rose hip tea

MID-MORNING SNACK
Silken Smoothie*

LUNCH
Black-eyed Peas and Barley Salad*
Mixed steamed vegetables

MID-AFTERNOON SNACK
Beneficial fruit or protein

DINNER
Turkey Burgers*
Mixed green salad

EVENING SNACK
Super Baby Smoothie*

DAY 11

BREAKFAST
Heidi's Early Morning Shake*
Banana spelt muffin

MID-MORNING SNACK
Sliced pear with walnuts and raisins
Cranberry seltzer

LUNCH
Salmon with Wakame Seaweed*
Rice crackers
Vegetable consumé

MID-AFTERNOON SNACK
Banana Yogurt Drink*

DINNER
Chicken Breasts with Artichoke
    Hearts*
Grilled Pepper Medley*
Baked Apple*

EVENING SNACK
Glass of soy milk

DAY 12

BREAKFAST
Tropical Salad*
Slice of Ezekiel toast with
    blackberry preserves

MID-MORNING SNACK
Banana-Papaya Smoothie*

LUNCH
Grilled Chicken Salad* on spelt bread
Spinach Salad*

MID-AFTERNOON SNACK
Beneficial fruit or protein

DINNER
Beef Stew with Green Beans and
    Carrots*
Baked sweet potato
Beneficial vegetable

EVENING SNACK
Super Baby Smoothie*

DAY 13

BREAKFAST
Zucchini-Carrot Omelet
Sautéed Pears
Rose hip tea

MID-MORNING SNACK
High-Energy Protein Shake*

LUNCH
Cuban Black Bean Soup*
Mixed green salad with Olive Oil and
    Lemon Dressing*

MID-AFTERNOON SNACK
Beneficial fruit or protein

DINNER
Old-Fashioned Yankee Pot Roast*
Pureed root vegetables
Braised Collards*

EVENING SNACK
Spelt bread with apple butter
Glass of calcium-enriched rice milk

DAY 14

BREAKFAST
Wheat-Free Waffles* with blackberry
preserves
Fresh Fig Salad*
Slippery elm tea

MID-MORNING SNACK
Sassy Smoothie*

LUNCH
Mushroom Barley Soup with Spinach*
Green Bean Salad with Walnuts and
Goat Cheese*

MID-AFTERNOON SNACK
Beneficial fruit or protein

DINNER
Baked Chicken with Plum Barbecue
Sauce*
Vegetable stir fry
Basmati rice

EVENING SNACK
Tofu Banana Pudding*
Glass of soy-rice milk

Third Trimester

Reduce Swelling and Edema

Some water retention can be expected toward the end of your pregnancy, the result of an estrogen spike prior to the delivery of your baby. Type Os are particularly susceptible to the swelling and puffiness of edema. If you have an inflammatory condition, it will increase your discomfort.

Here are some suggestions for reducing edema:

- Avoid Type O–reactive lectins, especially grains, in your diet.
- Elevate your legs when sitting or lying down.
- Drink six to eight 8-ounce glasses of water during the day.
- Wear comfortable clothing and avoid tight pantyhose. Support stockings may offer relief.
- Cut back on high-sodium foods; many processed foods are loaded with sodium.
- Make sure your shoes fit properly.
- Drink one to three cups of dandelion tea every day if you are experiencing mild water retention.
- Ask your partner to gently massage the area from your ankles to your thighs, with a very light touch.

WARNING
Do not use a diuretic to rid your body of excess water. Diuretics can cause dehydration and nutrient deficiency.

* You can find recipes for asterisk-marked items in appendix A.

Control Your Blood Pressure

Blood Type O is more susceptible than the other blood types to toxemia—also known as preeclampsia or pregnancy-induced hypertension. Left unchecked this can be an extremely dangerous condition.

Type O's risk factors for toxemia include:

- Inadequate hydration
- Carbohydrate intolerance
- Calcium deficiency
- Food allergies

Maintaining your blood type diet is especially critical during this time—especially the avoidance of foods that trigger allergies or raise your blood sugar. Drink plenty of water throughout the day. Get plenty of calcium in your diet and include a calcium supplement. (See Supplement Guidelines, page 89).

NATURAL BLOOD PRESSURE REDUCTION TONIC: One excellent method for enabling healthy blood pressure is to juice several stalks of celery, taking 6 to 8 ounces as fresh juice daily.

Third Trimester Menu Plans

During the third trimester you may feel full after eating very little. Smaller meals, eaten at regular intervals of 3 to 4 hours, may be required to get all the nutrients you need. The following menus offer a guide to healthy eating during the third trimester. They include some adjustments to account for the special emphasis of this period in your pregnancy.

- They place even greater emphasis on lean meats, fish, and fresh fruits and vegetables—all foods that help maintain metabolic balance.
- They provide an extra boost of calcium and protein with Type O–specific smoothies. This will help you prepare for the rigors of labor and delivery.
- Vitamin A– and C–rich foods are abundant, also in preparation for delivery.

The menus are flexible and can be mixed and reorganized according to your personal needs. I have purposely not included portion sizes for most dishes, since caloric needs vary depending upon your height and weight. You may need to divide up the meals and snacks further if you don't think you can finish them at one sitting. However, it's vital that you maintain your overall caloric level.

Note that although beverages are listed with some meals, I suggest you drink them half an hour before or after eating. Liquids consumed with solid foods dilute the digestive juices and fill you up faster. Don't forget to keep drinking water throughout the day.

Menus

DAY 1

BREAKFAST
Omelet with Fresh Spinach and Feta*
Mixed berries
Vegetable juice
Raspberry leaf tea

MID-MORNING SNACK
Banana-Papaya Smoothie*

LUNCH
Jerusalem Artichoke Soup*
Carrot Raisin Salad*

MID-AFTERNOON SNACK
Beneficial fruit or protein

DINNER
Cellophane Noodles with Grilled
    Sirloin and Green Vegetables*
Basmati rice
Beneficial vegetable

EVENING SNACK
Super Baby Smoothie*

DAY 2

BREAKFAST
Heidi's Early Morning Shake*
Banana Plum Bread*

MID-MORNING SNACK
Poached Fruit*
Glass of soy-rice milk

LUNCH
Salmon Salad* on a bed of greens
Speltberry and Rice Salad*

MID-AFTERNOON SNACK
Beneficial fruit or protein
Dandelion leaf tea

DINNER
Roast Turkey*
Braised Collards*
Brown Rice Pilaf with Carrots
    and Onions*

EVENING SNACK
Rice Pudding with Soy Milk*
Mint Tea

DAY 3

BREAKFAST
Poached egg
Slice of Ezekiel toast with black cherry
    preserves
Mixed berries
Raspberry leaf tea

MID-MORNING SNACK
Beneficial fruit or protein

LUNCH
Turkey Soup*
Super Broccoli Salad*
Crackers

MID-AFTERNOON SNACK
Type O Trail Mix-2*

DINNER
Broiled Salmon with Lemongrass*
Carrots and Parsnips with Garlic
    and Cilantro*
Millet Couscous*

EVENING SNACK
Super Baby Smoothie*

DAY 4

BREAKFAST
Scrambled eggs
Ezekiel toast with almond butter
Sliced pear
Glass of soy-rice milk
Rose hip tea

MID-MORNING SNACK
Cherry-Peach Smoothie*

LUNCH
Grilled goat cheese on Ezekiel bread*
Mesclun Salad*

MID-AFTERNOON SNACK
Beneficial fruit or protein

DINNER
Flank Steak*
Pureed root vegetables
Steamed asparagus

EVENING SNACK
Cranberry Biscotti*
Super Baby Smoothie*

DAY 5

BREAKFAST
Amaranth Pancakes*
Blackberry preserves
Mixed fruit salad
Dandelion tea

MID-MORNING SNACK
Beneficial fruit or protein

LUNCH
Sliced cold flank steak on a bed of
    Romaine
Mixed Roots Soup*

MID-AFTERNOON SNACK
Rice cakes with apple/prune butter
Cranberry seltzer

DINNER
Green Leafy Pasta*
Endive salad

EVENING SNACK
Super Baby Smoothie*

DAY 6

BREAKFAST
Spinach Frittata*
Spelt toast
Pineapple slices
Rose hip tea

MID-MORNING SNACK
Sassy Smoothie*

LUNCH
Grilled Chicken Salad*
Slice of spelt bread

MID-AFTERNOON SNACK
Sliced apple, raisins, and walnuts

DINNER
Braised Veal Shanks*
Glazed Turnips and Onions*
Steamed broccoli

EVENING SNACK
Super Baby Smoothie*

DAY 7

BREAKFAST
Wheat-free Waffles* with blueberry
   preserves
Pineapple slices
Soy-rice milk

MID-MORNING SNACK
Beneficial fruit or protein

LUNCH
Waldorf Salad*
Tomato, mozzarella, and basil on
   spelt bread

MID-AFTERNOON SNACK
Super Baby Smoothie*

DINNER
Baked Chicken with Plum Barbecue
   Sauce*
Basmati rice
Steamed broccoli

EVENING SNACK
Pineapple sherbet
Chamomile tea

DAY 8

BREAKFAST
Brown Rice–Spelt Pancakes* with
   maple syrup
Mixed fruit
Slippery elm tea

MID-MORNING SNACK
Beneficial fruit or protein

LUNCH
White Bean and Wilted Greens Soup*
Mixed Mushroom Salad*

MID-AFTERNOON SNACK
Super Baby Smoothie*

DINNER
Steamed Whole Red Snapper*
Steamed broccoli
Grilled Sweet Potato Salad*

EVENING SNACK
Spelt bread with apple butter
Glass of calcium-enriched rice milk

DAY 9

BREAKFAST
Heidi's Early Morning Shake*
Scrambled eggs
Plums

MID-MORNING SNACK
Beneficial fruit or protein

LUNCH
Broiled lean ground beef patty with
    melted goat cheese and raw
    spinach leaves
Spelt bread
Mixed green salad

MID-AFTERNOON SNACK
Toasted Tamari Pumpkin Seeds*
Carrot juice

DINNER
Sesame Chicken*
Braised Collards*
Grilled Pepper Medley*

EVENING SNACK
Super Baby Smoothie*

DAY 10

BREAKFAST
Banana Walnut Bread*
Stewed apricots
Pineapple juice
Slippery elm tea

MID-MORNING SNACK
High-Energy Protein Shake*

LUNCH
Sardine Salad*
Mushroom Barley Soup with Spinach*
Crackers

MID-AFTERNOON SNACK
Beneficial fruit

DINNER
Grilled sirloin steak
Steamed Artichoke*
Wild rice

EVENING SNACK
Walnut Cookies*
Glass of soy or rice milk

DAY 11

BREAKFAST
Poached eggs
Essene toast with almond butter
Stewed prunes
Rose hip tea

MID-MORNING SNACK
Silken Smoothie*

LUNCH
Grilled Chicken Salad* on spelt bread
    with lettuce and tomatoes

MID-AFTERNOON SNACK
Beneficial fruit or protein

DINNER
Grilled Loin of Lamb Chops*
Green beans
Sweet Potato Pancakes*

EVENING SNACK
Super Baby Smoothie*

DAY 12

BREAKFAST
Scrambled eggs
Slice of spelt toast with black cherry
    preserves
Pineapple juice
Rose hip tea

MID-MORNING SNACK
Beneficial fruit or protein

LUNCH
Black-eyed Peas and Barley Salad*
Mixed steamed vegetables

MID-AFTERNOON SNACK
Cherry-Peach Smoothie*

DINNER
Tempeh Kabobs*
Wild rice
2 Beneficial vegetables

EVENING SNACK
Super Baby Smoothie*

DAY 13

BREAKFAST
Spelt flakes with raisins and soy milk
Mixed berries
Pineapple juice
Type O Tea

MID-MORNING SNACK
Banana Yogurt Drink*

LUNCH
Mozzarella, tomato, and sprouts on
spelt bread
Mixed green salad

MID-AFTERNOON SNACK
Beneficial fruit or protein

DINNER
Pan-Fried Liver and Onions*
Grilled mixed vegetables
Black-eyed Peas with Leeks*

EVENING SNACK
Apple slices with walnuts and goat
cheese
Chamomile tea

DAY 14

BREAKFAST
Zucchini-Carrot Omelette*
Sautéed Pears*
Rose hip tea

MID-MORNING SNACK
Tofu Carob Protein Drink*

LUNCH
Spinach Salad*
Grilled peppers and goat cheese on
spelt toast

MID-AFTERNOON SNACK
Beneficial fruit

DINNER
Old-Fashioned Yankee Pot Roast*
Pureed root vegetables
Braised Collards*

EVENING SNACK
Super Baby Smoothie*

Exercise Guidelines

First Trimester

Maintenance for Healthy Type Os

If you are healthy and do not have a history of miscarriages, there is no reason why you cannot continue your regular exercise program during the first trimester. Type

* You can find recipes for asterisk-marked items in appendix A.

Os thrive on aerobic exercise. However, if your exercise of choice includes Rollerblading, contact sports, or skating, I strongly suggest that you replace it with a safer routine—such as running, brisk walking, low-impact aerobics, or swimming. Be sure to wear a good support bra and drink plenty of water throughout your exercise period.

Pregnancy is not the time to *begin* an exercise program. Ideally, you've already been engaged in a pre-pregnancy conditioning program, or, better still, have been following the Type O exercise guidelines for some time.

Choose from among the following Type O exercises for a minimum regimen of 45 minutes, three to four times a week.

EXERCISE	DURATION	FREQUENCY
Aerobics (low-impact)	40–50 minutes	3–4 × week
Weight training	25–35 minutes	3–4 × week
Running	40–45 minutes	3–4 × week
Calisthenics	30–45 minutes	3 × week
Treadmill	30 minutes	3 × week
Cycling	30 minutes	3 × week
Swimming	30 minutes	3 × week
Tennis (doubles)	45–50 minutes	1–2 × week
Brisk walking	45 minutes	3–4 × week

CAUTIONS FOR HIGH-RISK PREGNANCIES

Consult with your doctor before continuing your exercise regimen if you are in a high-risk pregnancy. Most doctors will discourage exercise if you:

- Have a history of miscarriages, or have had even one miscarriage, if it is recent.
- Have a history of recurrent pelvic or abdominal infections.
- Have an incompetent cervix. This condition causes the cervix to open early, usually in the second trimester, leading to miscarriage.
- Have had toxemia in a previous pregnancy.
- Have a history of premature deliveries.
- Have or have had a serious medical condition, such as cancer, heart disease, asthma, or kidney disease.

Second Trimester

Adaptations for Advancing Pregnancy

Your normal exercise regimen should change somewhat as you approach your sixth month. Replace any strenuous exercise with more controlled, less strenuous variations—for example, brisk walking instead of running. The following are second trimester guidelines:

- Spend more time on your warm-up and cool-down to fully warm and stretch your muscles. This will minimize the muscle cramps that are common as your pregnancy progresses.
- Look for opportunities to incorporate fitness into your daily routine. If feasible, walk to work instead of driving. Take the stairs instead of the elevator.
- You can continue to do a weight workout, but use extreme caution. Your center of gravity has shifted, and you may feel awkward. Lighter weights may be the answer. Experiment to find the right balance. Consistency is more important than the amount of weight you use.
- Swimming is an excellent exercise for the second and third trimesters. It places minimum stress on your joints and heart rate. You may even want to replace your regular aerobics class with a water aerobics class.
- If you haven't already started your Kegel exercises (see page 28), do so now.

Choose from among the following Type O exercises for a minimum regimen of 45 minutes, three to four times a week.

EXERCISE	DURATION	FREQUENCY
Aerobics (low impact)	40–50 minutes	3–4 × week
Weight training (light free weights)	25–35 minutes	3–4 × week
Calisthenics	30–45 minutes	3 × week
Treadmill	30 minutes	3 × week
Cycling (recumbent bike)	30 minutes	3 × week
Swimming	30 minutes	3 × week
Tennis (doubles)	45–50 minutes	1–2 × week
Brisk walking	45 minutes	3–4 × week
Kegel exercises	2 minutes	10–20 × daily

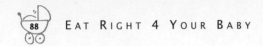

PREGNANCY-SAFE EXERCISE SUBSTITUTIONS

INSTEAD OF . . .	TRY . . .
Bicycling	indoor stationary bike (recumbent)
Running	brisk walking/treadmill
Aerobics	water aerobics
Weight machines	free weights (5 to 10 pounds)

Third Trimester

Adaptations for Late Pregnancy

Exercise is essential during the third trimester. It can help keep your blood pressure in check, combat fatigue, regulate your blood sugar, and reduce the effects of stress. It can also keep you limber and reduce some of the aches and pains you're probably experiencing. However, even if you have been exercising vigorously for years, you need to pay close attention to the signs that you may be pushing yourself too hard. If you feel light-headed or crampy during your workout routine, stop exercising. Avoid any exercises that place pressure on your abdominal area. Lay on your side for floor exercises. This position also helps your circulation and will decrease your blood pressure.

Type Os can benefit in the final months of pregnancy by replacing one or two of your weekly aerobic exercises with a prenatal yoga class. Also, begin your daily perineal massage to tone the vaginal canal (page 31).

An excellent third trimester exercise regimen for Type O would be the following:

THREE TIMES A WEEK, CHOOSE ONE:

EXERCISE	DURATION
Water aerobics	40–50 minutes
Treadmill	30 minutes
Cycling (recumbent bike)	30 minutes
Swimming	30 minutes
Brisk walking	45 minutes

TWO TIMES A WEEK, CHOOSE ONE:

EXERCISE	DURATION
Light yoga	40–50 minutes
Stretching and relaxation	30 minutes
Labor preparation class	40–50 minutes

DAILY, PERFORM BOTH:

EXERCISE	DURATION
Kegel exercises	2 minutes, 10–20 times.
Perineal massage	5 minutes, 1–2 times

Supplement Guidelines

First Trimester

Vitamins/Minerals

Take a standard prenatal vitamin supplement, choosing one made from whole food, not synthetic ingredients. Powder-in-capsule forms dissolve most efficiently. If you would like to use a prenatal supplement specifically formulated for Type O, see appendix B for information about Healthy Start ABO Prenatal. The following nutrient breakdown is the optimal formula for Type O:

PRENATAL SUPPLEMENT—TYPE O		% DAILY VALUE
Vitamin A (100% as natural beta-carotene from *Dunaliella salina*)	6,000 iu	120
Vitamin C (100% from acerola berry, *Malpighia puncifolia*)	75 mg	125
Vitamin D (Cholecalciferol)	100 iu	25
Vitamin K (Phytonadione)	35 mcg	–
Thiamin (from Thiamin HCl)	15 mg	1,000
Riboflavin	20 mg	1,176
Niacin and Niacinamide (vitamin B$_3$)	5 mg	25
Vitamin B$_6$ (from Pyridoxine HCl)	15 mg	750
Folic Acid	800 mcg	200

PRENATAL SUPPLEMENT—TYPE O		% DAILY VALUE
Vitamin B$_{12}$ (Methylcobalamin)	15 mcg	250
Biotin	600 mcg	200
Pantothenic Acid (from D-Calcium Pantothenate)	10 mg	100
Calcium (seaweed base, derived from *Lithothamnium corralliodes* and *Lithothamnium calcareum*)	300 mg	30
Iron (Ferrous Succinate)	18 mg	100
Iodine (Potassium Iodide)	150 mcg	100
Magnesium (Citrate and Oxide)	100 mg	25
Zinc (Picolinate)	20 mg	133
Selenium (L-Selenomethionine)	20 mcg	–
Copper (Gluconate)	1 mg	50

Herbal Remedies

HERB	FUNCTION	FORM AND DOSAGE
Chamomile	Calms; relieves heartburn	As tea, 1 to 2 cups daily; or add 2 to 4 drops of essential oil to bath
Horsetail	Contains silica, which supports healthy bones, skin, hair, and nails	250-mg capsule daily
Peppermint	Calms; relieves indigestion	As tea, 2 to 3 cups daily, after meals
Red raspberry leaf	Relieves morning sickness	As tea, 2 cups daily
Slippery elm bark	Relieves heartburn	250-mg capsule, twice daily; or as tea, 2 cups daily; or as Thayer's lozenges, 2 to 4 daily

Nutritional Supplements

NUTRITIONAL SUPPLEMENT	FUNCTION	FORM AND DOSAGE
Larch arabinogalactan	Relieves constipation	Soluble fiber supplement; 1 tablespoon mixed with water or juice, twice daily
Probiotic	For intestinal health	2 capsules, twice daily*
DHA	Provides essential nutrients for fetal development	300-mg capsule daily

* See appendix B for information on blood type–specific probiotics.

NOTE: Type O pregnant women should avoid the flu vaccine—especially if your baby's father is Type A or Type AB. The flu vaccine will boost the presence of anti-A antibodies in your system, which can attack your fetus.

Second Trimester

Vitamins/Minerals

Continue to take your prenatal supplement, preferably one formulated for Type O.

Herbal Remedies

HERB	FUNCTION	FORM AND DOSAGE
Bilberry	Relieves hemorrhoids and varicose veins	25 mg, 2 capsules daily
Chamomile	Calms; relieves heartburn; relieves hemorrhoids and varicose veins	As tea, 1 to 2 cups daily; or add 2 to 4 drops of essential oil to bath
Horsetail	Contains silica, which supports healthy bones, skin, hair, and nails	250-mg capsule daily
Peppermint	Calms; relieves indigestion	As tea, 2 to 3 cups daily, after meals
Red raspberry leaf	Treatment for bleeding gums	As tea, 2 cups daily
Rose hip	Treatment for varicose veins, bleeding gums, allergies	1 tablespoon concentrate every 30 minutes for allergy attack; as tea, 2 to 3 cups daily
Stinging nettle leaf	Allergy relief	As tea, 2 cups daily for symptoms
Witch hazel	Treatment for hemorrhoids	Use topically as needed

Nutritional Supplements

NUTRITIONAL SUPPLEMENT	FUNCTION	FORM AND DOSAGE
Larch arabinogalactan	Relieves constipation	Soluble fiber supplement: 1 tablespoon mixed with water or juice, twice daily

NUTRITIONAL SUPPLEMENT	FUNCTION	FORM AND DOSAGE
Probiotic	For intestinal health; prevention of candida infection	2 capsules, twice daily*
DHA	Provides essential nutrients for fetal development	300-mg capsule daily

* See appendix B for information on blood type–specific probiotics.

Third Trimester

Vitamins/Minerals

Continue to take your prenatal supplement, preferably one formulated for Type O.

Herbal Remedies

HERB	FUNCTION	FORM AND DOSAGE
Dandelion leaf/root	Lowers blood pressure; decreases edema	As tea, 2 cups daily; or 250-mg capsule, twice daily
Nettles	Rich in vitamin K, promotes blood clotting	As tea, 2 cups daily; or 250-mg capsule, twice daily
Raspberry leaf	Softens the cervix in preparation for birth; stimulates milk production	As tea, 2 cups daily; as tincture, 15 to 20 drops daily
Squaw vine	Prepares uterus for birth	As tincture, 10 drops in warm water, twice daily

Nutritional Supplements

NUTRITIONAL SUPPLEMENT	FUNCTION	FORM AND DOSAGE
Larch arabinogalactan	Relieves constipation	Soluble fiber supplement: 1 tablespoon mixed with water or juice, twice daily
Probiotic	For intestinal health	2 capsules, twice daily*
DHA	Provides essential nutrients for fetal development	300-mg capsule daily

* See appendix B for information on blood type–specific probiotics.

Labor and Delivery

In addition to the general guidelines for labor and delivery (page 32), you have some specific Type O needs.

Type O Blood-Building Needs

Type O has a limited amount of certain blood-clotting factors, making you more vulnerable in circumstances where surgical procedures are required. To guard against excessive bleeding in the event that a cesarean or other surgical procedure might be required, increase your blood-clotting factors. Follow these guidelines in the final weeks of pregnancy:

- Vitamin K is essential to blood clotting. Eat lots of leafy green vegetables, especially kale, spinach, and collard greens. Rye, oats, and nettle tea are also good sources of vitamin K.
- Make sure to include fish oils in your diet. They promote clotting factors.
- Avoid using aspirin, which has blood-thinning properties.
- Eat Natto: Natto is a cultured soy product from Japan made by fermenting boiled soy beans with *Bacillus natto*. It is similar to miso. Natto has substantial fibrinolytic activity—that is, the ability of factors in the blood to break down or dissolve thrombi.

Type O Energy Needs

In normal circumstances, Type Os maintain energy through diet and exercise. This can apply during labor, too. The first stage of labor can last many hours. Drink plenty of liquids and keep a light protein snack nearby. Stay hydrated. Be sure to discuss in advance with your doctor or midwife what the policy is about eating light foods or drinking liquids during labor.

Move around as much as possible during the early stages of labor. This will increase your energy and flexibility for the final stages.

Type O Emotional Needs

Type O does best in situations where you have a sense of control. That's a big challenge during labor, when it's easy to feel as if something is occurring that is well beyond your control. Visualization is helpful here. Focus on yourself bringing your baby to birth—controlling the pace and intensity of the process with your breathing.

Type Os can benefit from having a doula to assist in labor, since you feel stronger and more emotionally stable when you are working with others to achieve a common purpose. (See page 32 for a discussion of the role of a doula.)

Anxiety is enhanced by fear of the unknown. Arrange in advance for your doctor, nurse, midwife, and other providers to keep you informed about the process and apprised of any problems or complications. Well before your delivery date, establish a partnership with your birth team.

See page 35 for natural childbirth painkillers.

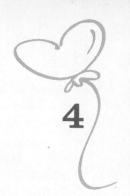

4

The Type A Pregnancy

A HEALTHY TYPE A WOMAN IS LEAN AND FIT, with a well-regulated metabolism and a strong immune system. However, when you don't follow the diet and lifestyle guidelines for your blood type, conditions can develop that may compromise your health and ability to pursue a successful pregnancy. Type A is particularly susceptible to stress-related health problems, such as colds and flu, high blood pressure, heart conditions, and even cancer. Stress has a weakening effect on body systems and hormonal activity and can also be an impediment to fertility. Gestational hypertension and diabetes are always potential risk factors for the Type A woman, and these tendencies can be countered by foods and supplements that maximize the most efficient use of your body's own healing mechanisms.

The adaptations that produced blood Type A were based on the need to fully utilize nutrients from plant sources. For this reason, Type A has difficulty digesting and metabolizing animal protein and fat. High-quality protein can be provided by increased consumption of legumes, fish, and small amounts of lean, organic poultry.

Following the blood type diet is an essential foundation, enabling you to optimize your health and prepare for an energetic and enjoyable pregnancy.

The Type A Diet

The following food lists comprise the Type A diet. Note that the values for certain foods change in preparation for pregnancy, during pregnancy, and/or while you are breast-feeding. I call these Chameleon Foods, and they are included in the following table. Use this table for quick reference. Specific Chameleon Foods are also marked with an asterisk (*).

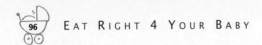

Values are calculated for secretors. If you are a non-secretor and want a higher level of compliance, refer to *Live Right 4 Your Type*.

Type A Chameleon Foods

Chameleons are foods whose values change before pregnancy, during pregnancy, and/or while breast-feeding.

FOOD	PRE-/POST-PREGNANCY	PREGNANCY	FACTORS
SEAFOOD			
Bass	Neutral	Avoid	Heightened risk of contamination
Carp	Beneficial	Avoid	Heightened risk of contamination
Mahimahi	Neutral	Avoid	Heightened risk of contamination
Salmon	Beneficial	Neutral	Some risk of contamination
Shark	Neutral	Avoid	High mercury content
Swordfish	Neutral	Avoid	High mercury content
Tilapia	Neutral	Avoid	Heightened risk of contamination
Tuna	Neutral	Avoid	High mercury content
Whitefish	Beneficial	Avoid	Heightened risk of contamination
DAIRY/EGGS			
Egg/chicken	Neutral	Beneficial	Good source of DHA
OIL			
Linseed (flaxseed)	Beneficial	Neutral	Limit intake; can be a uterine stimulant in large amounts*
Borage	Neutral	Avoid	Uterine stimulant
NUTS/SEEDS			
Flaxseed	Beneficial	Neutral	Limit intake; can be a uterine stimulant in large amounts
VEGETABLES			
Aloe	Beneficial	Avoid	Uterine stimulant
Parsley	Beneficial	Neutral	Limit intake; can be a uterine stimulant in large amounts
SPICES			
Chocolate	Neutral	Avoid	Contains caffeine
Fenugreek	Beneficial	Avoid	Uterine stimulant
Ginger	Beneficial	Avoid	May cause miscarriage in large amounts
Licorice	Neutral	Avoid	Can influence estrogen levels
Parsley	Beneficial	Neutral	Limit intake; can be a uterine stimulant in large amounts
Turmeric	Beneficial	Avoid	Uterine stimulant

FOOD	PRE-/POST-PREGNANCY	PREGNANCY	FACTORS
HERBAL TEAS			
Aloe	Beneficial	Avoid	Uterine stimulant
Dong quai	Neutral	Avoid	Can start uterine bleeding
Fenugreek	Beneficial	Avoid	Uterine stimulant
Ginger	Beneficial	Avoid	May cause miscarriage in large amounts
Goldenseal	Neutral	Avoid	Potentially harmful to fetus
Licorice	Neutral	Avoid	Can influence estrogen levels
Parsley	Beneficial	Neutral	Limit intake; can be a uterine stimulant in large amounts
Raspberry leaf	Neutral	Beneficial	Supports the pregnancy
St. John's wort	Beneficial	Avoid	Can influence estrogen levels
Yarrow	Neutral	Avoid	Uterine stimulant
BEVERAGES			
Coffee, regular	Beneficial	Avoid	Contains caffeine
Tea, green	Beneficial	Avoid	Contains caffeine; start weaning yourself before pregnancy, and avoid during pregnancy
Wine, red	Beneficial	Avoid	Alcohol should be completely avoided during pregnancy
Wine, white	Neutral	Avoid	Alcohol should be completely avoided during pregnancy

Meats and Poultry

To receive the greatest benefits, Type As should eliminate all meats from your diet. While neutral meats like chicken or turkey are acceptable, to maximize your pregnancy fitness, you should limit them to occasional consumption. Be sure to choose organic meats. Stay away from processed meat products like ham, frankfurters, and cold cuts. They contain nitrates, which are toxic for you and your fetus.

HIGHLY BENEFICIAL
None

NEUTRAL
Chicken   Ostrich
Cornish hen   Squab
Grouse   Turkey
Guinea hen

AVOID

All commercially processed meats	Liver
	Mutton
Bacon	Partridge
Beef	Pheasant
Buffalo	Pork
Duck	Quail
Goose	Rabbit
Ham	Squirrel
Heart	Turtle
Horse	Veal
Lamb	Venison

Seafood

Seafood is an excellent source of protein for Type As, but pregnant women must use special caution to avoid fish that may contain PCBs or that are otherwise potentially toxic. Check with your local health department about the safety of fish caught in local waters. In addition, avoid certain fish that are especially vulnerable to contamination by environmental pollutants, such as pesticides and PCBs. These include bass, bluefish, grouper, mahimahi, fresh salmon, tilapia, and whitefish. Also avoid fish that may contain a high level of mercury—halibut, swordfish, shark, and fresh tuna.

HIGHLY BENEFICIAL

Carp*	Salmon*
Cod	Sardine
Mackerel	Sea trout
Monkfish	Silver perch
Pickerel	Snail
Pollack	Whitefish*
Red snapper	Whiting
Rainbow trout	Yellow perch

NEUTRAL

Abalone	Bullhead
Bass*	Chub
Butterfish	Croaker
Brook trout	Cusk

Food with different values than the standard Type A diet are indicated with an asterisk (*).

Drum
Halfmoon fish
Mahimahi*
Mullet
Muskellunge
Ocean perch
Orange roughy
Parrot fish
Pike
Pompano
Porgy
Rosefish
Sailfish
Salmon roe

Scrod
Shark*
Smelt
Snapper
Sturgeon
Sucker
Sunfish
Swordfish*
Tilapia*
Tuna*
Weakfish
White Perch
Yellowtail

AVOID

Anchovy
Barracuda
Beluga
Bluefish
Bluegill bass
Catfish
Caviar (sturgeon)
Clam
Conch
Crab
Crayfish
Eel
Flounder
Frog
Gray sole
Grouper
Haddock
Hake

Halibut
Harvest fish
Herring (fresh)
Herring (pickled)
Lobster
Mussels
Octopus
Opaleye
Oyster
Scallop
Scup
Shad
Shrimp
Smoked salmon
Sole
Squid (calamari)
Tilefish

Eggs and Dairy

Type As can tolerate small amounts of fermented dairy products, but you should avoid anything made with whole milk, and also limit egg consumption to occasional organically grown eggs.

Food with different values than the standard Type A diet are indicated with an asterisk (*).

Your Type A choices should be yogurt, kefir, nonfat sour cream, and cultured dairy products. Raw goat's milk is a good substitute for whole milk.

If you are a Type A allergy sufferer or are experiencing respiratory problems, be aware that dairy products greatly increase the amount of mucus you secrete. Type As normally produce more mucus than the other blood types, but an over-abundance of mucus means a greater risk of infection and respiratory problems. This is another good reason to limit your intake of dairy foods.

HIGHLY BENEFICIAL
None

NEUTRAL

Egg, chicken*	Goat's milk
Egg, duck	Kefir
Egg, goose	Mozzarella
Egg, quail	Paneer
Farmer cheese	Ricotta
Feta	Sour cream
Ghee (clarified butter)	Yogurt
Goat cheese	

AVOID

American cheese	Half & half
Blue cheese	Ice cream
Brie	Jarlsberg
Butter	Milk (cow)
Buttermilk	Monterey jack
Camembert	Muenster
Casein	Neufchâtel
Cheddar	Parmesan
Colby	Provolone
Cottage cheese	Quark cheese
Cream cheese	Sherbet
Edam	String cheese
Emmenthal	Swiss
Gouda	Whey
Gruyère	

Food with different values than the standard Type A diet are indicated with an asterisk (*).

Oils and Fats

When cooking, give preference to the healthful monounsaturated olive oil. Linseed (flaxseed) oil, normally beneficial for Type A, should be limited during pregnancy; in large quantities, it can be a uterine stimulant. Borage oil should be eliminated.

HIGHLY BENEFICIAL

Black currant seed	Olive
Linseed (flaxseed)*	Walnut

NEUTRAL

Almond	Safflower
Borage*	Sesame
Canola	Soy
Cod liver	Sunflower
Evening primrose	Wheat germ

AVOID

Castor	Cottonseed
Coconut	Peanut
Corn	

Nuts and Seeds

Since Type As eat very little animal protein, nuts and seeds supply an important protein component to your diet. If you have gallbladder problems or are suffering from pregnancy-related digestive problems limit yourself to small amounts of nut butters instead of whole nuts. Again, limit flaxseeds during pregnancy.

HIGHLY BENEFICIAL

Flaxseed*	Pumpkin seed
Peanut	Walnut
Peanut butter	

NEUTRAL

Almond	Beechnut
Almond butter	Butternut
Almond cheese	Chestnut
Almond milk	Filbert (Hazelnut)

Food with different values than the standard Type A diet are indicated with an asterisk (*).

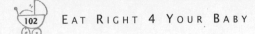

Hickory nut
Litchi
Macadamia nut
Pecan
Pignolia (pine nut)
Poppy seed

Safflower
Sesame butter (tahini)
Sesame seed
Sunflower butter
Sunflower seed

AVOID

Brazil nut
Cashew

Pistachio

Beans and Legumes

Type As thrive on the vegetable proteins found in beans and legumes. Many beans and legumes provide a nutritious source of protein. Be aware, however, that not *all* beans and legumes are good for you. Some, like kidney, lima, navy, and garbanzo, can contain a lectin that produces a decrease in insulin production. This can be a factor in both obesity and diabetes—and during pregnancy can place you at risk of gestational diabetes.

Soy beans and their products—tofu, tempeh, soy milk, soy cheese—are highly recommended as Type A diet staples. Many supermarkets now carry these products, and they are available in health-food stores.

HIGHLY BENEFICIAL

Adzuki bean
Black bean
Black-eyed pea
Fava (broad) bean
Green bean
Lentil bean
Pinto bean

Soy bean
Soy cheese
Soy milk
Soy, miso
Soy, tempeh
Soy, tofu
String bean

NEUTRAL

Cannellini bean
Green pea
Jicama bean
Mung bean, sprouts

Northern bean
Snap bean
White bean

AVOID

Copper bean
Garbanzo bean
Kidney bean

Lima bean
Navy bean
Tamarind bean

Grains, Pastas, and Cereals

Type As generally do well on most cereals and grains, as long as you select the more concentrated whole grains instead of instant and processed cereals. If you have a pronounced mucus condition caused by asthma, or frequent respiratory infections, limit your wheat consumption, as wheat causes mucus production. You'll have to experiment for yourself to determine how much wheat you can eat.

HIGHLY BENEFICIAL

Amaranth
Artichoke pasta
Buckwheat
Essene (manna) bread
Ezekiel 4:9 bread
Oat bread
Oat flour
Rice

Rice bran
Rice cake
Rice flour
Rice milk
Rice (puffed)
Rye flour
Soba noodles

NEUTRAL

Barley
Cornflakes
Cornmeal
Corn muffin
Couscous
Cream of rice
Fin crisp
Gluten flour
Grits
Ideal flat bread
Kamut
Millet
Oat bran
Oatmeal

Popcorn
Quinoa
Rye bread
Ry-krisp
Sorghum
Spelt
Tapioca
Wheat (gluten flour products)
Wheat (refined, unbleached)
Wheat (semolina flour
   products)
Wheat (white flour products)
Wheat bread (sprouted/
   commercial)

AVOID

Cream of wheat
English muffin
Familia
Farina
Grape-Nuts
Matzo

Wheat (whole wheat
   products)
Wheat bran
Wheat germ
Shredded wheat

Vegetables

Vegetables are vital to the Type A diet, providing minerals, enzymes, and antioxidants. Eat your vegetables in as natural a state as possible (raw or steamed) to preserve their full benefits.

Most vegetables are available to Type As, but there are a few caveats: Peppers aggravate the delicate Type A stomach, as do the molds in fermented olives. Domestic potatoes, sweet potatoes, yams, and cabbage contain proteins that may interfere with the proper absorption of essential nutrients. Avoid tomatoes, as their lectins have a negative effect on the Type A digestive tract. Broccoli is highly recommended for its antioxidant benefits. Antioxidants strengthen the immune system and prevent abnormal cell division. Other vegetables that are excellent for Type As are carrots, collard greens, kale, pumpkin, and spinach. Yellow onions are very good immune boosters, too. They contain a substance called quercetin, which is a powerful antioxidant.

Aloe, normally beneficial for Type A, should be avoided during pregnancy, as it is a uterine stimulant. Limit parsley and fennel. Also note that although onions and garlic are beneficial for Type A, you may want to avoid or limit them while you're breast-feeding. Some babies experience colic when moms eat these foods.

Values for whole vegetables apply to their juices, unless otehwise noted.

HIGHLY BENEFICIAL

Alfalfa sprouts	Leek
Aloe*	Lettuce (Romaine)
Artichoke (domestic, globe, Jerusalem)	Mushroom (maitake, silver dollar)
Beet greens	Okra
Broccoli	Onion (green, red, Spanish, yellow)
Carrot	
Celery	Parsley*
Chicory	Parsnip
Collard greens	Pumpkin
Escarole	Rappini (broccoli rabe)
Garlic	Spinach
Horseradish	Swiss chard
Kale	Turnip
Kohlrabi	

Food with different values than the standard Type A diet are indicated with an asterisk (*).

NEUTRAL

Arugula
Asparagus
Asparagus pea
Bamboo shoot
Beet/beet greens
Bok choy
Brussels sprouts
Cabbage juice
Caraway
Cauliflower
Celeriac
Chervil
Cilantro (coriander leaf)
Corn
Cucumber
Daikon
Endive
Fennel
Fiddlehead fern
Lettuce (bibb, Boston,
   butter, iceberg,
   mesclun)
Mushroom (abalone,
   enoki, portabello,
   straw, tree oyster)

Mustard greens
Olive, green
Oyster plant
Pea, green
Pea, pod
Pickles (in brine)
Pimiento
Poi
Radicchio
Radish
Radish sprouts
Rutabaga
Scallion
Seaweeds
Shallot
Snow pea
Squash (all types)
String bean
Taro
Water chestnut
Watercress
Zucchini

AVOID

Cabbage (not juice)
Eggplant
Juniper
Mushroom, shiitake
Olive (black, Greek,
   Spanish)
Peppers (all types)
Pickles (in vinegar)

Potato (all types)
Rhubarb
Sauerkraut
Sweet potato
Tomato
Yam
Yucca

Fruits

Type As should eat fruits at least three times a day. Most fruits are allowable, although you should try to emphasize the more alkaline fruits, such as berries and melons, which can help to balance the acid-forming grains. Type As don't do well on tropical fruits like mangoes, oranges, and papaya. Grapefruit is closely related to oranges, but it has positive effects on the Type A stomach. Pineapple is an excellent digestive for Type As. Lemons are also excellent for Type As, helping to aid digestion and clear mucus from the system. Unless noted separately, all values of the whole fruit apply to the juice as well.

HIGHLY BENEFICIAL

Apricot	Grapefruit
Blackberry	Lemon
Blueberry	Lime
Boysenberry	Pineapple
Cherry (all types)	Plum (all types)
Fig (fresh or dried)	Prune

NEUTRAL

Apple	Kumquat
Apple cider	Loganberry
Asian pear	Musk melon
Avocado	Nectarine
Breadfruit	Peach
Canang melon	Pear
Cantaloupe	Persian melon
Casaba melon	Persimmon
Christmas melon	Pomegranate
Cranberry	Prickly pear
Crenshaw melon	Quince
Currant (black and red)	Raisin
Date	Raspberry
Dewberry	Sago palm
Elderberry (dark blue, purple)	Spanish melon
Gooseberry	Star fruit (carambola)
Grape (all types)	Strawberry
Guava	Watermelon
Kiwi	Youngberry

AVOID

Banana	Orange
Bitter melon	Papaya
Coconut	Plantain
Honeydew melon	Tangerine
Mango	

Spices and Sweeteners

Spices can be either helpful or dangerous, and this is especially true during pregnancy. A number of spices are uterine stimulants and should be avoided—especially if you have a high-risk pregnancy or a history of miscarriage. Ginger can be an excellent remedy for digestive ailments. However, it can cause miscarriage in high amounts, so limit its use to pre- and post-pregnancy. Chocolate contains caffeine and should also be avoided. Type As should also limit the consumption of sugars.

Certain spices, normally used in small amounts for cooking, should be used sparingly during pregnancy. These include cinnamon, marjoram, nutmeg, oregano, parsley, rosemary, sage, and thyme.

If you have problems with heartburn, nausea, or morning sickness, which occur mostly in the first trimester, you may find it helpful to eliminate strong spices such as curry and horseradish. However, if you don't experience digestive problems, go ahead and use them.

HIGHLY BENEFICIAL

Barley malt	Horseradish
Blackstrap molasses	Parsley*
Fenugreek*	Soy sauce
Garlic	Tamari
Ginger*	Turmeric*

NEUTRAL

Agar	Brown rice syrup
Allspice	Caraway
Almond extract	Cardamon
Anise	Carob
Arrowroot	Chervil
Basil	Chive
Bay leaf	Chocolate*
Bergamot	Cinnamon

Food with different values than the standard Type A diet are indicated with an asterisk (*).

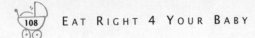

Clove   Oregano
Coriander   Paprika
Cornstarch   Peppermint
Corn syrup   Rice syrup
Cream of tartar   Rosemary
Cumin   Saffron
Curry   Sage
Dextrose   Savory
Dill   Sea salt
Fructose   Senna
Guarana   Spearmint
Honey   Stevia
Licorice root*   Sugar (brown, white)
Mace   Tamarind
Maple syrup   Tapioca
Marjoram   Tarragon
Mint (all kinds)   Thyme
Mustard (dry)   Vanilla
Nutmeg   Yeast (baker's and brewer's)

AVOID

Aspartame   MSG
Capers   Pepper (all types)
Carrageenan   Sucanat
Chili powder   Vinegar (all types)
Gelatin (plain)   Wintergreen
Guar gum (gum arabic)

Condiments

You can eat small quantities of jam and low-fat salad dressing if it's made without vinegar. Vinegar-pickled foods have been linked to stomach cancer in people with low levels of stomach acid. Eliminate ketchup from your diet. Type As react badly to tomato and vinegar.

HIGHLY BENEFICIAL

Mustard (prepared, no wheat or vinegar)

Food with different values than the standard Type A diet are indicated with an asterisk (*).

NEUTRAL

Jam (from acceptable fruits)

Jelly (from acceptable fruits)

Salad dressing (low-fat, from
acceptable ingredients)

AVOID

Ketchup

Mayonnaise

Pickles (all types)

Pickle relish

Vinegar-pickled vegetables
and fruit

Worcestershire sauce

Herbal Teas

Herbal teas can deliver strong doses of herbs, and for this reason many are not advised for pregnant women. However, certain teas are particularly beneficial, especially late in pregnancy. Raspberry leaf is rich in vitamins and nourishes the uterus. Chamomile is excellent as a calming tea and sleep aid. Dandelion tea aids digestion. Rose hip tea is a good source of vitamin C. Slippery elm tea is an excellent remedy for intestinal problems.

HIGHLY BENEFICIAL

Alfalfa

Aloe*

Ashwagandha

Burdock

Chamomile

Dandelion

Echinacea

Fenugreek*

Gentian

Ginger*

Gingko biloba

Ginseng, siberian

Hawthorn

Holy basil

Milk thistle

Parsley*

Rose hip

Slippery elm

St. John's wort*

Stone root

Valerian

NEUTRAL

Chickweed

Coltsfoot

Dong quai*

Elderberry

Goldenseal*

Hops

Horehound

Licorice root*

Linden

Mulberry

Mullein

Peppermint

Food with different values than the standard Type A diet are indicated with an asterisk (*).

Raspberry leaf*
Sage
Sarsparilla
Senna
Shepherd's purse
Skullcap

Spearmint
Strawberry leaf
Thyme
White birch
White oak bark
Yarrow*

AVOID

Catnip
Cayenne
Chaparral
Comfrey
Corn silk

Red clover
Rhubarb
Sassafras
Yellow dock

Miscellaneous Beverages

Start eliminating caffeine and alcohol three to six months before pregnancy, and continue until you are no longer breast-feeding. The common caffeine withdrawal symptoms—headache, fatigue, and irritability—won't occur if you wean yourself gradually.

HIGHLY BENEFICIAL

Coffee, decaf
Coffee, regular*

Tea, green*
Wine, red*

NEUTRAL

Wine, white*

AVOID

Beer
Liquor, all distilled
Soda, all types

Seltzer water
Tea, black (regular and decaf)

Before You Get Pregnant

The best guarantee for a healthy pregnancy is to be in top condition before you get pregnant. Start getting ready at least six months before you conceive.

Food with different values than the standard Type A diet are indicated with an asterisk (*).

Pre-pregnancy Diet Strategies

Get Serious About the Type A Diet

Begin to increase your compliance to the Type A diet at least six months before you attempt to conceive. The most efficient approach is to add to the number of Type A beneficial foods you consume. These foods exert a powerful medicinal influence on your system, creating the optimal atmosphere for conception. Simultaneously, make an effort to eliminate those foods that are "avoids" for Type A.

Check the Type A Chameleon Foods in the chart on page 96. Some of these show different values for the pre-pregnancy period.

Control Your Weight

The most effective way for Type A to control weight gain is to reduce your intake of animal protein. Poorly digested by Type A, animal protein has the effect of slowing down your metabolism and promoting water retention and increased body fat.

TYPE A HEALTHY WEIGHT-LOSS GUIDELINES
1. Eat a low-fat, largely plant-based diet.
2. Avoid red meats and non-cultured dairy.
3. Derive your primary protein from soy-based foods, fresh seafoods, and beans.
4. Limit grains, especially wheat, if you have a weight problem.
5. Eat plenty of fiber derived from fresh fruits and vegetables.
6. Reduce your stress levels. High stress hormones contribute to weight gain.
7. Engage in regular moderate exercise, with an emphasis on stress-reducing exercises, such as Hatha yoga and T'ai chi.

Type A

THESE FOODS PROMOTE WEIGHT LOSS	THESE FOODS PROMOTE WEIGHT GAIN
Cultured soy foods	Meat
Olive and flaxseed oil	Dairy foods (uncultured)
Green vegetables	Wheat (in overabundance)
Pineapple	

Incorporate Detoxifiers into Your Diet

Toxins are the by-products of bacterial activity on unabsorbed foods that grow in your intestinal tract. Most often these toxins are the result of eating foods that are poorly digested by your blood type—including foods that are overly processed and chemically treated.

SIGNS OF TOXICITY IN TYPE A

- Skin problems, such as acne, eczema, and psoriasis
- Headaches
- Mental agitation
- Bad breath
- Low blood sugar
- Odiferous stools
- Blurred vision

To aid in detoxification before pregnancy, follow this protocol for one week:

TYPE A DETOXIFICATION PROTOCOL
(Do not use during pregnancy.)

- Milk thistle (*Silymarin*). 250 mg daily.
- Dandelion (*Taraxacum officinale*). One 250-mg capsule, twice daily.
- Fig powder or dried figs. One tablespoon fig powder or three figs before bed with an 8-oz. glass of water.
- Dry skin brushing. See page 171.

Detoxifying foods that are especially effective for Type A include cultured dairy foods, such as yogurt and kefir, and soy products, such as miso, natto, okara, soy sauce, and tempeh.

Pre-pregnancy Supplement Guidelines

VITAMINS	MINERALS	HERBS
Vitamin B complex— daily, with: 400–600 mcg folic acid 500 mcg vitamin B_{12}	Calcium citrate— 1,000 mg daily	Chamomile—1 to 3 cups daily
Vitamin C from rose hip or acerola cherry—500 mg daily	Iron—45–60 mg daily	Dandelion—250-mg capsule, daily: also use fresh in salads or as tea

VITAMINS	MINERALS	HERBS
Vitamin E—400 iu daily	Zinc—15–25 mg daily	Green tea—1 to 3 cups daily *before* pregnancy
		Holy Basil—50 mg twice daily

The Type A diet offers abundant quantities of important nutrients. It's vital to get as many nutrients as possible from fresh foods, and only use supplements to fill in the minor blanks in your diet. In addition to vitamins, minerals, protein, carbohydrates, and fats, many grains, beans, vegetables, and fruits are excellent sources of fiber, which is necessary for proper digestion. Also, fresh vegetables are an important source of phytochemicals, the substances in foods that strengthen the immune system and help prevent cancer and heart disease.

VITAMINS

VITAMIN B. Type As may need extra amounts of B_1, B_5, and B_6 to have an optimal stress response. B_{12} is vital if you are strictly a vegetarian Type A. Vitamins B_1 and B_6 help improve the cortisol function of the adrenal gland (an area of stress-related weakness for Type As) and simultaneously normalize the rhythmic activity of the gland. Stress in virtually all forms places extra demands on your B_5 status, increasing overreaction and exhaustion in the face of stress. I advise all Type As to take a well-rounded vitamin B supplement. Be sure it provides at least 400 to 600 micrograms of folic acid.

VITAMIN C. Vitamin C in amounts greater than 500 milligrams per day provides a buffer against high levels of the stress hormone cortisol. Look for food-derived vitamin C preparations, such as those found from rose hip or acerola cherry.

VITAMIN E. A daily supplement of no more than 400 international units will help enhance the immune system and cardiac health for Type A.

MINERALS

IRON. The Type A diet is naturally low in iron, which is found in the greatest abundance in red meats. If you take an iron supplement, I recommend Floradix, a liquid iron and herb supplement, found in most health-food stores. Floradix is well assimilated by Type As.

ZINC. About 15 to 25 milligrams per day of supplemental zinc can reduce cortisol and offer protection against infection. Be aware that in high doses zinc can be dangerous. Do not exceed 50 milligrams per day.

HERBS

CHAMOMILE. This is an effective antistress remedy.

DANDELION (*Taraxacum officinale*). It is very effective for mild water retention. It can be used in salads or as a tea. Dandelion is also a good source of potassium.

GREEN TEA (*Camellia sinensis*). Regular consumption of green tea appears to enhance chances of conception.

HOLY BASIL. Holy basil is another excellent antistress remedy.

Improve Your Emotional Health

Your emotional well-being—especially your ability to adapt to stress—is every bit as important to your overall health as your physical well-being. Indeed, the two are inextricably linked. As a Type A, you are particularly sensitive to an overreaction to stress, due to your naturally high levels of the stress hormone cortisol. High cortisol levels are implicated in a wide range of health conditions, including insulin resistance, metabolic imbalances, heart disease, chronic fatigue, and susceptibility to infections.

It is crucial that you take steps to regulate your stress levels before you become pregnant. Here are some suggestions:

- Reduce stress in your environment. The following factors are known to increase cortisol levels and mental exhaustion for Type A individuals. Be aware of them and limit your exposure.

Crowds of people	Smoking
Long telephone calls	Too much sugar and starch
Cold or hot weather conditions	Strong smells or perfumes
	Too much exercise
Coffee (more than 1 cup)	Financial concerns
High-carbohydrate breakfast	Anxiety for others
Strong chemicals	Lack of sleep
Overwork	Dieting (low calories)
Unproductive meetings	Violent movies
Negative emotions	Loud noise
Sunbathing	Arguments

- If you are being treated for an anxiety disorder, ask your doctor about taking a melatonin supplement. People with high anxiety often have low levels of melatonin.

Some of my Type A patients who have had difficulty sleeping through the night because of anxiety have benefited from the installation of a small, diochromatic green light. You can find it on the Internet or from a theater lighting supplier.

If you are experiencing anxiety or sleep deprivation, I also recommend a technique called alternate nostril breathing. Left nostril breathing generates a more relaxing effect. Right nostril breathing generates a more energized effect. Switching back and forth tends to balance your nervous system. Holding your right nostril closed, breathe slowly through the left nostril to the count of 10. Switch nostrils and repeat. Perform the exercise five times.

Pre-pregnancy Exercise Guidelines

MAINTENANCE FOR HEALTHY TYPE As

For Type A, stress regulation and overall fitness depend on engaging in regular exercise, with an emphasis on calming exercises such as hatha yoga and t'ai chi, as well as light aerobic exercise such as walking.

Hatha yoga has become increasingly popular in Western countries as a method for coping with stress, and in my experience it is an excellent form of exercise for Type As.

T'ai chi, a martial art that is basically a form of moving meditation, has also been studied for its antistress effects. T'ai chi helps reduce stress, lowers blood pressure, and improves mood.

Walking or brisk walking is the ideal aerobic exercise for Type A, especially when you walk outdoors in a quiet, natural setting. Walking promotes the type of stress-balancing effect you need, along with cardiovascular, immune, and other health benefits.

The following comprises the ideal exercise regimen for Type A:

THREE TO FOUR TIMES A WEEK, CHOOSE ONE:

EXERCISE	DURATION
Hatha yoga	40–50 minutes
T'ai chi	40–50 minutes

TWO TO THREE TIMES A WEEK, CHOOSE ONE:

EXERCISE	DURATION
Aerobics (low-impact)	40–50 minutes
Treadmill	30 minutes
Weight training (5–10 lb free weights)	15 minutes
Cycling (recumbent bike)	30 minutes
Swimming	30 minutes
Brisk walking	45 minutes
Pilates	40–50 minutes

Your Pregnancy:
Type A Three-Trimester Plan

Diet Strategies

First Trimester

Choose Type A Beneficial Foods

Continue your compliance with the Type A diet, paying special attention to the Type A Chameleon Foods in the table on page 96. These are foods whose normal values are different during pregnancy. If you are new to the Type A diet, your most important first steps are the replacement of animal proteins with soy and other high-quality vegetable proteins, and the elimination of dairy products, except for cultured dairy foods such as yogurt and kefir.

The first trimester is such a critical time that you should emphasize highly beneficial foods whenever possible. These foods act as medicine for Type A. While many foods are good choices of important nutrients, your power foods offer an extra benefit. For example:

Choose tofu over chicken.
Choose soy cheese and soy milk over beans and bean sprouts.
Choose walnuts over almonds.
Choose oat flour over wheat flour.
Choose artichokes and fennel over asparagus and Brussels sprouts.
Choose blackberries and blueberries over apples and melons.

Emphasize Pregnancy Power Foods

There are some nutrients that have special importance. These include protein, calcium, iron, and folic acid.

Blood Type A Pregnancy Power Foods			
PROTEIN	**CALCIUM**	**IRON**	**FOLIC ACID**
Cultured soy (miso, natto, okara, soy sauce, tempeh) Fish (cod, mackerel, red snapper, salmon)	Yogurt, kefir, soy milk Sardines (unboned) Canned salmon	Whole grains Beans (adzuki, black, black-eyed peas) Figs Blackstrap molasses	Whole grains Fish Dark green leafy vegetables Lentil beans Sunflower seeds

A special note for vegetarians: You may be concerned about getting enough protein in your diet to meet the increased needs of your pregnancy. Be sure to consume a varied diet and eat adequate amounts of soy protein. If you use rice- and soy-based protein supplements, avoid those containing added sugar.

Enhance Digestive Enzymes

Type As have low levels of stomach acid, which can contribute to digestive problems common early in pregnancy. By improving digestive efficiency, you'll experience far less heartburn, nausea, and "morning sickness."

- Avoid meat, which requires high levels of digestive enzymes to consume.
- Use a plant-derived enzyme formula, such as bromelain. Heartburn can be a persistent problem in the first trimester of the Type A pregnancy. Enzymes help break down foods and help transport nutrients across the intestinal walls for your body to use. (See Supplement Guidelines, page 148.)
- Avoid carbonated beverages, such as mineral water, seltzer, and soda. The carbonation decreases gastrin production, which decreases stomach acidity and makes it difficult to properly digest food. Type A is also at greater risk of developing celiac disease, a digestive condition linked to wheat. If you have digestive distress, it's best to avoid wheat.
- Morning sickness results from excessive liver activity, a condition that Type A has a tendency toward. Vitamin B_6 is a good remedy because it impacts the metabolic cycle directly. (See Supplement Guidelines, page 148).

Fight Fatigue and Mood Swings

It is common to feel especially fatigued during the first trimester of pregnancy, as your body adapts to the tremendous changes taking place. Elevated stress hormones also contribute to fatigue and mood swings. Try to establish a regular sleep schedule and adhere to it as closely as possible. When you have a normal sleep-wake rhythm, it reduces cortisol levels. During the day, schedule at least two breaks of 20 minutes each for complete relaxation. Combat sleep disturbances with regular exercise and a relaxing pre-bedtime routine. A light snack before bedtime will help raise your blood sugar levels and improve sleep.

A contributing factor to Type A fatigue—especially if you are on a vegetarian diet—is the increased susceptibility to iron-deficiency anemia. Ask your doctor about taking an iron supplement and increase your consumption of foods high in folic acid, vitamin C, iron, selenium, and zinc. These include coldwater fish (salmon, mackerel, herring, and sardines), eggs, green beans, tahini, beets, spinach, kelp, green vegetables, parsley, lettuce, prunes, currants, peaches, and mulberries.

BEST TYPE A IRON SOURCES
Seaweed
Brewer's yeast
Molasses
Prunes
Raisins
Mushrooms
Chard
Spinach
Nuts and seeds

Handle Your Cravings and Aversions

If you crave foods that are not beneficial for your blood type, find healthy blood type–friendly substitutes. For example:

WHEN YOU CRAVE ...	EAT ...
Sugar	Fresh berries; pineapple slices
Salty foods	Miso soup; soy sauce
Ice cream	Frozen yogurt; soy- or rice-based ice cream
Fatty foods	Peanut butter; almond butter on spelt or Essene bread
Creamy foods	Soy shakes; soy and fruit smoothies

First Trimester Menu Plans

The following menus offer a guide to healthy eating during the first trimester of your pregnancy. They are designed to offer well-balanced, delicious meals that include the primary values critical for Type A:

- They emphasize a variety of delicious soy-food preparations, fish, pasta, and beneficial beans, fresh fruits, and vegetables.
- They provide an extra boost of calcium and protein with Type A–specific smoothies.
- They provide many foods to help overcome first trimester problems, such as constipation, fatigue, and morning sickness.

They break the daily diet into six meals/snacks a day—aiding digestion and reducing fatigue by avoiding an empty stomach. The menus are flexible and can be mixed and reorganized according to your personal needs. I have purposely not included portion sizes for most dishes, since caloric needs vary depending on your height and weight. However, try to eat about 300 calories a day more than normal during the first trimester.

Although beverages are listed with some meals, I suggest you drink them half an hour before or after eating. Liquids consumed with solid foods dilute the digestive juices. Don't forget to keep drinking water throughout the day.

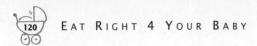

Menus

DAY 1

BREAKFAST
Silken Scramble with Fresh Spinach
   and Feta*
Spelt toast
Pineapple juice
Rose hip tea

MID-MORNING SNACK
Super Baby Smoothie*

LUNCH
Artichoke and Vidalia Onion Tart*
Mixed green salad

MID-AFTERNOON SNACK
Beneficial fruit

DINNER
Steamed Whole Red Snapper*
Basmati rice
Steamed broccoli

EVENING SNACK
Fresh Fig Salad*
Chamomile tea

DAY 2

BREAKFAST
Spelt flakes with raisins and soy milk
Ezekiel toast
Mixed berries
Slippery elm tea

MID-MORNING SNACK
Beneficial fruit or protein

LUNCH
Farmer's Vegetable Soup*
Mesclun Salad*

MID-AFTERNOON SNACK
Type A Trail Mix-1*

DINNER
Tofu-Sesame Fry*
Faro Pilaf*
Braised leeks

EVENING SNACK
Super Baby Smoothie*

DAY 3

BREAKFAST
Millet-Spelt-Soy Pancakes* with
   blueberry syrup
2 plums
Slippery elm tea

MID-MORNING SNACK
Silken Smoothie*

LUNCH
Grilled soy cheese on Ezekiel bread
Apple

MID-AFTERNOON SNACK
Super Baby Smoothie*

DINNER
Baked chicken breast
Brown rice
Green Bean Salad with Walnuts and
   Goat Cheese*

EVENING SNACK
Sliced strawberries with soy milk
Chamomile tea

DAY 4

BREAKFAST
Silken Scramble*
Pumpkin Almond Bread*
Pineapple juice
Rose hip tea

MID-MORNING SNACK
Beneficial fruit or protein

LUNCH
Salmon with Wakame Seaweed*
Cuban Black Bean Soup*

MID-AFTERNOON SNACK
Oatmeal Cookies*

DINNER
Spicy Stir-fried Tofu with Apricots and
   Almonds*
Braised shiitake mushrooms
Braised greens with garlic
Raw Enzyme Relish*

EVENING SNACK
Super Baby Smoothie*

DAY 5

BREAKFAST
Scrambled eggs
Rice cakes with almond butter and
    cherry preserves
Grapefruit juice
Rose hip tea

MID-MORNING SNACK
Beneficial fruit or protein

LUNCH
Turkey sandwich on spelt bread with
    Romaine lettuce and mustard

MID-AFTERNOON SNACK
Peanut butter on Essene bread

DINNER
Quinoa Tortillas with Pureed Pinto
    Beans*
Steamed spinach
Braised escarole

EVENING SNACK
Tofu Pumpkin Pudding*
Chamomile tea

DAY 6

BREAKFAST
Silken Scramble*
Mixed berries
Slippery elm tea

MID-MORNING SNACK
Sliced apple with walnuts and raisins

LUNCH
Mushroom Barley Soup with Spinach*
Mesclun Salad*

MID-AFTERNOON SNACK
Beneficial fruit

DINNER
Fried Monkfish*
Steamed Artichoke*
Apple and Onion Confit*

EVENING SNACK
Super Baby Smoothie*

DAY 7

BREAKFAST
Wheat-free Waffles*
Mixed berries
Rose hip tea

MID-MORNING SNACK
High-Energy Protein Shake*

LUNCH
Sardine Salad*
Rye vita crackers
Mixed green salad

MID-AFTERNOON SNACK
Type A Trail Mix-2*

DINNER
Quinoa Pasta with Rappini
2 Beneficial vegetables

EVENING SNACK
Super Baby Smoothie*

DAY 8

BREAKFAST
Kasha with brown sugar and soy milk
Grapefruit juice
Rose hip tea

MID-MORNING SNACK
Pineapple Protein Shake*

LUNCH
Adzuki Bean and Pumpkin Soup*
Spinach Salad*

MID-AFTERNOON SNACK
Beneficial fruit or protein

DINNER
Broiled Salmon Steak*
Grilled Portabello Mushrooms*
Steamed Artichoke*
Raw Enzyme Relish*

EVENING SNACK
Rice Pudding with Soy Milk*
Chamomile Tea

DAY 9

BREAKFAST
Poached egg on toasted Ezekiel bread
Pineapple juice
Rose hip tea

MID-MORNING SNACK
Beneficial fruit or protein

LUNCH
Leftover salmon on a bed of Romaine
Miso soup*
Spelt bread

MID-AFTERNOON SNACK
Type A Trail Mix-1*

DINNER
Teriyaki Tofu Steak*
Brown Rice Pilaf* with carrots and
    onions
Beneficial vegetable

EVENING SNACK
Super Baby Smoothie*

DAY 10

BREAKFAST
Pumpkin Almond Bread*
½ grapefruit
Vegetable juice
Rose hip tea

MID-MORNING SNACK
Super Baby Smoothie*

LUNCH
Grilled chicken salad* on bed of
    Romaine
Simple Fish Soup*

MID-AFTERNOON SNACK
Raisins and chopped walnuts
Glass of soy-rice milk

DINNER
Fried Monkfish*
Wild rice
Steamed broccoli

EVENING SNACK
Glass of soy milk

DAY 11

BREAKFAST
Spelt flakes with fresh berries and soy
    milk
Essene bread with almond butter
Slippery elm tea

MID-MORNING SNACK
Pineapple-Apricot Silken Smoothie*

LUNCH
Jerusalem Artichoke Soup*
Mesclun Salad*

MID-AFTERNOON SNACK
Beneficial fruit or protein

DINNER
Spicy Stir-fried Tofu with Apricots
    and Almonds*
Braised Swiss chard*
Wild rice

EVENING SNACK
Super Baby Smoothie*

DAY 12

BREAKFAST
Poached egg
Tropical Salad*
Ezekiel toast with cherry preserves
Slippery elm tea

MID-MORNING SNACK
Beneficial fruit or protein

LUNCH
Black-eyed Peas with Leeks*
Carrot-Raisin Salad*

MID-AFTERNOON SNACK
Type A Trail Mix-2*

DINNER
Cornish game hen roasted with
    onions and parsnips
Green vegetables

EVENING SNACK
Super Baby Smoothie*

DAY 13

BREAKFAST
Blueberry Buckwheat Muffin*
Fresh pineapple
Raspberry-leaf tea

MID-MORNING SNACK
Super Baby Smoothie*

LUNCH
Super Broccoli Salad*
Sliced chicken on a bed of Romaine

MID-AFTERNOON SNACK
Beneficial fruit

DINNER
Steamed Whole Red Snapper*
Glazed Turnips and Onions*
Steamed asparagus
Raw Enzyme Relish*

EVENING SNACK
Sliced strawberries with soy milk
Mint tea

DAY 14

BREAKFAST
Brown Rice–Spelt Pancakes*
Mixed fruit
Slippery elm tea

MID-MORNING SNACK
Super Baby Smoothie*

LUNCH
Carrot-Tofu Soup with Dill*
Mesclun Salad*

MID-AFTERNOON SNACK
Type A Trail Mix-1*

DINNER
Butternut Squash and Tofu with
    Mixed Vegetables*
Spinach Salad*

EVENING SNACK
Rice cakes with apple butter
Chamomile tea

Second Trimester

Adjust to an Increased Appetite

Fetal growth is rapid during the second trimester, and you may experience a greater appetite, especially if you no longer suffer from the nausea that may have plagued you during the first three months. Use your extra calories to maximum benefit.

EMPHASIS FOR EXTRA CALORIES
• High-quality protein—soy, fish, beans
• Calcium-rich foods—sardines, unboned canned salmon, soy milk
• Vitamin C–rich foods—dark green leafy vegetables, plums, pineapple

Keep Your Blood Sugar in Check

Type A's susceptibility to blood sugar irregularities can be increased by elevated stress levels and high cholesterol, especially if your diet includes too much animal protein and fat. Gestational diabetes, a dangerous condition late in pregnancy, can place you and your baby in serious jeopardy. The following symptoms should alert you to blood sugar imbalances:

Sweating
Palpitations
Extreme hunger
Restlessness

---

* You can find recipes for asterisk-marked items in appendix A.

Anxiety

Dizziness and light-headedness

To restore a proper balance:

- Reduce the amount of fat in your diet.
- Eliminate refined sugars and starches.
- Eat fiber-rich foods every day.
- Never skip meals. Preferably, eat six small meals a day.
- Reduce your stress levels. There is a direct connection between high cortisol and blood sugar irregularities.

Build Your Immunity

Type A often struggles with compromised immune function, which can make you more vulnerable to colds and flus. Your overall immune health is critical to your ability to carry a fetus to term, since your immune system is suppressed during pregnancy to accept the fetus. If you have a history of miscarriages, immune health should be your top priority. Many dietary factors have been linked to immune function. Failure to eat breakfast, irregular eating habits, low vegetable intake, inadequate protein, excessive wheat intake, and high-fat diets (especially those with excessive amounts of polyunsaturated fatty acids) have all been associated with lowered immune function.

Deficiencies in a range of nutrients can result in decreased immune function, so keep your nutrient levels high. In particular, selenium, zinc, vitamin C, beta-carotene, vitamin A, vitamin E, and vitamin D deficiencies should be addressed.

Check the nutrient chart below to be sure your diet contains plenty of these nutrient-rich foods.

SELENIUM	ZINC	VITAMIN C	BETA-CAROTENE
Whole grains	Turkey	Citrus fruit	Dark green
Seafood	Dried beans	Strawberries	vegetables
	and peas	Brussels sprouts	Carrots
		Dark green	Pumpkin
		vegetables	Peaches

VITAMIN A	VITAMIN E	VITAMIN D
Chicken liver	Spinach	Fatty fish
Eggs	Safflower oil	Egg yolk

Eliminate Excess Mucus Production

Type A has a tendency to suffer from excessive mucus production, which can cause a stuffy nose, respiratory problems, and ear infections. I recommend that all Type As begin the day with a glass of room temperature water mixed with the juice of a quarter to half a lemon. This will reduce mucus production. Two to three cups of stinging nettle tea every day can also minimize mucus.

If you have problems with mucus, you should also avoid dairy products, which are known to increase mucus.

Second Trimester Menu Plans

The following menus offer a guide to healthy eating during the second trimester of your pregnancy. They include some adjustments from the first trimester, taking into account the special emphasis on this period in your pregnancy.

- The menu suggestions place an even greater emphasis on soy, fish, grains, and fresh fruits and vegetables—all foods that help regulate Type A blood sugar.
- They include more calories than the first trimester menus, to accommodate the growing nutritional needs of your fetus.
- They provide an extra boost of calcium and protein with Type A–specific smoothies.
- They provide additional foods that will help to overcome second-trimester problems, such as hemorrhoids, varicose veins, and mucus production.

The menus are flexible and can be mixed and reorganized according to your personal needs. I have purposely not included portion sizes for most dishes, since caloric needs vary depending upon your height and weight. However, these menus do offer more foods than the first trimester—and you should try to increase your intake by 100 to 300 calories per day.

Note that although beverages are listed with some meals, I suggest you drink them half an hour before or after eating. Liquids consumed with solid foods dilute the digestive juices. Don't forget to keep drinking water throughout the day.

Menus

DAY 1

BREAKFAST
Fruit Silken Scramble*
Ezekiel toast
Fresh vegetable juice
Rose hip tea

MID-MORNING SNACK
Peanut butter on Essene bread

LUNCH
Salmon Salad* on a bed of Romaine
    lettuce
Rice crackers
Raisins and walnuts

MID-AFTERNOON SNACK
Type A Trail Mix-1*

DINNER
Sesame Chicken*
Glazed Turnips and Onions*
Brown Rice Pilaf*

EVENING SNACK
Super Baby Smoothie*

DAY 2

BREAKFAST
Silken Scramble* with brown rice and
    vegetables
Date-Prune Smoothie*
Rose hip tea

MID-MORNING SNACK
Pineapple Yogurt Drink*

LUNCH
Cold Buckwheat Noodles with Peanut
    Sauce*
Mixed steamed vegetables

MID-AFTERNOON SNACK
Beneficial fruit or protein

DINNER
Broiled Salmon Steaks*, marinated in
    Tamari Dipping Sauce*
Kasha*
Stewed okra and onion

EVENING SNACK
Baked Apple*
Glass of soy-rice milk

DAY 3

BREAKFAST
Wheat-Free Waffles*
Cherry preserves
Fresh blueberries
Slippery elm tea

MID-MORNING SNACK
Beneficial fruit or protein

LUNCH
Grape Ice*
Tofu, avocado, alfalfa sprouts, on
    spelt bread
Vidalia Onion Vinaigrette*

MID-AFTERNOON SNACK
Super Baby Smoothie*

DINNER
Tofu Vegetable Stir-fry*
Steamed broccoli
Wild rice

EVENING SNACK
Peanut Butter Cookies*
Chamomile Tea

DAY 4

BREAKFAST
Scrambled eggs
Poached Fruit*
Raspberry leaf tea

MID-MORNING SNACK
Sassy Smoothie*

LUNCH
Peanut butter and blueberry jam on
    soy-flour bread
Glass of goat's milk
2 apricots

MID-AFTERNOON SNACK
Beneficial fruit

DINNER
Tofu and Black Bean Chili*
2 Beneficial vegetables

EVENING SNACK
Super Baby Smoothie*

DAY 5

BREAKFAST
Amaranth Pancakes* with maple syrup
Fresh blueberries

MID-MORNING SNACK
Beneficial fruit or protein

LUNCH
Jerusalem Artichoke Soup*
Super Broccoli Salad*

MID-AFTERNOON SNACK
Type A Trail Mix-1*

DINNER
Broiled rainbow trout
Basmati rice
Carrots and Parsnips with Garlic
    and Cilantro*

EVENING SNACK
Chocolate soy pudding (available in
    health food stores)
Chamomile tea

DAY 6

BREAKFAST
Poached egg
Blueberry Muffin*
Fresh pineapple slices
Slippery elm tea

MID-MORNING SNACK
Date-Prune Smoothie*

LUNCH
Grilled mozzarella and zucchini
    sandwich
Miso Soup*

MID-AFTERNOON SNACK
Raisin Peanut Balls*

DINNER
Green Leafy Pasta*
Romaine salad with Olive Oil and
    Lemon Dressing*

EVENING SNACK
Super Baby Smoothie*

DAY 7

BREAKFAST
Silken Scramble*
Sautéed Pears*
Raspberry leaf tea

MID-MORNING SNACK
Beneficial fruit or protein

LUNCH
Lentil Soup*
Mesclun Salad*

MID-AFTERNOON SNACK
Pineapple-Apricot Silken Smoothie*

DINNER
Peter's Escargot*
Faro Pilaf*
Steamed artichoke
Pureed root vegetables

EVENING SNACK
Rice cakes with apple butter
Mint tea

DAY 8

BREAKFAST
Spelt flakes with soy milk
Stewed plums
Pineapple juice
Rose hip tea

MID-MORNING SNACK
Beneficial fruit or protein

LUNCH
Sardine Salad*
Rice crackers
Apple slices

MID-AFTERNOON SNACK
Super Baby Smoothie*

DINNER
Kung Pao Tofu and Chicken*
Braised dandelion greens
   with garlic
Steamed broccoli

EVENING SNACK
Frozen yogurt
Chamomile tea

DAY 9

BREAKFAST
Tofu Carob Protein Drink*
Mixed berries
Raspberry leaf tea

MID-MORNING SNACK
Beneficial fruit or protein

LUNCH
Greek Salad*
Salmon Salad* on a bed of Romaine
   lettuce

MID-AFTERNOON SNACK
Carrot-Cucumber-Apple Smoothie*

DINNER
Sauteed Monkfish*
Millet Couscous*
Steamed broccoli and carrots

EVENING SNACK
Super Baby Smoothie*

DAY 10

BREAKFAST
Fresh blueberries and yogurt
Ezekiel toast
Vegetable juice
Rose hip tea

MID-MORNING SNACK
Super Baby Smoothie*

LUNCH
Black-eyed Peas and Barley Salad*
Mixed steamed vegetables

MID-AFTERNOON SNACK
Beneficial fruit or protein

DINNER
Tasty Tofu-Pumpkin Stir-Fry*
Brown rice
Green beans

EVENING SNACK
Rice crackers with almond butter
Grapes

DAY 11

BREAKFAST
Pineapple Yogurt Drink*
Ezekiel toast with almond butter

MID-MORNING SNACK
Super Baby Smoothie*

LUNCH
Tofu-Vegetable Stir Fry*
Rice crackers

MID-AFTERNOON SNACK
Peanut Butter Cookies*

DINNER
Turkey Cutlets*
Black-eyed Peas, Okra, and Leek
    Melange*
Baked Apple*

EVENING SNACK
Glass of soy milk

DAY 12

BREAKFAST
Tropical Salad*
Ezekiel toast with blackberry preserves
Vegetable juice
Type A Tea

MID-MORNING SNACK
Silken Smoothie* with peaches and
    mixed berries

LUNCH
Grilled Chicken Salad* on spelt bread
Spinach Salad*

MID-AFTERNOON SNACK
Beneficial fruit or protein

DINNER
Butternut Squash and Tofu with
    Mixed Vegetables*
Braised greens

EVENING SNACK
Poached Fruit*
Glass of soy-rice milk
Mint tea

DAY 13

BREAKFAST
Zucchini-carrot omelet
Sautéed Pears*
Spelt toast

MID-MORNING SNACK
High-Energy Protein Shake*

LUNCH
Adzuki Bean and Pumpkin Soup*
Mixed green salad with Olive Oil and
    Lemon Dressing*

MID-AFTERNOON SNACK
Beneficial fruit or protein

DINNER
Roast Turkey*
Pureed root vegetables
Braised Collards*

EVENING SNACK
Super Baby Smoothie*

DAY 14

BREAKFAST
Wheat-Free Pancakes* with blackberry
 preserves
Pineapple juice
Slippery elm tea

MID-MORNING SNACK
Cherry-Peach Smoothie*

LUNCH
Miso Soup*
Green Bean Salad with Walnuts and
 Goat Cheese*
Rice crackers

MID-AFTERNOON SNACK
Beneficial fruit or protein

DINNER
Pan-Fried Grouper with Peanut Sauce*
Steamed broccoli
Wild rice

EVENING SNACK
Chocolate soy pudding (available at
 health-food stores)
Glass of soy-rice milk
Mint tea

Third Trimester

Increase Healthy Blood Flow

Pregnancy places extra stress on your blood vessels as your blood volume increases to support your fetus. Type A has naturally "thicker" blood, making you more susceptible to pulmonary embolisms and clots. To keep your blood flowing efficiently:

- Drink a glass of water with the juice of one quarter to one half a fresh lemon every morning upon rising.
- Get serious about reducing stress. There is good evidence that Type As react to stress by increasing the viscosity (thickness) of your blood. Deep breathing, long walks, and stretching are all wonderful.

Control Your Blood Pressure

Type As need to be particularly careful to keep blood pressure under control during pregnancy. Preeclampsia, or pregnancy-induced hypertension, is a very serious condition that afflicts some women in the late stages of pregnancy.

Maintaining your blood type diet is essential.

---

* You can find recipes for asterisk-marked items in appendix A.

NATURAL BLOOD PRESSURE REDUCTION TONIC. One excellent method for ensuring healthy blood pressure is to juice several stalks of celery, taking 6 to 8 ounces as fresh juice daily.

Fight Fatigue and Stress

Many women experience great fatigue toward the end of pregnancy, which is perfectly understandable. For Type As, fatigue is often the result of a buildup of stress, sleep disruptions, and digestive problems—all of which cause a weakening of your immune system. Your focus as you prepare for delivery is to strengthen your immune system.

- Don't undereat or skip meals. Use appropriate blood type snacks between meals if you get hungry.
- If you haven't already, cut down on your work hours during the final months of pregnancy.
- Get extra sleep. Try to add an extra hour or two to your nightly sleep. If possible, take a restorative 30-minute nap during the afternoon. If you have trouble falling asleep because of discomfort, a body pillow might be helpful. A neutral (body temperature) bath with lavender oil is a good remedy for insomnia.

Third Trimester Menu Plans

During the third trimester you may feel full after eating very little. Smaller meals, eaten at 3- or 4-hour intervals, may be required to get all the nutrients you need. The following menus offer a guide to healthy eating during the third trimester of your pregnancy. They include some adjustments to account for the special emphasis of this period in your pregnancy.

- They place even greater emphasis on soy foods, fish, and fresh fruits and vegetables—all foods that help maintain metabolic balance.
- They provide an extra boost of calcium and protein with Type A–specific smoothies. This will help you prepare for the rigors of labor and delivery.
- Vitamin A– and C–rich foods are abundant, also in preparation for delivery.

The menus are flexible and can be mixed and reorganized according to your personal needs. I have purposely not included portion sizes for most dishes, since caloric needs vary depending upon your height and weight. You may need to divide up the meals and snacks further if you don't think you can finish them at one sitting. However, it's vital that you maintain your overall caloric level.

Note that although beverages are listed with some meals, I suggest you drink them half an hour before or after eating. Liquids consumed with solid foods dilute the digestive juices and fill you up faster. Don't forget to keep drinking water throughout the day.

Menus

DAY 1

BREAKFAST
Silken Scramble* with spinach and feta
Spelt toast
Mixed fruit
Raspberry leaf tea

MID-MORNING SNACK
Glass of soy-rice milk
Essene bread with peanut butter

LUNCH
Jerusalem Artichoke Soup*
Carrot-Raisin Salad*
Crackers

MID-AFTERNOON SNACK
Beneficial fruit or protein

DINNER
Tasty Tofu-Pumpkin Stir-fry*
Basmati rice
2 Beneficial vegetables

EVENING SNACK
Super Baby Smoothie*

DAY 2

BREAKFAST
Spelt flakes with raisins and soy milk
½ grapefruit
Ezekiel toast with soy spread
Rose hip tea

MID-MORNING SNACK
Poached Fruit*
Glass of soy-rice milk

LUNCH
Salmon Salad* on a bed of greens
2 slices spelt or Ezekiel bread
Tofu, avocado, and sprouts on spelt bread

MID-AFTERNOON SNACK
Beneficial fruit or protein
Chamomile tea

DINNER
Sesame Chicken*
Brown Rice Pilaf* with carrots and onions
Raw Enzyme Relish*

EVENING SNACK
Super Baby Smoothie*

DAY 3

BREAKFAST
Oatmeal with soy milk
Ezekiel toast with black cherry
    preserves
Mixed berries
Raspberry leaf tea

MID-MORNING SNACK
Beneficial fruit or protein

LUNCH
Lentil Soup*
Super Broccoli Salad*

MID-AFTERNOON SNACK
Type A Trail Mix-2*

DINNER
Broiled Salmon with Lemongrass*
Carrots and Parsnips with Garlic
    and Cilantro*
Black-eyed Peas with Leeks*

EVENING SNACK
Fresh sliced peaches, nectarines,
    figs, and plums
or
Super Baby Smoothie*

DAY 4

BREAKFAST
Scrambled eggs
Sliced pear
Essene toast
Glass of soy-rice milk
Raspberry leaf tea

MID-MORNING SNACK
Cherry-Peach Smoothie*

LUNCH
Vegetable Fritters*
Mesclun Salad*

MID-AFTERNOON SNACK
Beneficial fruit

DINNER
Spicy Stir-fried Tofu with Apricots and
    Almonds
Pureed root vegetables
Steamed asparagus

EVENING SNACK
Super Baby Smoothie*

DAY 5

BREAKFAST
Amaranth Pancakes*
Blackberry preserves
Mixed fruit salad
Rose hip tea

MID-MORNING SNACK
Beneficial fruit or protein

LUNCH
Sardines on a bed of Romaine lettuce
Mixed Roots Soup*
Crackers

MID-AFTERNOON SNACK
Super Baby Smoothie*

DINNER
Green Leafy Pasta*
Endive salad
Beneficial vegetable

EVENING SNACK
Tofu-Pumpkin Pudding*
Glass of soy milk

DAY 6

BREAKFAST
Spinach Frittata*
Pineapple slices
Raspberry leaf tea

MID-MORNING SNACK
Silken Smoothie*

LUNCH
Grilled Chicken Salad*
2 slices of spelt bread

MID-AFTERNOON SNACK
Raisin Peanut Balls*

DINNER
Tofu Vegetable Stir-fry*
Steamed broccoli
Raw Enzyme Relish*

EVENING SNACK
Poached Fruit*
Type A Tea

DAY 7

BREAKFAST
Poached egg
Spelt flakes with soy-rice milk
Mixed berries
Rose hip tea

MID-MORNING SNACK
Beneficial fruit or protein

LUNCH
Waldorf Salad*
Spelt bread with peanut butter and
    jam

MID-AFTERNOON SNACK
Rye crisp snack with prune butter
Chamomile-mint tea

DINNER
Broiled Salmon Steak, Marinated in
    Tamari Dipping Sauce*
Brown rice
Mixed green salad with Seaweed
    Dressing*

EVENING SNACK
Super Baby Smoothie*

DAY 8

BREAKFAST
Amaranth Pancakes* with maple
    syrup
Mixed fruit
Slippery elm tea

MID-MORNING SNACK
Beneficial fruit or protein

LUNCH
White Bean and Wilted Greens Soup*
Mixed green salad
Crackers

MID-AFTERNOON SNACK
Rice cakes with prune butter

DINNER
Steamed Whole Red Snapper*
Steamed broccoli
Brown Rice Pilaf*

EVENING SNACK
Super Baby Smoothie*

DAY 9

BREAKFAST
Silken Scramble
Sauteed Pears*
Ezekiel toast
Pineapple juice

MID-MORNING SNACK
Beneficial fruit or protein
Slippery elm tea

LUNCH
Broiled ground turkey patty with
    melted goat cheese and raw
    spinach leaves
Spelt or wheat toast

MID-AFTERNOON SNACK
Toasted Tamari Pumpkin Seeds*
Carrot juice

DINNER
Pasta with Rappini*
Mixed steamed vegetables

EVENING SNACK
Peanut Butter Cookies*
Glass of soy-rice milk

DAY 10

BREAKFAST
Wheat-free Waffles*
Berry preserves
Stewed apricots
Vegetable juice
Slippery elm tea

MID-MORNING SNACK
Pineapple-Apricot Silken Smoothie*

LUNCH
Sardine Salad*
Farmer's Vegetable Soup*
Crackers

MID-AFTERNOON SNACK
Beneficial fruit or protein

DINNER
Sesame Chicken*
Steamed Artichoke*
Black-Eyed Peas with Leeks*

EVENING SNACK
Super Baby Smoothie*

DAY 11

BREAKFAST
Scrambled eggs
Stewed prunes
Essene toast with peanut butter
Raspberry leaf tea

MID-MORNING SNACK
Heidi's Early Morning Shake

LUNCH
Grilled Chicken Salad on Spelt Bread*
Mixed green salad
Slippery elm tea

MID-AFTERNOON SNACK
Type A Trail Mix-1*

DINNER
Grilled Wild Rice Tempeh*
Broccoli rabe
Turkey Soup*

EVENING SNACK
Walnut Cookies*
Glass of soy-rice milk

DAY 12

BREAKFAST
Silken Scramble*
Ezekiel toast with blueberry preserves
Raspberry leaf tea

MID-MORNING SNACK
Beneficial fruit or protein

LUNCH
Black-eyed Peas and Barley Salad*
Mixed steamed vegetables

MID-AFTERNOON SNACK
Raisins and chopped walnuts
Glass of soy-rice milk

DINNER
Tofu Vegetable Stir-fry*
Basmati rice

EVENING SNACK
Super Baby Smoothie*

DAY 13

BREAKFAST
Poached egg
Blueberry Muffin*
Mixed fruit
Rose hip tea

MID-MORNING SNACK
Rye krisp with prune butter
Pineapple-Apricot Silken Smoothie*

LUNCH
Farmer's Vegetable Soup*
Mesclun Salad*

MID-AFTERNOON SNACK
Beneficial fruit or protein

DINNER
Peanut Chicken*
Brown rice
Steamed broccoli

EVENING SNACK
Super Baby Smoothie*

DAY 14

BREAKFAST
Spelt flakes with mixed fruit and soy-
    rice milk
Ezekiel toast
Raspberry leaf tea

MID-MORNING SNACK
Tofu Carob Protein Shake*

LUNCH
Greek Salad*
Rye krisp
Apple
Lemon chamomile tea

MID-AFTERNOON SNACK
Super Baby Smoothie*

DINNER
Broiled Salmon Steak*
Brown rice
Sesame Broccoli*

EVENING SNACK
Peanut butter cookies*
Valerian-chamomile tea

Exercise Guidelines

First Trimester

Maintenance for Healthy Type As

Since Type A is particularly susceptible to high levels of stress hormones causing anxiety and mood swings, it is particularly important that you employ stress-reducing strategies during this period. The best way for Type A to accomplish that is to continue a program of regular aerobic exercise, incorporated with meditative and stretching exercises, such as Hatha yoga and T'ai Chi.

Do not begin an exercise program during your pregnancy. Hopefully, you've already been engaged in a pre-pregnancy conditioning program, or, better still, have been following the Type A exercise guidelines for some time. The following comprises the ideal exercise regimen for Type A, which is safe for healthy Type As during the first trimester:

THREE TO FOUR TIMES A WEEK, CHOOSE ONE:

EXERCISE	DURATION
Hatha yoga	40–50 minutes
T'ai Chi	40–50 minutes

* You can find recipes for asterisk-marked items in appendix A.

TWO TO THREE TIMES A WEEK, CHOOSE ONE:

EXERCISE	DURATION
Aerobics (low-impact)	40–50 minutes
Treadmill	30 minutes
Weight training (5–10 lb free weights)	15 minutes
Cycling	30 minutes
Swimming	30 minutes
Brisk walking	45 minutes

TYPE A NOTE: A healthy lifestyle that includes exercise, adequate rest, and good nutrition can help to reduce the impact of anxiety attacks. Rhythmic aerobic and yoga exercise programs lasting for more than fifteen weeks have been found to help reduce anxiety. Strength, or resistance, training does not seem to help anxiety, although it is not to be discouraged, as it has many positive benefits.

CAUTIONS FOR HIGH-RISK PREGNANCIES
Consult with your doctor before continuing your exercise regimen if you are in a high-risk pregnancy. Most doctors will discourage exercise if you:

- Have a history of miscarriages, or have had even one miscarriage, if it is recent.
- Have a history of recurrent pelvic or abdominal infections.
- Have an incompetent cervix. This condition causes the cervix to open early, usually in the second trimester, leading to miscarriage.
- Have had toxemia in a previous pregnancy.
- Have a history of premature deliveries.
- Have or have had a serious medical condition, such as cancer, heart disease, asthma, or kidney disease.

Second Trimester

Adaptations for Advancing Pregnancy

Continue your regular program of exercise during the second trimester, with an additional emphasis on gentle stretching and calming exercises.

- Join a yoga class specifically designed for pregnant women.
- Spend more time on your warm-up and cooldown to fully warm and stretch your muscles. This will minimize the muscle cramps that are common as your pregnancy progresses.

- Look for opportunities to incorporate fitness into your daily routine. If feasible, walk to work instead of driving. Take the stairs instead of the elevator.
- Limit your weight workouts to very light weights—no more than 10 pounds. Your center of gravity has shifted, and you may feel awkward. Lighter weights may be the answer. Experiment to find the right balance. Consistency is more important than the amount of weight you use.
- Swimming is an excellent exercise for the second and third trimesters. It places minimum stress on your joints and heart rate. A water aerobics class is an ideal substitution for more strenuous aerobics.
- If you haven't already started your Kegel exercises (see page 28), do so now.

The following comprises a good mix for your second trimester.

THREE TO FOUR TIMES A WEEK, CHOOSE ONE:

EXERCISE	DURATION
Hatha yoga	40–50 minutes
T'ai Chi	40–50 minutes

ONE TO THREE TIMES A WEEK, CHOOSE ONE:

EXERCISE	DURATION
Water aerobics	40 minutes
Treadmill	30 minutes
Weight training (5–10 lb free weights)	15 minutes
Cycling (recumbent)	30 minutes
Swimming	30 minutes
Brisk walking	30–45 minutes

DAILY:

EXERCISE	DURATION
Kegel exercises	2 minutes, 10 to 20 times

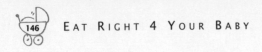

PREGNANCY-SAFE EXERCISE SUBSTITUTIONS

INSTEAD OF . . .	TRY . . .
Bicycling	Indoor stationary bike (recumbent)
Running	Brisk walking/treadmill/ stair climbing
Aerobics	Water aerobics

Third Trimester

Adaptations for Late Pregnancy

Your focus during the final months of pregnancy should be on stress reduction. Not only is this a particularly stressful time, but Type A has a heightened tendency to produce excess cortisol in response to even minor stress. These calming exercises can help:

MEDITATION. Calming yourself through the process of meditation is a wonderful way to reduce your stress level. Quieting the mind will help you eliminate stress-causing thoughts and help you to approach your day in a more positive and efficient manner.

MEDITATION EXERCISE
- Choose a quiet place.
- Sit in a comfortable chair.
- Close your eyes.
- Relax your muscles.
- Become aware of your breathing.
- Choose a pleasant word or visual image that you can hear and see in your imagination. Think of this word or image every time you exhale, for about 15 minutes each day. If you have an intrusive thought or feeling during your meditation, return to the repetition of your relaxing word or image.

DEEP BREATHING. Many of us breathe too fast for the conditions in which we find ourselves; that is, we hyperventilate. This fast, shallow breathing expels carbon dioxide too quickly and can have damaging effects on physical and emotional health. However, when our breathing is deep (using not only the respiratory muscles of the chest but also the belly, lower rib cage, and lower back) it slows the breathing. This slower, deeper breathing, combined with the rhythmical pumping of the diaphragm, abdomen, and belly, helps turn on our parasympathetic nervous system—our "relaxation response." Such breathing helps to harmonize our nervous system and reduce the amount of stress in our lives. And this, of course, has a positive impact on our overall health.

Breathing Exercise

The art of deep breathing is rather simple. Begin by lying on your back in a quiet room. Place your fingers below your rib cage and feel your abdomen rise and fall while you breathe. It should rise up as you breathe in and fall as you breathe out. Now try a deep breath, always keeping the same pattern. Breathe in through your nose and out through your mouth. Inhale for a count of 4 and exhale for a count of 4 with a slight pause in the middle.

Begin daily perineal massage to tone the vaginal canal (page 31). An excellent third trimester exercise regimen for Type A would be the following.

THREE TO FIVE TIMES A WEEK, CHOOSE ONE:

EXERCISE	DURATION
Light yoga	40–50 minutes
Stretching, relaxation, breathing	30 minutes
Meditation	30–40 minutes
Labor preparation class	40–50 minutes

ONE TO THREE TIMES A WEEK, CHOOSE ONE:

EXERCISE	DURATION
Water aerobics	40 minutes
Cycling (recumbent)	30 minutes
Swimming	30 minutes
Brisk walking	30–45 minutes

DAILY, PERFORM BOTH:

EXERCISE	DURATION
Kegel exercises	2 minutes, 10–20 times
Perineal massage	5 minutes, 1–2 times

Supplement Guidelines

First Trimester

Vitamins/Minerals

Take a standard prenatal vitamin supplement, choosing one made from whole food, not synthetic ingredients. Powder-in-capsule forms dissolve most efficiently. If you would like to use a prenatal supplement specifically formulated for Type A, see appendix B for information about Healthy Start ABO Prenatal. The following nutrient breakdown is the optimal formula for Type A.

PRENATAL SUPPLEMENT TYPE A		% DAILY VALUE
Vitamin A (100% as natural beta-carotene from *Dunaliella salina*)	2,500 iu	50
Vitamin C (100% from acerola berry, *Malpighia puncifolia*	75 mg	125
Vitamin D (cholecalciferol)	125 iu	31
Vitamin E (natural d,alpha-tocopheryl succinate)	75 iu	250
Vitamin K (phytonadione)	25 mcg	–
Thiamin (from thiamin HCl)	7.5 mg	500
Riboflavin	10 mg	588
Niacin and niacinamide (vitamin B_3)	10 mg	50
Vitamin B_6 (from pyridoxine HCl)	10 mg	500
Folic acid	800 mcg	200
Vitamin B_{12} (methylcobalamin)	10 mcg	166
Biotin	600 mcg	200
Pantothenic acid (from D-calcium pantothenate)	20 mg	200
Calcium (seaweed base, derived from *Lithothamnium corralliodes* and *Lithothamnium calcareum*)	300 mg	30
Iron (ferrous succinate)	25 mg	138
Iodine (potassium iodide)	100 mcg	66
Zinc (picolinate)	25 mg	166
Selenium (L-selenomethionine)	30 mcg	–
Copper (gluconate)	1 mg	50

Herbal Remedies

HERB	FUNCTION	FORM AND DOSAGE
Chamomile	Calms; relieves heartburn	As tea, 1 to 2 cups daily; or add 2–4 drops of essential oil to bath
Peppermint	Calms; relieves indigestion	As tea, 2 to 3 cups daily, after meals
Red raspberry leaf	Relieves morning sickness	As tea, 2 cups daily
Slippery elm bark	Relieves heartburn	250-mg capsule, twice daily; or as tea, 2 cups daily; or as Thayer's lozenges, 2–4 daily
Stinging nettle leaf	Rich in iron	As tea, 2 cups daily

Nutritional Supplements

NUTRITIONAL SUPPLEMENT	FUNCTION	FORM AND DOSAGE
Digestive enzymes	Aid digestion	Bromelain, 500-mg capsule before meals
Larch arabinogalactan	Relieves constipation	Soluble fiber supplement: 1 tablespoon mixed with water or juice, once daily
Probiotic	For intestinal health	2 capsules, twice daily*
DHA	Provides essential nutrients for fetal development	300-mg capsule daily

* See appendix B for information on blood type–specific probiotics.

Second Trimester

Vitamins/Minerals

Continue to take your prenatal supplement, preferably one formulated for Type A.

Herbal Remedies

HERB	FUNCTION	FORM AND DOSAGE
Bilberry	Relieves hemorrhoids and varicose veins	25-mg capsule, twice daily
Chamomile	Calms; relieves heartburn; relieves hemorrhoids and varicose veins	As tea, 1 to 2 cups daily; or add 2–4 drops of essential oil to bath
Horsetail	Contains silica, which supports healthy bones, skin, hair, and nails	250-mg capsule daily
Peppermint	Calms; relieves indigestion	As tea, 2 to 3 cups daily, after meals
Red raspberry leaf	Treatment for bleeding gums	As tea, 2 cups daily
Rose hip	Treatment for varicose veins, bleeding gums, allergies	1 tablespoon concentrate every 30 minutes for allergy attack; as tea, 2 to 3 cups daily
Stinging nettle leaf	Allergy relief	As tea, 2 cups daily for symptoms
Witch hazel	Treatment for hemorrhoids	Use topically as needed

Nutritional Supplements

NUTRITIONAL SUPPLEMENT	FUNCTION	FORM AND DOSAGE
Larch arabinogalactan	Relieves constipation	Soluble fiber supplement: 1 tablespoon mixed with water or juice, twice daily
Probiotic	For intestinal health	2 capsules, twice daily*
DHA	Provides essential nutrients for fetal development	300-mg capsule daily

* See appendix B for information on blood type–specific probiotics.

Third Trimester

Vitamins/Minerals

Continue to take your prenatal supplement, preferably one formulated for Type A.

Herbal Remedies		
HERB	**FUNCTION**	**FORM AND DOSAGE**
Dandelion leaf/root	Lowers blood pressure; decreases edema	As tea, 2 cups daily; or 250-mg capsule, twice daily
Raspberry leaf	Softens the cervix in preparation for birth; stimulates milk production	As tea, 2 cups daily; as tincture, 15–20 drops daily
Squaw vine	Prepares uterus for birth	As tincture, 10 drops in warm water, twice daily

Nutritional Supplements		
NUTRITIONAL SUPPLEMENT	**FUNCTION**	**FORM AND DOSAGE**
Larch arabinogalactan	Relieves constipation	Soluble fiber supplement: 1 tablespoon mixed with water or juice, twice daily
Probiotic	For intestinal health	2 capsules, twice daily*
DHA	Provides essential nutrients for fetal development	300-mg capsule daily

* See appendix B for information on blood type–specific probiotics.

Labor and Delivery

In addition to the general guidelines for labor and delivery (page 32), you have some specific Type A needs.

Type A Energy Needs

Begin several weeks before your delivery date to prepare yourself for the stress of labor and delivery. Try to get more sleep than usual and eat plenty of nutrient-rich foods. Type As have a tendency to let stress levels build, and you don't want to reach the point of labor with all of your energy resources depleted.

The first stage of labor can last many hours. Drink plenty of liquids and eat a small amount of nourishing food—a vegetable broth, soy milk, or yogurt. Stay hydrated. Be sure to discuss in advance with your doctor or midwife what the policy is about eating light foods or drinking liquids during labor.

Type A Emotional Needs

Type As are extremely sensitive to environmental factors. Try to arrange for your labor room to be in a quiet area; use soothing music if that helps.

Your partner and coach can help you here by encouraging you to focus on your rhythmic breathing and offering encouragement and support. Relaxation techniques can be essential during this period. Some facilities allow women to shower or relax in a warm tub. You might also find it helpful to practice a form of visualization or meditation.

Creative Visualization

This exercise helps to reduce stress by imagining a very calm and relaxing scene in your mind. Some people picture themselves at the beach, feeling the warmth of the sun and the sound of the waves crashing on the shore. Others think of being in the mountains, with eagles soaring overhead, as they breathe in the cool clean air. Others imagine being a leaf floating on the water. The goal is to replace negative, stressful thoughts with more relaxing ones. As your mind relaxes, so does your body.

See page 35 for natural childbirth painkillers.

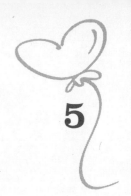

The Type B Pregnancy

A HEALTHY TYPE B WOMAN IS PHYSICALLY FIT and mentally focused. Type B carries the genetic potential for great adaptability and the ability to thrive in changeable conditions. This can give you a substantial advantage during pregnancy. However, to fully realize these benefits, you must adhere to the blood type diet. Type Bs are susceptible to the effects of high stress, such as chronic viral and bacterial infections. Stress has a weakening effect on body systems and hormonal activity and can also be an impediment to fertility. Your digestive tract tends to be sensitive to the protein lectins in certain foods. Dietary lectins can induce inflammation, cause water retention, and influence the control of your blood sugar.

Following the blood type diet is an essential foundation, enabling you to optimize your health and prepare for an energetic and enjoyable pregnancy.

The Type B Diet

The following food lists comprise the Type B diet. Note that the values for certain foods change in preparation for pregnancy, during pregnancy, and/or while you are breast-feeding. I call these Chameleon Foods, and they are contained in the following table. Use this table for quick reference. Chameleon Foods are also marked with an asterisk (*) in the specific food lists.

Values are calculated for secretors. If you are a non-secretor and want a higher level of compliance, refer to *Live Right 4 Your Type*.

Type B Chameleon Foods

Chameleons are foods whose values change before pregnancy, during pregnancy, and/or while breastfeeding.

FOOD	PRE-/POST-PREGNANCY	PREGNANCY	FACTORS
SEAFOOD			
Bass	Neutral	Avoid	Heightened risk of contamination
Bluefish	Neutral	Avoid	Heightened risk of contamination
Carp	Neutral	Avoid	Heightened risk of contamination
Catfish	Neutral	Avoid	Heightened risk of contamination
Flounder	Beneficial	Avoid	Heightened risk of contamination
Grouper	Beneficial	Avoid	Heightened risk of contamination
Halibut	Beneficial	Avoid	High mercury content
Mahimahi	Beneficial	Avoid	Heightened risk of contamination
Salmon	Beneficial	Neutral	Some risk of contamination
Shark	Neutral	Avoid	High mercury content
Swordfish	Neutral	Avoid	High mercury content
Tilapia	Neutral	Avoid	Heightened risk of contamination
Tuna	Neutral	Avoid	High mercury content
Whitefish	Neutral	Avoid	Heightened risk of contamination
DAIRY/EGGS			
Egg/chicken	Neutral	Beneficial	Good source of DHA
SPICES			
Cayenne pepper	Beneficial	Neutral	May cause digestive difficulties
Chocolate	Neutral	Avoid	Contains caffeine
Ginger	Beneficial	Avoid	May cause miscarriage in large amounts
Parsley	Beneficial	Neutral	Limit intake; can be a uterine stimulant in large amounts
Turmeric	Neutral	Avoid	Uterine stimulant
HERBAL TEAS			
Catnip	Neutral	Avoid	Uterine stimulant
Chamomile	Neutral	Beneficial	A calmative and sleep aid
Dandelion	Neutral	Beneficial	Aids digestion
Dong quai	Neutral	Avoid	Can start uterine bleeding
Ginger	Beneficial	Avoid	May cause miscarriage in large amounts
Goldenseal	Neutral	Avoid	Potentially harmful to fetus
Licorice	Beneficial	Avoid	Can influence estrogen levels

FOOD	PRE-/POST-PREGNANCY	PREGNANCY	FACTORS
Parsley	Beneficial	Neutral	Limit intake; can be a uterine stimulant in large amounts
Sage	Beneficial	Neutral	Limit intake; can be a uterine stimulant in large amounts
St. John's wort	Neutral	Avoid	Can be harmful to fetus
Vervain	Neutral	Avoid	Uterine stimulant
Yarrow	Neutral	Avoid	Uterine stimulant
BEVERAGES			
Beer	Neutral	Avoid	Alcohol should be completely avoided during pregnancy
Coffee, regular	Neutral	Avoid	Contains caffeine
Tea, black regular	Neutral	Avoid	Contains caffeine
Tea, green	Neutral	Avoid	Contains caffeine; start weaning yourself before pregnancy, and avoid during pregnancy
Wine, red	Neutral	Avoid	Alcohol should be completely avoided during pregnancy
Wine, white	Neutral	Avoid	Alcohol should be completely avoided during pregnancy

Meats and Poultry

Eat only lean, organic meat of the highest grade available. If you are fatigued or suffer from immune deficiencies, you should eat a red meat such as lamb, mutton, or rabbit several times a week, in preference to beef or turkey.

Avoid chicken altogether. Chicken contains a blood Type B agglutinating protein in its muscle tissue. If you're accustomed to eating more poultry than red meat, you can eat other poultry, such as turkey.

HIGHLY BENEFICIAL
Goat
Lamb
Mutton

Rabbit
Venison

NEUTRAL
Beef
Buffalo

Liver
Ostrich

Pheasant   Veal
Turkey

AVOID

All commercially   Ham
    processed meats   Heart
Bacon   Horse
Chicken   Partridge
Cornish hen   Pork
Duck   Quail
Goose   Squab
Grouse   Squirrel
Guinea hen   Turtle

Seafood

Seafood is an excellent source of protein for Type B, but pregnant women must use special caution to avoid fish that may contain PCBs or that are otherwise potentially toxic. Check with your local health department about the safety of fish caught in local waters. In addition, avoid certain fish that are especially vulnerable to contamination by environmental pollutants, such as pesticides and PCBs. These include bass, bluefish, flounder, grouper, halibut, mahimahi, fresh salmon, tilapia, and whitefish. Also avoid fish that may contain a high level of mercury—halibut, swordfish, shark, and fresh tuna.

Avoid all shellfish—crab, lobster, shrimp, mussels, etc.

HIGHLY BENEFICIAL

Caviar (sturgeon)   Monkfish
Cod   Ocean perch
Croaker   Pickerel
Flounder*   Pike
Grouper*   Porgy
Haddock   Salmon*
Hake   Sardine
Halibut*   Shad
Harvest fish   Sole
Mackerel   Sturgeon
Mahimahi*

Food with different values than the standard Type B diet are indicated with an asterisk (*).

NEUTRAL

Abalone
Bass*
Bluefish*
Bullhead
Carp*
Catfish*
Chub
Cusk
Drum
Grey sole
Herring (fresh, pickled)
Mullet
Muskellunge
Opaleye fish
Orange roughy
Parrot fish
Perch (silver, white, yellow)
Pompano
Red snapper

Rainbow trout
Rosefish
Sailfish
Scallop
Scup
Scrod
Shark*
Smelt
Smoked salmon
Snapper
Squid (calamari)
Swordfish*
Tilapia*
Tilefish
Tuna*
Weakfish
Whitefish*
Whiting

AVOID

Anchovy
Barracuda
Beluga
Butterfish
Clam
Conch
Crab
Crayfish
Eel
Frog

Lobster
Mussels
Octopus
Oysters
Pollack
Shrimp
Snail
Trout (all)
Yellowtail

Eggs and Dairy

Type B is the only blood type that can fully enjoy a variety of dairy foods. If you are of Asian descent, you may initially have a problem adapting to dairy foods—

Food with different values than the standard Type B diet are indicated with an asterisk (*).

not because your system is resistant to them, but because your *culture* has typically been resistant. See page 168 for advice on introducing unfamiliar foods.

Eggs can be consumed in moderation. They are a good source of DHA, which is a beneficial nutrient for your health and the health of your developing fetus. Choose organic eggs only.

HIGHLY BENEFICIAL

Cottage cheese   Mozzarella
Farmer cheese   Paneer
Feta   Ricotta
Goat cheese   Milk (cow)
Goat's milk   Yogurt
Kefir

NEUTRAL

Brie   Gruyère
Butter   Half & half
Buttermilk   Jarlsberg
Camembert   Monterey jack
Casein   Muenster
Cheddar   Neufchatel
Colby   Parmesan
Cream cheese   Provolone
Edam   Quark
Egg, chicken*   Sherbet
Emmenthal   Sour cream (low, nonfat)
Ghee (clarified butter) Swiss
Gouda   Whey

AVOID

American cheese   Egg, quail
Blue cheese   Ice cream
Egg, duck   String cheese
Egg, goose

Oils and Fats

When cooking, give preference to the healthful monounsaturated olive oil. Linseed (flaxseed) oil is neutral for Type B, but limit its use during pregnancy.

Food with different values than the standard Type B diet are indicated with an asterisk (*).

HIGHLY BENEFICIAL
Olive

NEUTRAL

Almond	Linseed (flaxseed)
Black currant seed	Walnut
Cod liver	Wheat germ
Evening primrose	

AVOID

Borage	Peanut
Canola	Safflower
Castor	Sesame
Coconut	Soy
Corn	Sunflower
Cottonseed	

Nuts and Seeds

Most nuts and seeds are not advised for Type Bs. Peanuts, sesame seeds, and sunflower seeds, among others, contain lectins that can cause inflammation and upset the digestive tract.

HIGHLY BENEFICIAL
Walnut (black)

NEUTRAL

Almond	Flaxseed
Almond butter	Hickory
Beechnut	Litchi
Brazil	Macadamia
Butternut	Pecan
Chestnut	Walnut (English)

AVOID

Cashew	Poppy seed
Filbert	Pumpkin seed
Peanut	Sesame butter (tahini)
Peanut butter	Sesame seed
Pignolia (pine nut)	Sunflower butter
Pistachio	Sunflower seed

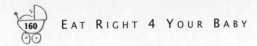

Beans and Legumes

Type Bs can eat some beans and legumes, but many beans, such as lentils, garbanzos, pintos, and black-eyed peas, contain lectins that can cause inflammation and upset the digestive tract. Generally, Type B Asians tolerate beans and legumes better than other Type Bs because they are culturally accustomed to them.

HIGHLY BENEFICIAL

Kidney bean	Navy bean
Lima bean	

NEUTRAL

Cannellini bean	Northern bean
Copper bean	Snap bean
Fava (broad) bean	Soy bean
Green bean	String bean
Green pea	Tamarind bean
Jicama bean	White bean

AVOID

Adzuki bean	Soy cheese
Black bean	Soy flakes
Black-eyed pea	Soy granules
Garbanzo bean (chickpea)	Soy milk
Lentil	Soy, miso
Mung bean, sprouts	Soy, tempeh
Pinto bean	Soy, tofu

Grains, Breads, and Pasta

I've encountered some Type Bs who can tolerate wheat products, but overall, they are more like Type O in their intolerance. Type Bs should also avoid rye, which is a common allergen in your system.

I would advise that you moderate your intake of breads, pasta, and rice. You won't need much of these nutrients if you're consuming the meat, seafood, and dairy products advised.

HIGHLY BENEFICIAL

Essene (manna) bread	Oat bran
Ezekiel 4:9 bread	Oatmeal
(100% sprouted)	Rice milk

Millet
Rice
Rice bran

Rice cake
Rice (puffed)
Spelt (whole)

NEUTRAL

Barley
Cream of rice
Familia
Farina
Gluten-free bread
Granola
Grape-Nuts
Quinoa
Rice (white, brown, basmati)
Rice bread

Rice flour
Soy flour bread
Spelt flour products
Spinach pasta
Wheat (refined, unbleached)
Wheat (semolina flour
  products)
Wheat (white flour products)
Wheat bread, sprouted (not
  Essene/Ezekiel)

AVOID

Amaranth
Artichoke pasta (pure)
Buckwheat/kasha
Corn (white, yellow, blue)
Cornflakes
Cornmeal
Couscous (cracked wheat)
Cream of wheat
Gluten flour
Grits
Kamut
Kasha popcorn
Rice (wild)
Rye

Rye bread (100%)
Rye flour
Seven-grain bread/cereal
Shredded wheat
Soba noodles
  (100% buckwheat)
Sorghum
Tapioca
Teff
Wheat bran
Wheat germ
Wheat (gluten flour products)
Wheat (whole-wheat
  products)

Vegetables

There are many high-quality, nutritious vegetables available for Type Bs. Take full advantage of them with three to five servings a day. There is only a handful of vegetables that Type Bs should avoid, but take these guidelines to heart. Corn is filled with lectins that negatively affect your blood and digestion. Radishes and artichokes are also bad for Type B digestion. Tomatoes should be eliminated by Type Bs. Also avoid olives, as their molds can trigger allergic reactions.

Fennel and parsley should be limited during pregnancy, as these are uterine stimulants in large amounts. Also note that although onions and garlic are allowed for Type B, you may want to avoid or limit them while you're breast-feeding. Some babies experience colic when moms eat these foods.

Values for whole vegetables apply to their juices, unless otherwise noted.

HIGHLY BENEFICIAL

Beets

Beet greens

Broccoli

Brussels sprouts

Cabbage (all types)

Carrot

Cauliflower

Collard greens

Eggplant

Kale

Mushroom (shiitake)

Mustard greens

Parsnip

Peppers (all types)

Potato (sweet)

Yam

NEUTRAL

Alfalfa sprouts

Arugula

Asparagus

Asparagus pea

Bamboo shoots

Bok choy

Caraway

Carrot juice

Celeriac

Celery

Chervil

Chicory

Chili peppers

Cilantro (coriander leaf)

Cucumber

Daikon radish

Dandelion

Dill

Endive

Radicchio

Rappini (broccoli rabe)

Escarole

Fennel

Fiddlehead fern

Garlic

Horseradish

Kohlrabi

Leek

Lettuce (all types)

Mushroom (abalone, silver
    dollar, enoki, maitake,
    oyster, portabello)

Okra

Onion (all types)

Oyster plant

Pea (green, pod)

Pickle (in brine or vinegar)

Poi

Potato (all white-fleshed
    types)

String bean

Swiss chard

Food with different values than the standard Type B diet are indicated with an asterisk (*).

Rutabaga
Sauerkraut
Scallion
Seaweeds
Shallot
Snow pea
Spinach
Squash (all types,
    except pumpkin)

Taro
Turnip
Water chestnut
Watercress
Yucca
Zucchini

AVOID

Aloe
Artichoke (domestic, globe,
    Jerusalem)
Corn
Olive (all types)

Pumpkin
Radish
Rhubarb
Sprouts (mung bean, radish)
Tomato

Fruits

There are very few fruits a Type B must avoid and a wide range of beneficial fruits to choose from. Pineapple is an especially good digestive for Type Bs. Bromelain, an enzyme in the pineapple, helps you to more easily digest your food. On the whole, you can choose your fruits liberally from the following lists.

Unless noted separately, all values of the whole fruits apply to their juices as well.

HIGHLY BENEFICIAL

Banana
Cranberry
Grape (all types)
Papaya

Pineapple
Plum (all types)
Watermelon

NEUTRAL

Apple/cider
Apricot
Asian pear
Blackberry
Blueberry
Crenshaw melon
Currant (black, red)

Boysenberry
Breadfruit
Canang melon
Cherry (all types)
Christmas melon
Musk melon
Nectarine

Date
Dewberry
Elderberry
Fig (fresh, dried)
Gooseberry
Grapefruit
Guava
Honeydew melon
Kiwi
Kumquat
Lemon
Lime
Loganberry
Mango
Mulberry

Orange
Peach
Pear
Persian melon
Plantain
Prune
Quince
Raisin
Raspberry
Sago plum
Spanish melon
Strawberry
Tangerine
Youngberry

AVOID

Avocado
Bitter melon
Coconut
Persimmon

Pomegranate
Prickly pear
Star fruit (carambola)

Spices and Sweeteners

Spices can be either helpful or dangerous, and this is especially true during pregnancy. A number of spices are uterine stimulants and should be avoided—especially if you have a high-risk pregnancy or a history of miscarriage. Ginger can be an excellent remedy for digestive ailments. However, it can cause miscarriage in high amounts. Chocolate contains caffeine and should also be avoided. Type Bs should also limit their consumption of sugars.

Certain spices, normally used in small amounts for cooking, should be minimized during pregnancy. These inclulde marjoram, nutmeg, oregano, parsley, rosemary, sage, and thyme.

If you have problems with heartburn, nausea, or morning sickness, which occur mostly in the first trimester, you may find it helpful to eliminate strong spices such as curry and horseradish. However, if you have no digestive problems, go ahead and use these spices.

HIGHLY BENEFICIAL

Cayenne pepper*
Curry
Ginger*

Horseradish
Molasses (blackstrap)
Parsley*

NEUTRAL

Agar
Anise
Apple pectin
Arrowroot
Basil
Bay leaf
Bergamot
Caper
Caraway
Cardamom
Carob
Chervil
Chili powder
Chive
Chocolate*
Cilantro (coriander leaf)
Clove
Coriander
Cream of tartar
Cumin
Dill
Dulse
Fructose
Garlic
Honey
Kelp
Mace

Maple syrup
Marjoram
Molasses
Mustard (dry)
Nutmeg
Oregano
Paprika
Pepper (peppercorn,
    red flakes)
Peppermint
Rice syrup
Rosemary
Saffron
Sage
Savory
Sea salt
Spearmint
Sugar (white, brown)
Tamarind
Tarragon
Thyme
Turmeric*
Vanilla
Vinegar (all types)
Wintergreen
Yeast (bakers, brewer's)

AVOID

Allspice
Almond extract
Aspartame

Barley malt
Carrageenan
Cinnamon

Food with different values than the standard Type B diet are indicated with an asterisk (*).

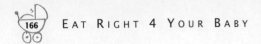

Cornstarch	MSG
Corn syrup	Pepper (black, white)
Gelatin (plain)	Soy sauce
Guarana	Stevia
Gums (acacia, Arabic)	Sucanat
Juniper	Tapioca
Maltodextrin	

Condiments

There are no highly beneficial condiments for Type Bs. If you must have mustard, mayonnaise, or salad dressing on your foods, use them in moderation and stick to the low-fat, low-sugar varieties. Another option is to make your own from okay ingredients. My recommendation is that you try to wean yourself from condiments or replace them with healthier seasonings like olive oil, lemon juice, and garlic. There are a number of recipes in appendix A for healthy, delicious dressings.

HIGHLY BENEFICIAL
None

NEUTRAL

Jam (from acceptable fruits)	Pickles (all types)
Jelly (from acceptable fruits)	Pickle relish
Mayonnaise	Salad dressing (from
Mustard	acceptable ingredients)

AVOID

Ketchup	Worcestershire sauce

Herbal Teas

Herbal teas can deliver strong doses of herbs, and for this reason many are not advised for pregnant women. However, certain teas are particularly beneficial, especially late in pregnancy. Raspberry leaf is rich in vitamins and nourishes the uterus. Chamomile is excellent as a calming tea and sleep aid. Dandelion tea aids digestion. Rose hip tea is a good source of vitamin C. Slippery elm tea is an excellent remedy for intestinal problems.

HIGHLY BENEFICIAL

Ginger*

Ginseng*

Licorice root*

Parsley*

Peppermint

Raspberry leaf

Rose hip

Sage*

NEUTRAL

Alfalfa

Burdock

Chamomile*

Catnip*

Chickweed

Dandelion*

Dong quai*

Echinacea

Elder

Goldenseal*

Hawthorn

Horehound

Mulberry

Rosemary

Sarsaparilla

Slippery elm

Spearmint

St. John's wort*

Strawberry leaf

Thyme

Valerian

Vervain*

White birch

White oak bark

Yarrow*

Yellow dock

AVOID

Aloe

Coltsfoot

Corn silk

Fenugreek

Gentian

Hops

Linden

Mullein

Red clover

Rhubarb

Senna

Shepherd's purse

Skullcap

Miscellaneous Beverages

Start eliminating caffeine and alcohol three to six months before pregnancy, and continue until you are no longer breast-feeding. The common caffeine withdrawal symptoms—headache, fatigue, and irritability—won't occur if you wean yourself gradually. Consumption of alcohol during pregnancy can cause miscarriage, birth defects, and fetal alcohol syndrome.

Food with different values than the standard Type B diet are indicated with an asterisk (*).

HIGHLY BENEFICIAL
Tea, green*

NEUTRAL

Beer*

Coffee, decaf

Coffee, regular*

Tea, black regular*

Tea, black decaf

Wine, red*

Wine, white*

AVOID

Liquor

Seltzer water

Soda (all types)

Before You Get Pregnant

The best guarantee for a healthy pregnancy is to be in top condition before you get pregnant. Start getting ready at least six months before you conceive.

Pre-pregnancy Diet Strategies

Get Serious About the Type B Diet

Begin to increase your compliance with the Type B diet at least six months prior to attempting to conceive. The most efficient approach is to add to the number of Type B super foods you consume. These beneficial foods exert a powerful medicinal influence on your system, creating the optimal atmosphere for conception. At the same time, make an effort to eliminate those foods that are obviously detrimental to Type B. Check the Type B Chameleon Foods in the table on page 154. Some of these foods show different values for the pre-pregnancy period.

Introduce Yourself Gradually to Unfamiliar Foods

Many new subscribers to the Type B diet are not accustomed to eating dairy foods. In fact, a high percentage of people of Asian ancestry are Type B, and these cultures emphasize soy over dairy—especially that derived from cows. These intolerances are not classic food intolerances but, rather, deeply ingrained cultural values. If you are not used to dairy foods, you will need to proceed more slowly in

Food with different values than the standard Type B diet are indicated with an asterisk (*).

adapting to the Type B diet. The same holds true for Type Bs who have been vegetarians and are introducing red meat.

- Introduce dairy foods gradually, after you have been on the Type B diet for several weeks. Begin with cultured dairy products, such as yogurt and kefir, which are more easily tolerated than fresh dairy products. Be sure to choose hormone-free, organic dairy foods.
- Take a digestive enzyme with your main meal until you adapt to eating meat and dairy. Bromelain, an enzyme found in pineapple, is available in supplemental form.
- Keep in mind that some Type Bs can have problems with milk that are not related to blood type, such as lactose intolerance. In these cases, you will have to navigate through the diet with that knowledge guiding your final choices.

Control Your Weight

If you are overweight prior to becoming pregnant, it's important to gain control of your weight before you conceive. Overweight women are at increased risk for elevated blood pressure, diabetes, joint aches and pains, and muscle spasms during pregnancy.

TYPE B HEALTHY WEIGHT-LOSS GUIDELINES
1. Eliminate foods that slow your metabolism—in particular, chicken, corn, buckwheat, peanuts, and lentils.
2. Derive your primary proteins from highly beneficial meats, seafood, and dairy.
3. Limit grains, especially those that impair your metabolism, such as wheat.
4. Make sure you are ingesting plenty of fiber derived from fresh fruits and vegetables.
5. Engage in a regular exercise program. Type B does very well with a combination of cardiovascular, weight training, deep breathing, and meditation. Walking, easy running, hiking, swimming, and cycling can all provide potent metabolic boosts for the Type B woman.

Type B

THESE FOODS PROMOTE WEIGHT LOSS	THESE FOODS PROMOTE WEIGHT GAIN
Low-fat and cultured dairy foods	Chicken
Lean, organic venison	Corn
Green vegetables	Peanuts
	Buckwheat
	Wheat

Incorporate Detoxifiers into Your Diet

Toxins are the by-products of bacterial activity on unabsorbed foods that grow in your intestinal tract. Most often these toxins are the result of eating foods that are poorly digested by your blood type—including foods that are overly processed and chemically treated.

SIGNS OF TOXICITY IN TYPE B
- Diminished sex drive
- Circulation problems
- Sensitivity to light
- Bad breath
- Feelings of fullness in lower intestine
- Cystic breasts

To aid in detoxification before pregnancy, follow this protocol for one week.

TYPE B DETOXIFICATION PROTOCOL
(Do not use during pregnancy.)

- Flaxseed (*Linum usitatissimum*). Take 1 tablespoon added to 8 ounces of water; allow to soak overnight and drink in morning.
- L-glutathione. Take a 100-mg capsule, twice daily.
- Epsom salt bath. Take a shower first, then start with a very clean tub; fill the tub with the hottest water you can stand. Begin with ¼ cup of Epsom salts, work up gradually to 4 cups, and soak as long as half an hour. If you experience light-headedness, drain the tub and hold a cold cloth on your brow until you feel steady enough to leave the tub.
- Probiotic supplement (friendly bacteria). Take twice daily (preferably blood type specific—see appendix B).

- Larch arabinogalactan (soluble fiber supplement). Take 1 tablespoon mixed with water or juice, twice daily.
- Dry skin brushing. Do this once a day.

About Dry Skin Brushing

Dry skin brushing is a method of daily hygiene that has many benefits and has been around for a long time. The skin is a major organ of the body that functions as protection and as a means of elimination. Daily skin brushing will:

- Remove dried, dead cells that block the pores of the skin, allowing the skin to breathe easier and increasing its ability to protect and eliminate the waste products of metabolism.
- Increase circulation of the blood and lymph vessels that lie close to the surface just under the skin. The blood, fluid, and its contents are returned to the heart for redistribution and/or elimination.
- Increase the nutrients to the skin. By clearing out stagnant materials, there is an increased oxygen/carbon dioxide exchange, and other nutrients, vitamins, minerals, enzymes, etc., are also brought to the area.
- Remove waste products of cellular metabolism through the blood vessels and sweating.
- Decrease the workload on the rest of the body in regard to circulation and elimination.
- Warm the skin.

PROCEDURE

Skin brushing should be done with a natural or nylon bristle body brush before the bath or shower. It is suggested that the brushing be done toward the heart; start with the lower limbs, arms, and back, and then the front of the body, using a moderate pressure with short strokes upward and inward. If you have a soft complexion brush, the face can be done as well using more circular motions. Strokes should bring a slight pink color or slight tingling sensation to the skin—never bruising, scraping, bleeding, or pain. One time through for each body area is sufficient.

AVOID SKIN BRUSHING IF:

- You have delicate skin.
- You have easily damaged skin.
- You have an open wound.
- You have known malignancies of the skin or lymph system.

Pre-pregnancy Supplement Guidelines

VITAMINS	MINERALS	HERBS
Vitamin B complex, daily, with: 400–600 mcg folic acid 500 mcg vitamin B$_{12}$	Magnesium citrate— 500 mg, once daily	Bromelain—500-mg capsule before meals
Vitamin C from rose hip or acerola cherry— 250 mg daily		Dandelion—250-mg capsule daily; also use fresh in salads or as tea
		Green tea—1 to 3 cups daily *before* pregnancy
		Licorice (DGL)—150-mg capsule or chewable tablet as needed

The Type B diet is extremely well balanced and offers abundant quantities of important nutrients. It's important to get as many nutrients as possible from fresh foods and only use supplements to address minor additional needs. In addition to vitamins, minerals, protein, carbohydrates, and fats, many grains, beans, vegetables, and fruits are excellent sources of fiber, which is necessary for proper digestion. In addition, fresh vegetables are an important source of phytochemicals, the substances in foods that strengthen the immune system and help prevent cancer and heart disease.

MINERALS

MAGNESIUM. While Type B gets a substantial amount of calcium from dairy foods, you can risk magnesium/ calcium imbalance. Magnesium is essential to the metabolism of calcium and aids in the proper metabolism of foods. A supplement of 500 milligrams may be necessary if you experience the symptoms of sluggish metabolism. Magnesium can occasionally cause a loosening of the stool. If you notice this, just cut back until it disappears.

HERBS

BROMELAIN (Pineapple enzyme). Aids digestion.

DANDELION (*Taraxacum officinale*). This is very effective for mild water retention. It can be used in salads or as a tea. It is also a good source of potassium.

GREEN TEA (*Camellia sinensis*). Regular consumption of green tea appears to enhance chances of conception. (Do not use during pregnancy.)

LICORICE (DGL). Many Type B women complain about stomach acidity (heartburn). This common form of licorice is very helpful. Do not use "whole herb" forms of licorice: They can encourage water retention. (Do not use during pregnancy.)

Improve Your Emotional Health

Your emotional well-being—especially your ability to adapt to stress—is every bit as important to your overall health as is your physical well-being. Indeed, the two are inextricably linked. Studies show that when Type B is in "balance" emotionally and physically, you are able to block stress, anxiety, and depression, using your powerful gift for relaxation and visualization. I have always noted these qualities in my Type B patients, and current research supports my observations.

Out of balance, Type B can suffer from the effects of high cortisol (a stress hormone manufactured by the adrenal gland), and a susceptibility to viral infections, chronic fatigue, mental fogginess, and autoimmune diseases. Your focus in achieving emotional balance needs to be on balancing your cortisol levels and increasing your mental acuity.

Type Bs have a remarkable ability to reduce stress through meditation and visualization. Of all the meditation techniques, transcendental meditation (TM) has been the most thoroughly studied for its antistress effects. Evidence indicates that cortisol decreases during meditation, especially for long-term practitioners, and remains somewhat lower after meditation.

Pre-pregnancy Exercise Guidelines

For Type B, stress regulation and overall fitness is achieved with a balance of moderate aerobic activity and mentally soothing exercise. Below is a list of exercises that are recommended for Type Bs. Choose from among these exercises for a minimum regimen of 45 minutes, three to four times a week. Later, I'll give you the appropriate adjustments for each trimester of pregnancy.

EXERCISE	DURATION	FREQUENCY
Tennis	45–60 minutes	2–3 × week
Martial arts	30–60 minutes	3 × week
Cycling	45–60 minutes	3 × week
Hiking	30–60 minutes	3 × week
Golf (no cart!)	60–90 minutes	2 × week

Your Pregnancy:
Type B Three-Trimester Plan

Diet Strategies

First Trimester

Choose Type B Beneficial Foods

Continue your compliance with the Type B diet, paying special attention to the Type B Chameleon Foods in the table on page 154. These are foods whose normal values are different during pregnancy. If you are new to the Type B diet, your most important first steps are inclusion of high-quality protein found in lean, organic meat and the avoidance of chicken, buckwheat, and corn.

The first trimester is such a critical time that you should emphasize your beneficial foods whenever possible. These foods act as medicine for Type B. While many foods are good choices for important nutrients, your beneficial foods offer an extra benefit. For example:

> Choose lamb over beef.
> Choose goat cheese over cheddar.
> Choose yogurt over cow's milk.
> Choose broccoli and greens over carrots and mushrooms.
> Choose bananas over apples.

Emphasize Pregnancy Power Foods

There are some nutrients that have special importance. These include protein, calcium, iron, and folic acid.

Blood Type B Pregnancy Power Foods			
PROTEIN	**CALCIUM**	**IRON**	**FOLIC ACID**

Lean, organic lamb
Beef liver
Lean, organic
  venison
	Low-fat dairy
	  foods, including
	  cultured dairy
	Sardines
	  (unboned)
		Lean, organic
		  mutton
			Liver, kidney,
			  muscle meats
			Fish
			Dark green leafy
			  vegetables

Minimize Digestive Discomfort

Type B normally doesn't have many digestive problems, as long as you are eating right for your blood type. However, the first trimester of pregnancy brings some digestive challenges. In addition to following your diet, here are some ways to minimize common digestive complaints.

HEARTBURN
- Eat frequent small meals—five to six a day instead of three.
- Eat slowly and chew thoroughly.
- Bend at the knees, not at the waist, when picking up objects.
- Avoid acid-stimulating foods, such as oranges, tangerines, and strawberries.
- Avoid coffee, chocolate, mints, and black tea, all of which can provoke heartburn.
- Avoid sugars and sweets.
- Don't lie down directly after meals.

CONSTIPATION
- Get plenty of exercise.
- Drink lots of water between meals.
- Include dietary sources of inulin, a form of soluble fiber found in over 30,000 plants, such as cabbage, chicory, onion, and asparagus. Inulin helps increase stool volume and intestinal motility.
- Take a daily probiotic supplement to keep your intestines healthy. (See appendix B for blood type–specific probiotics.)
- Get plenty of fiber from fresh fruits and vegetables.

MORNING SICKNESS
- Adhere to the blood type diet.
- Drink plenty of water and nonacidic juices (no caffeine—it dehydrates).

- Eat small, frequent meals throughout the day.
- Do not mix fluids with meals. Drink 30 minutes before or after.
- Dry carbohydrates are usually well tolerated (such as spelt, rice, millet, oat breads or crackers, brown rice).
- Exercise to reduce stress, which can promote nausea.
- Avoid the sight and smell of offensive foods.
- Avoid secondhand smoke.
- Wear an acupressure wristband, used by travelers to prevent motion sickness.
- There is some evidence that vitamin B_6 minimizes nausea. Foods rich in vitamin B_6 include fish and bananas.

Fight Fatigue and Mood Swings

It is common for women to feel especially fatigued during the first trimester of pregnancy, as your body adapts to the tremendous changes that are taking place. That is one reason it's so important for you to be in optimal condition before you get pregnant. A Type B who is run down and stressed out is extremely vulnerable to exhaustion, depression, and inertia.

You need to get at least 1 to 2 hours of additional sleep every night. Establish a regular sleep schedule and adhere to it as closely as possible. During the day, schedule at least two breaks of 20 minutes each for complete relaxation. Combat sleep disturbances with regular exercise and a relaxing pre-bedtime routine. A neutral bath (room temperature) with lavender oil prior to bedtime will help you sleep. (See page 22.)

Type Bs may also benefit from the daily consumption of what I call the Membrane Fluidizer Cocktail, which improves the health of your immune and nervous systems:

MEMBRANE FLUIDIZER COCKTAIL

1 tablespoon flaxseed oil
1 tablespoon high-quality lecithin granules
6 to 8 ounces fruit juice

Shake well and drink.

Handle Your Cravings and Aversions

If you crave foods that are not beneficial for your blood type, find healthy blood type–friendly substitutes. For example:

WHEN YOU CRAVE . . .	EAT . . .
Sugar	Raisins or a plum; any suitable fruit
Salty foods	Nori (seaweed) snack; peppers; celery
Ice cream	Frozen yogurt; frozen fruit ice
Fatty foods	A banana or walnuts
Creamy foods	Yogurt; vegetable puree—sweet potato, onion, parsnip, or carrot; a fruit smoothie

First Trimester Menu Plans

The following menus offer a guide to healthy eating during the first trimester of your pregnancy. They are designed to offer well-balanced, delicious meals that include the primary values critical for Type B:

- They emphasize lean meats, fish, dairy, and fresh fruits and vegetables.
- They provide an extra boost of protein and vital nutrients with Type B–specific smoothies.
- They provide many foods to help overcome first trimester problems, such as constipation, fatigue, and morning sickness.
- They break the daily diet into six meals/snacks a day—aiding digestion and reducing fatigue by avoiding an empty stomach.

The menus are flexible and can be mixed and reorganized according to your personal needs. I have purposely not included portion sizes for most dishes, since caloric needs vary depending on your height and weight. However, try to eat about 300 calories a day more than normal during the first trimester.

Although beverages are listed with some meals, I suggest you drink them half an hour before or after eating. Liquids consumed with solid foods dilute the digestive juices. Don't forget to keep drinking water throughout the day.

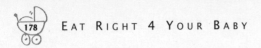

Menus

DAY 1

BREAKFAST
One-Egg Omelet with Fresh Spinach
   and Feta*
1 slice of Essene toast with apple
   butter
Papaya juice
Slippery elm tea

MID-MORNING SNACK
Apricot-Yogurt Drink*

LUNCH
Caesar Salad*
Cream of Lima Bean Soup*

MID-AFTERNOON SNACK
Beneficial fruit or protein

DINNER
Pan-Fried Liver and Onions*
Baked sweet potato
Steamed broccoli

EVENING SNACK
Walnut Cookies*
Chamomile tea

DAY 2

BREAKFAST
Poached egg
Spelt flakes with raisins and cow's milk
Mixed berries
Slippery elm tea

MID-MORNING SNACK
Beneficial fruit or protein

LUNCH
Farmer's Vegetable Soup*
Mesclun Salad*

MID-AFTERNOON SNACK
Type B Trail Mix-1*

DINNER
Broiled Lamb Chops*
Wild rice
Braised leeks

EVENING SNACK
Super Baby Smoothie*

DAY 3

BREAKFAST
Spinach Frittata*
2 plums
Essene toast
Slippery elm tea

MID-MORNING SNACK
Apricot Yogurt Drink*

LUNCH
Grilled Goat Cheddar on Spelt Bread*
Spinach Salad*

MID-AFTERNOON SNACK
Toasted Tamari Pumpkin Seeds*

DINNER
Broiled Salmon Steak*
Steamed Brussels sprouts with butter,
    lemon, and parsley*
Green Bean Salad with Walnuts and
    Goat Cheese*

EVENING SNACK
Sliced banana with cow's milk
Chamomile tea

DAY 4

BREAKFAST
Omelet with feta cheese
    and chopped parsley
Pineapple juice
Rose hip tea

MID-MORNING SNACK
Beneficial fruit or protein

LUNCH
Smoked Mackerel Salad*
Rice crackers*

MID-AFTERNOON SNACK
Super Baby Smoothie*

DINNER
Braised Rabbit*
Pureed sweet potato
Braised greens with garlic

EVENING SNACK
Poached Fruit*
Chamomile tea

DAY 5

BREAKFAST
Rice cereal with milk and berries
Spelt toast
Rose Water Lassi*
Rose hip tea

MID-MORNING SNACK
Beneficial fruit or protein

LUNCH
Turkey sandwich on spelt bread with
   Romaine lettuce and mustard or
   chutney
Mixed green salad

MID-AFTERNOON SNACK
Super Baby Smoothie*

DINNER
Fried Monkfish*
Steamed spinach
Grilled Pepper Medley*

EVENING SNACK
Tofu Banana Pudding*
Glass of milk

DAY 6

BREAKFAST
2 scrambled eggs
Essene toast with butter
½ grapefruit

MID-MORNING SNACK
Banana Plum Bread*

LUNCH
Cream of Lima Bean Soup*
Mesclun Salad*

MID-AFTERNOON SNACK
Beneficial fruit

DINNER
Fettucine with Grilled Lamb Sausages
   and Vegetables*
Mixed green salad

EVENING SNACK
Rice Pudding*
Chamomile tea

DAY 7

BREAKFAST
Poached egg
Cottage cheese with fresh pineapple
    and papaya
Slice of spelt bread with grape jelly
Rose hip tea

MID-MORNING SNACK
High-Energy Protein Shake*

LUNCH
Sardine Salad*
Rye vita crackers
Turkey soup*

MID-AFTERNOON SNACK
Rice cakes with prune butter

DINNER
Pasta with Rappini*
2 Beneficial vegetables

EVENING SNACK
Super Baby Smoothie*

DAY 8

BREAKFAST
Zucchini and Mushroom Frittata*
Spelt toast
Cranberry juice
Slippery elm tea

MID-MORNING SNACK
Glass of kefir
Banana Walnut Muffin*
Grapes

LUNCH
White Bean and Wilted Greens Soup*
Mesclun Salad*

MID-AFTERNOON SNACK
Beneficial fruit or protein

DINNER
Grilled lamb chops
Grilled Portabello Mushrooms*
Steamed broccoli

EVENING SNACK
Walnut Cookies*
Mint tea

DAY 9

BREAKFAST
Poached egg on toasted Ezekiel bread
Fresh figs with goat cheese
Pineapple juice
Rose hip tea

MID-MORNING SNACK
Beneficial fruit or protein

LUNCH
Grilled peppers and goat cheese on
    spelt toast
Mixed green salad

MID-AFTERNOON SNACK
Type B Trail Mix-1*

DINNER
Roast Turkey*
Brown Rice Pilaf* with carrots and
    onions
Braised greens with garlic

EVENING SNACK
Super Baby Smoothie*

DAY 10

BREAKFAST
High-Protein Energy Shake*
Banana Walnut Bread*

MID-MORNING SNACK
Slice of spelt bread with apple butter
Rose hip tea

LUNCH
Fresh Cherries and Yogurt Soup*
Rice cakes with almond butter
2 plums

MID-AFTERNOON SNACK
Raisins and chopped walnuts
Glass of cow's milk

DINNER
Fried Monkfish*
Mashed potatoes with butter
Tossed salad with olive oil and
    balsamic vinegar
Mineral water

EVENING SNACK
Super Baby Smoothie*

DAY 11

BREAKFAST
Spelt flakes with fresh berries and
    cow's milk
Ezekial toast with melted cheese
Slippery elm tea

MID-MORNING SNACK
Banana Yogurt Drink*

LUNCH
Mushroom Barley Soup with Spinach*
Mesclun Salad*

MID-AFTERNOON SNACK
Beneficial fruit

DINNER
Pan-Fried Liver and Onions*
Braised Swiss chard
Wild rice

EVENING SNACK
Super Baby Smoothie*

DAY 12

BREAKFAST
Tropical Salad*
Ezekiel toast with cherry preserves
Rose hip tea

MID-MORNING SNACK
Beneficial fruit or protein

LUNCH
Turkey Soup*
Carrot Raisin Salad*
Crackers

MID-AFTERNOON SNACK
Type B Trail Mix-2*

DINNER
Stuffed Shells with Pesto*
Braised Collards*
Mixed green salad

EVENING SNACK
Super Baby Smoothie*

DAY 13

BREAKFAST
Scrambled eggs
Ezekiel bread with plum preserves
Red raspberry tea

MID-MORNING SNACK
Super Baby Smoothie*

LUNCH
Super Broccoli Salad*
Grilled goat cheese sandwich on spelt
    bread

MID-AFTERNOON SNACK
Beneficial fruit or protein

DINNER
Steamed Whole Red Snapper*
Braised Collards*
Steamed asparagus

EVENING SNACK
Sliced banana with cow's milk
Mint tea

DAY 14

BREAKFAST
Banana Plum Bread*
Mixed fruit
Slippery elm tea

MID-MORNING SNACK
Rice cakes with apple butter

LUNCH
Simple Fish Soup*
Cole Slaw*
Mixed green salad

MID-AFTERNOON SNACK
Type B Trail Mix-1*

DINNER
Grilled Loin of Lamb Chops*
Sautéed greens
Romaine-feta salad

EVENING SNACK
Super Baby Smoothie*

Second Trimester

Adjust to an Increased Appetite

Fetal growth is rapid during the second trimester, and you may experience a
greater appetite, especially if you no longer suffer from nausea or "morning sickness." Use your extra calories to maximum benefit.

---

* You can find recipes for asterisk-marked items in appendix A.

EMPHASIS FOR EXTRA CALORIES
- High-quality protein—organic lean red meat, fish, low-fat dairy
- Calcium-rich foods—organic cow's milk, goat's milk, yogurt, sardines
- Vitamin C–rich foods—dark green leafy vegetables, plums, pineapple, bananas

Keep Your Blood Sugar in Check

For Type B, blood sugar irregularities are usually the result of carbohydrate intolerance—especially if you're eating too many grains, beans, and potatoes. While some increase in blood sugar is normal during pregnancy, be aware that severely elevated blood sugar leads to a dangerous condition called gestational diabetes, which can cause premature birth and even birth defects. The following symptoms should alert you to blood sugar imbalances:

Fatigue
Extreme hunger
Dry skin
Anxiety
Dizziness and light-headedness

To restore a proper balance:

- Increase the protein and decrease the carbohydrates in your diet.
- Eliminate refined sugars and starches.
- Eat fiber-rich foods every day.
- Never skip meals, especially breakfast. Preferably, eat six small meals a day.

Avoid Urinary Tract Infections

Many women are susceptible to urinary tract infections (UTI) during the second trimester. As a Type B, you need to be aware of this tendency, because Type Bs typically have an extremely high risk factor for UTIs. In addition to following the Type B diet, you can guard against UTIs with the following:

- Eat cranberries and blueberries—effective UTI fighters.
- Eat plenty of cultured dairy foods, such as yogurt and kefir.
- Urinate frequently to avoid a buildup of urine in the bladder.
- Continue taking your probiotic supplement. It will help keep the colon flora, vaginal flora, and urinary tract healthy.

Help Your Body Resist Infection

Type Bs have the weakest defense of all the blood types against the most common influenza viruses. Since your immune system is suppressed during pregnancy, you need to be particularly alert. I highly recommend that you take regular doses of elderberry extract—1 teaspoon once or twice daily during the flu season. Elderberry has been used by herbalists for centuries, and it has been shown to inhibit replication of all strains of influenza virus. Don't exceed the recommended dosage, since it can make you slightly nauseated. You can also build your immune system with the following strategies:

- *Reduce stress.* There is ample evidence of a connection between stress and lowered immunity. Get away from the computer and the bill paying, at least for 30 minutes every day to get a few moments of fresh air and sunshine. Try to go for a quick walk during lunch. Practice deep breathing while you walk.
- *Adopt good dietary habits.* Failure to eat breakfast, irregular eating habits, low vegetable intake, inadequate protein, excessive wheat intake, and high-fat diets (especially those with excessive amounts of polyunsaturated fatty acids) have all been associated with lowered immune function.
- *Eat exotic mushrooms.* Shiitake, maitake, and reishi mushrooms are very effective in supporting long-term antiviral resistance.

Control Food Intolerance

Blood Type B can be intolerant to many common foods. Note that research shows that upward of 55 percent of our immune function is located in the digestive system. Avoid foods that trigger allergies for Type B:

Bitter melon
Coconut/milk
Persimmon
Avocado
Artichoke
Corn
Olive
Tomato
Black bean
Chickpea
Lentil
Soy bean/milk/tofu
Peanut

Wheat germ
Whole wheat

Second Trimester Menu Plans

The following menus offer a guide to healthy eating during the second trimester of your pregnancy. They include some adjustments from the first trimester, taking into account the special emphasis on this period in your pregnancy.

- The menu suggestions place an even greater emphasis on lean meats, fish, dairy, and fresh fruits and vegetables—all foods that help regulate blood sugar.
- They include more calories than the first trimester menus, to accommodate the growing nutritional needs of your fetus.
- They provide an extra boost of protein and vital nutrients with Type B–specific smoothies.
- They provide additional foods that will help to overcome second trimester problems, such as hemorrhoids, varicose veins, bleeding gums, and allergic sensitivities. The menus are flexible and can be mixed and reorganized according to your personal needs. I have purposely not included portion sizes for most dishes, since caloric needs vary depending upon your height and weight. However, these menus do offer more foods than the first trimester—and you should try to increase your intake by 100 to 300 calories per day.

Note that although beverages are listed with some meals, I suggest you drink them half an hour before or after eating. Liquids consumed with solid foods dilute the digestive juices. Don't forget to keep drinking water throughout the day.

Menus

DAY 1

BREAKFAST
Oatmeal with raisins, warm milk,
    and maple syrup
Poached Fruit*
Cranberry juice
Slippery elm tea

MID-MORNING SNACK
Super Baby Smoothie*

LUNCH
Mackerel Salad* on a bed of Romaine
    lettuce
Rice crackers
Fruit salad

MID-AFTERNOON SNACK
Type B Trail Mix-1*

DINNER
Broiled cod
Tossed green salad with Balsamic
    Mustard Vinaigrette*
Brown Rice Pilaf*

EVENING SNACK
Sliced apple and walnuts
Chamomile tea

DAY 2

BREAKFAST
Scrambled eggs
Spelt flakes with raisins and cow's
    milk
Prune Whip*
Rose hip tea

MID-MORNING SNACK
Pineapple Yogurt Drink*

LUNCH
Mushroom Barley Soup with Spinach*
Mixed green salad
Crackers

MID-AFTERNOON SNACK
Beneficial fruit or protein

DINNER
Braised Rabbit*
Mixed Mushroom Salad*
Grilled Pepper Medley*

EVENING SNACK
Super Baby Smoothie*

DAY 3

BREAKFAST
Wheat-free Waffles*
Cherry preserves
Banana
Vegetable juice
Rose hip tea

MID-MORNING SNACK
Beneficial fruit or protein

LUNCH
Grilled Peppers and Goat Cheddar on
    Ezekiel Bread*
Carrot and celery sticks
Grape Ice*

MID-AFTERNOON SNACK
Type B Trail Mix-2*

DINNER
Pan-Fried Liver and Onions*
Steamed broccoli
Pureed sweet potato

EVENING SNACK
Super Baby Smoothie*

DAY 4

BREAKFAST
Omelet
Spelt toast
Poached Fruit*
Raspberry leaf tea

MID-MORNING SNACK
Mango-Lime Smoothie*

LUNCH
Broiled lean ground beef patty with
    lettuce and onion
Ezekiel bread
Mixed green salad

MID-AFTERNOON SNACK
Beneficial fruit or protein

DINNER
Broiled sole
Lima beans with goat cheese and
    scallions
Steamed spinach

EVENING SNACK
Super Baby Smoothie*

DAY 5

BREAKFAST
Pineapple Yogurt Drink*
Spinach Frittata*

MID-MORNING SNACK
Beneficial fruit or protein

LUNCH
Sardines and lettuce on Wasa bread
Super Broccoli Salad*
Mixed fruit

MID-AFTERNOON SNACK
Type B Trail Mix-1*

DINNER
Roast Turkey*
Brown rice
Carrots and Parsnips with Garlic
    and Cilantro*

EVENING SNACK
Banana Pudding*
Chamomile tea

DAY 6

BREAKFAST
Poached eggs on toasted spelt bread
Fresh pineapple slices
Slippery elm tea

MID-MORNING SNACK
Date-Prune Smoothie*

LUNCH
Spinach Salad*
Fresh mozzarella and sautéed
    zucchini on spelt bread

MID-AFTERNOON SNACK
Beneficial fruit

DINNER
Green Leafy Pasta*
Romaine salad with Olive Oil and
    Lemon Dressing*

EVENING SNACK
Super Baby Smoothie*

DAY 7

BREAKFAST
Cream of rice with dried cherries and
    milk
Essene toast
Fresh pineapple
Raspberry leaf tea

MID-MORNING SNACK
Beneficial fruit or protein

LUNCH
Farmer's Vegetable Soup*
Mesclun Salad*

MID-AFTERNOON SNACK
Strawberry-Banana Smoothie*

DINNER
Broiled Lamb Chops*
Braised leeks
Pureed root vegetables

EVENING SNACK
Rice cakes with apple butter
Mint tea

DAY 8

BREAKFAST
Banana Plum Bread*
Stewed plums
Pineapple juice
Type B Tea

MID-MORNING SNACK
Beneficial fruit or protein

LUNCH
Grilled cheese sandwich
    on spelt bread
Apple slices

MID-AFTERNOON SNACK
Super Baby Smoothie*

DINNER
Steamed Whole Red Snapper*
Grilled Sweet Potato Salad*
Steamed broccoli

EVENING SNACK
Banana Pudding*
Chamomile tea

DAY 9

BREAKFAST
Scrambled eggs
Ezekiel toast with cherry preserves
Mixed berries
Raspberry leaf tea

MID-MORNING SNACK
Beneficial fruit or protein

LUNCH
Greek Salad*
Spelt pita
Figs with goat cheese and walnuts

MID-AFTERNOON SNACK
Type B Trail Mix-2*

DINNER
Pan-Fried Liver and Onions*
Vegetable Fritters*
Sauteed greens in olive oil

EVENING SNACK
Super Baby Smoothie*

DAY 10

BREAKFAST
Scrambled eggs
Sautéed Bananas* with ricotta
Papaya juice
Slippery elm tea

MID-MORNING SNACK
Banana Yogurt Drink*

LUNCH
Simple Fish Soup*
Mesclun Salad*

MID-AFTERNOON SNACK
Beneficial fruit or protein

DINNER
Turkey Cutlets*
Brown rice
Steamed broccoli

EVENING SNACK
Super Baby Smoothie*

DAY 11

BREAKFAST
Apricot Yogurt Drink*
Brown Rice–Spelt Pancakes*
Berry preserves

MID-MORNING SNACK
Sliced pear with walnuts and raisins

LUNCH
Salmon with Wakame Seaweed*
Rice crackers
Vegetable consommé

MID-AFTERNOON SNACK
Super Baby Smoothie*

DINNER
Steamed Whole Red Snapper*
Brown Rice Pilaf*
Steamed broccoli

EVENING SNACK
Rice pudding

DAY 12

BREAKFAST
Tropical Salad*
Ezekiel toast with blackberry preserves

MID-MORNING SNACK
Cottage cheese and fresh fruit
Peppermint tea

LUNCH
Sardine Salad* on spelt bread
Spinach Salad*

MID-AFTERNOON SNACK
Beneficial fruit or protein

DINNER
Beef Stew with Green Beans and
  Carrots*
Braised greens

EVENING SNACK
Super Baby Smoothie*

DAY 13

BREAKFAST
One-Egg Omelet* with grated carrots
Sautéed Pears*
Rose hip tea

MID-MORNING SNACK
High-Energy Protein Shake*

LUNCH
Lima Beans with Goat Cheese and
    Scallions*
Mixed green salad with Olive Oil and
    Lemon Dressing*

MID-AFTERNOON SNACK
Beneficial fruit or protein

DINNER
Fried Monkfish*
Faro Pilaf*
Braised Collards*

EVENING SNACK
Spelt bread with apple butter
Mint tea

DAY 14

BREAKFAST
Wheat-free Pancakes* with plum
    preserves
Mixed berries
Slippery elm tea

MID-MORNING SNACK
Super Baby Smoothie*

LUNCH
Cucumber-Yogurt Soup*
Green Bean Salad with Walnuts and
    Goat Cheese*

MID-AFTERNOON SNACK
Beneficial fruit

DINNER
Grilled Curried Leg of Lamb*
Mixed vegetable stir-fry
Basmati rice

EVENING SNACK
Banana Pudding*
Glass of milk

Third Trimester

Reduce Swelling and Edema

Some water retention can be expected toward the end of your pregnancy, the result of an estrogen spike prior to the delivery of your baby. Type Bs will experience edema as the result of a sluggish metabolism.

---

* You can find recipes for asterisk-marked items in appendix A.

SIGNS OF SLUGGISH METABOLISM

- Fatigue
- Dry skin
- Cold hands and feet
- Light-headedness
- Constipation and water retention
- Depression

AVOID REACTIVE LECTINS IN THESE FOODS

- Chicken
- Buckwheat
- Corn
- Lentil beans
- Peanuts

Here are some additional suggestions for reducing edema:

- Elevate your legs when sitting or lying down.
- Drink six to eight 8-ounce glasses of water during the day.
- Wear comfortable clothing and avoid tight pantyhose. Support stockings may offer relief.
- Cut back on high-sodium foods; many processed foods are loaded with sodium.
- Make sure your shoes fit properly.
- Drink 1 to 3 cups of dandelion tea every day for mild water retention.
- Ask your partner to gently massage the area from your ankles to your thighs with a very light touch.

> **WARNING:** Only use a diuretic on the advice of your doctor. Diuretics can cause dehydration and nutrient deficiency.

Control Your Blood Pressure

Pregnancy-induced hypertension, also known as toxemia or preeclampsia, can be extremely dangerous and can lead to miscarriage. Fortunately, Type Bs appear to have a special ability to control blood pressure using relaxation and visualization. This is something I have observed in my own practice. Take advantage of this ability to keep your blood pressure under control at this critical time. (See the visualization exercise on page 152.)

NATURAL BLOOD PRESSURE REDUCTION TONIC. One excellent method for ensuring healthy blood pressure is to juice several stalks of celery, taking 6 to 8 ounces as fresh juice daily.

Ward Off Infections

Continue to make immune system health a top priority in the third trimester. Many bacterial infections attack Type Bs with special force. There's a reason. Many common bacteria-producing infections are B-like in nature, and you don't produce antibodies against them.

A particular risk for Type Bs that also has grave implications for your offspring is streptococcal disease. This disease occurs more often in Type Bs than other blood types, resulting in strep throat, or more serious illnesses such as bacteremia and heart valve malformation and damage.

Follow the standard Type B guidelines for building your immune system. In addition, you need to take preventive measures to avoid food-borne bacterial infections, such as *E. coli*, which favors Type B:

- Never serve hamburger or other foods containing ground beef that is rare or raw. When properly cooked, the inside of ground beef should be brown rather than pink, with an internal temperature of 160 degrees, and the juices should run clear.
- Do not eat raw sprouts.
- Hands, utensils, and food-contact surfaces must be washed with warm, soapy water between contact with raw meat and foods that have already been cooked or foods that will be served raw.

Third Trimester Menu Plans

During the third trimester you may feel full after eating very little. Smaller meals, eaten at regular intervals of 3 to 4 hours, may be required to get all the nutrients you need. The following menus offer a guide to healthy eating during the third trimester of your pregnancy. They include some adjustments to account for the special emphasis of this period in your pregnancy.

- They place even greater emphasis on lean meats, fish, dairy, and fresh fruits and vegetables—all foods that help maintain metabolic balance.
- They provide an extra boost of protein and vital nutrients with Type B–specific smoothies. This will help you prepare for the rigors of labor and delivery.
- Vitamin A– and C–rich foods are abundant, also in preparation for delivery.

The menus are flexible and can be mixed and reorganized according to your personal needs. I have purposely not included portion sizes for most dishes, since caloric needs vary depending upon your height and weight. You may need to divide up the meals and snacks further if you don't think you can finish them at one sitting. However, it's vital that you maintain your overall caloric level.

Note that although beverages are listed with some meals, I suggest you drink them half an hour before or after eating. Liquids consumed with solid foods dilute the digestive juices and fill you up faster. Don't forget to keep drinking water throughout the day.

DAY 1

BREAKFAST
Omelet* with fresh spinach and feta
1 slice of Essene toast with plum
    preserves
Grapes

MID-MORNING SNACK
Banana Yogurt Drink*

LUNCH
Farmer's Vegetable Soup*
Carrot Raisin Salad*
Crackers

MID-AFTERNOON SNACK
Beneficial fruit or protein
Raspberry leaf tea

DINNER
Pan-Fried Liver and Onions*
Baked sweet potato
Steamed broccoli

EVENING SNACK
Super Baby Smoothie*

DAY 2

BREAKFAST
Oatmeal with raisins, maple syrup,
    and milk
Fresh pineapple
Slippery elm tea

MID-MORNING SNACK
Super Baby Smoothie*

LUNCH
Mackerel Salad* on a bed of greens
Rice cakes
Mixed fruit

MID-AFTERNOON SNACK
Beneficial fruit or protein
Raspberry leaf tea

DINNER
Roast Turkey*
Brown Rice Pilaf* with carrots and
    onions
Brussels sprouts

EVENING SNACK
Banana Pudding*
Chamomile tea

DAY 3

BREAKFAST
Ezekiel toast with black cherry
   preserves
Yogurt with mixed berries
Raspberry leaf tea

MID-MORNING SNACK
Beneficial fruit or protein

LUNCH
Turkey Soup*
Super Broccoli Salad*

MID-AFTERNOON SNACK
Type B Trail Mix-2*

DINNER
Fried Monkfish*
Carrots and Parsnips with Garlic
   and Cilantro*
Millet Tabbouleh*

EVENING SNACK
Super Baby Smoothie*

DAY 4

BREAKFAST
Scrambled eggs
Brown rice bread with plum preserves
Glass of milk
Rose hip tea

MID-MORNING SNACK
Cherry-Peach Smoothie*

LUNCH
Grilled eggplant and feta on spelt
   bread
Mesclun Salad*

MID-AFTERNOON SNACK
Beneficial fruit or protein
Peppermint tea

DINNER
Flank Steak*
Pureed root vegetables
Steamed broccoli

EVENING SNACK
Cranberry Biscotti*
Glass of milk

DAY 5

BREAKFAST
Brown Rice–Spelt Pancakes*
    with maple syrup
Grapes
Vegetable juice

MID-MORNING SNACK
Beneficial fruit or protein

LUNCH
Sliced cold flank steak on a bed of
    Romaine lettuce
Mixed Roots Soup*

MID-AFTERNOON SNACK
Super Baby Smoothie*

DINNER
Green Leafy Pasta*
Endive salad

EVENING SNACK
Banana Pudding*
Type B Tea

DAY 6

BREAKFAST
Spinach Frittata*
Essene toast
Pineapple slices
Rose hip tea

MID-MORNING SNACK
Banana Yogurt Drink*

LUNCH
Sardines
Rice cakes
Cucumber Yogurt Soup*

MID-AFTERNOON SNACK
Sliced apple, raisins, and walnuts

DINNER
Grilled Curried Leg of Lamb*
Steamed broccoli
Wild rice

EVENING SNACK
Super Baby Smoothie*

DAY 7

BREAKFAST
Spelt flakes with mixed fruit and milk
Banana Plum Bread*

MID-MORNING SNACK
Beneficial fruit or protein

LUNCH
Waldorf Salad*
Grilled cheese sandwich
   on spelt bread

MID-AFTERNOON SNACK
Super Baby Smoothie*

DINNER
Fried Monkfish*
Brown rice
Mixed green salad

EVENING SNACK
Lemon sorbet with pineapple chunks
Rose hip tea

DAY 8

BREAKFAST
Brown Rice–Spelt Pancakes*
   with maple syrup
Stewed prunes

MID-MORNING SNACK
Beneficial fruit or protein

LUNCH
White Bean and Wilted Greens Soup*
Mixed green salad with Seaweed
   Dressing*

MID-AFTERNOON SNACK
Rice cakes with plum preserves

DINNER
Fettuccine with Grilled Lamb Sausages
   and Vegetables*
Mixed green salad

EVENING SNACK
Banana Yogurt Drink*
Type B Bar

DAY 9

BREAKFAST
Poached egg on toasted Ezekiel bread
Poached Fruit*
Pineapple juice
Rose hip tea

MID-MORNING SNACK
Beneficial fruit or protein

LUNCH
Cole Slaw*
Broiled lean ground beef patty with
    melted goat cheese and raw
    spinach leaves
Spelt bread

MID-AFTERNOON SNACK
Toasted Tamari Pumpkin Seeds*
Carrot juice

DINNER
Broiled Salmon Steak*
Steamed broccoli
Brown rice

EVENING SNACK
Super Baby Smoothie*

DAY 10

BREAKFAST
Banana Walnut Bread*
Stewed prunes
Red raspberry leaf tea

MID-MORNING SNACK
Banana Yogurt Drink*

LUNCH
Grilled peppers on Rye Crackers with
    Chèvre*
Spinach Salad*

MID-AFTERNOON SNACK
Beneficial fruit or protein

DINNER
Grilled sirloin steak with shiitake
    mushrooms
Baked sweet potato
Braised Collards*

EVENING SNACK
Super Baby Smoothie*

DAY 11

BREAKFAST
Spelt flakes with sliced banana and
    cow's milk
Essene toast with butter
2 plums
Rose hip tea

MID-MORNING SNACK
Banana Yogurt Drink*

LUNCH
Sliced turkey on spelt bread
Mixed green salad

MID-AFTERNOON SNACK
Beneficial fruit or protein

DINNER
Grilled Loin of Lamb Chops*
2 Beneficial vegetables
Apple and Onion Confit*

EVENING SNACK
Super Baby Smoothie*

DAY 12

BREAKFAST
Scrambled eggs
Ezekiel toast with grape jam
Pineapple slices
Chamomile tea

MID-MORNING SNACK
Beneficial fruit or protein

LUNCH
Lima Beans with Goat Cheese and
    Scallions*
Mixed steamed vegetables

MID-AFTERNOON SNACK
Rice cakes with plum preserves
Grapes

DINNER
Indian Lamb Stew with Spinach*
Basmati rice
Beneficial vegetable

EVENING SNACK
Super Baby Smoothie*

DAY 13

BREAKFAST
Poached egg
Tropical Salad*
Ezekiel toast with plum preserves
Rose hip tea

MID-MORNING SNACK
Banana Yogurt Drink*

LUNCH
Turkey Soup*
Mesclun Salad*

MID-AFTERNOON SNACK
Beneficial fruit

DINNER
Pan-Fried Liver and Onions*
Brown rice
Broccoli

EVENING SNACK
Super Baby Smoothie*

DAY 14

BREAKFAST
Spelt flakes with mixed fruit and cow's
    milk
Essene toast
Raspberry leaf tea

MID-MORNING SNACK
Strawberry-Banana Smoothie*

LUNCH
Greek Salad*
Speltberry and Rice Salad*
Lemon-chamomile tea

MID-AFTERNOON SNACK
Raisins and walnuts
Super Baby Smoothie*

DINNER
Steamed Whole Red Snapper*
Brown rice
Steamed asparagus

EVENING SNACK
Beneficial fruit or protein
Chamomile tea

Exercise Guidelines

First Trimester

Maintenance for Healthy Type Bs

Since Type B is particularly susceptible to high levels of stress hormones causing anxiety and mood swings, you can benefit by continuing to incorporate relaxation and meditation exercises into your daily routine.

---

* You can find recipes for asterisk-marked items in appendix A.

Type Bs usually do best with moderate aerobic exercise, so this is not the time to engage in contact sports or in-line skating. I'd suggest you forgo them during pregnancy, to avoid any potential injury to the abdominal area.

Choose from among the following Type B exercises for a minimum regimen of 45 minutes, three to four times a week.

EXERCISE	DURATION
Tennis	45–60 minutes
Martial arts	30–60 minutes
Cycling	45–60 minutes
Hiking	30–60 minutes
Treadmill	30–40 minutes
Golf (no cart)	60 minutes
Swimming	30–45 minutes

CAUTIONS FOR HIGH-RISK PREGNANCIES
Consult with your doctor before continuing your exercise regimen if you are in a high-risk pregnancy. Most doctors will discourage exercise if you:

- Have a history of miscarriages, or have had even one miscarriage, if it is recent.
- Have a history of recurrent pelvic or abdominal infections.
- Have an incompetent cervix. This condition causes the cervix to open early, usually in the second trimester, leading to miscarriage.
- Have had toxemia in a previous pregnancy.
- Have a history of premature deliveries.
- Have or have had a serious medical condition, such as cancer, heart disease, asthma, or kidney disease.

Second Trimester

Adaptations for Advancing Pregnancy

As your pregnancy progresses, you'll need to shift the emphasis of your exercise regimen. Discontinue exercises that require speed and balance—such as tennis, biking, and martial arts (with the exception of T'ai Chi). Swimming is a very good exercise at this point in your pregnancy. Supplement your aerobic activity with a prenatal yoga class.

An ideal second trimester regimen for Type B includes the following.

THREE TIMES A WEEK, CHOOSE ONE:

EXERCISE	DURATION
Water aerobics	40–50 minutes
Treadmill	30 minutes
Cycling (recumbent bike)	30 minutes
Swimming	30 minutes
Brisk walking	45 minutes

TWO TIMES A WEEK, CHOOSE ONE:

EXERCISE	DURATION
Light yoga	40–50 minutes
T'ai Chi	30 minutes
Labor preparation class	40–50 minutes

DAILY:

EXERCISE	DURATION
Kegel exercises	2 minutes, 10–20 times

- Spend more time on your warm-up and cooldown to fully warm and stretch your muscles. This will minimize the muscle cramps that are common as your pregnancy progresses.
- Look for opportunities to incorporate fitness into your daily routine. If feasible, walk to work instead of driving. Take the stairs instead of the elevator.
- Swimming is an excellent exercise for the second and third trimesters. It places minimum stress on your joints and heart rate. You may even want to replace your regular aerobics class with a water aerobics class.
- If you haven't already started your Kegel exercises (see page 28), do so now.

PREGNANCY-SAFE EXERCISE SUBSTITUTIONS

INSTEAD OF . . .	TRY . . .
Bicycling	Indoor stationary bike (recumbent)
Tennis	Brisk walking/treadmill
Aerobics	Water aerobics

Third Trimester

Adaptations for Late Pregnancy

Your focus during the final months of pregnancy should be on stress reduction. Not only is this a particularly stressful time, but Type B has a heightened tendency to produce excess cortisol in response to even minor stress.

Avoid any exercises that place pressure on your abdominal area. Lay on your side for floor exercises. This position also helps your circulation and will decrease your blood pressure.

Type Bs can benefit in the final months of pregnancy by replacing one of your weekly aerobic exercises with a relaxation exercise. Also begin your daily perineal massage to tone the vaginal canal (page 31).

An excellent third trimester exercise regimen for Type B would be the following.

TWO TIMES A WEEK, CHOOSE ONE:

EXERCISE	DURATION
Water aerobics	40–50 minutes
Treadmill	30 minutes
Cycling (recumbent bike)	30 minutes
Swimming	30 minutes
Brisk walking	45 minutes

THREE TIMES A WEEK, CHOOSE ONE:

EXERCISE	DURATION
Light yoga	40–50 minutes
Meditation	30 minutes
Labor preparation class	40–50 minutes

DAILY, PERFORM BOTH:

EXERCISE	DURATION
Kegel exercises	2 minutes, 10–20 times
Perineal massage	5 minutes, 1–2 times

MEDITATION. Calming yourself through the process of meditation is a wonderful way to reduce your stress level. Quieting the mind will help you eliminate stress-causing thoughts and help you to approach your day in a more positive and efficient manner.

Meditation Exercise

- Choose a quiet place.
- Sit in a comfortable chair.
- Close your eyes.
- Relax your muscles.
- Become aware of your breathing.
- Choose a pleasant word or visual image that you can hear and see in your imagination. Think of this word or image every time you exhale for about 15 minutes each day. If you have an intrusive thought or feeling during your meditation, return to the repetition of your relaxing word or image.

Supplement Guidelines

First Trimester

Vitamins/Minerals

Take a standard prenatal vitamin supplement, choosing one made from whole food, not synthetic ingredients. Powder-in-capsule forms dissolve most efficiently. If you would like to use a prenatal supplement specifically formulated for Type B, see appendix B for information about Healthy Start ABO Prenatal. The following nutrient breakdown is the optimal formula for Type B.

PRENATAL SUPPLEMENT—TYPE B		% DAILY VALUE
Vitamin A (100% as natural beta-carotene from *Dunaliella salina*)	3,000 iu	60
Vitamin C (100 % from acerola berry, *Malpighia puncifolia*)	75 mg	125
Vitamin D (*cholecalciferol*)	75 iu	18
Vitamin E (natural d,alpha-tocopheryl succinate)	150 iu	500
Vitamin K (phytonadione)	15 mcg	–
Thiamin (from thiamin HCl)	20 mg	1,333
Riboflavin	20 mg	1,176
Niacin and niacinamide (vitamin B_3)	15 mg	75
Vitamin B_6 (from pyridoxine HCl)	10 mg	500

PRENATAL SUPPLEMENT—TYPE B		% DAILY VALUE
Folic acid	800 mcg	200
Vitamin B$_{12}$ (methylcobalamin)	15 mcg	250
Biotin	400 mcg	133
Pantothenic acid (from D-calcium pantothenate)	10 mg	100
Calcium (seaweed base, derived from *Lithothamnium corralliodes* and *Lithothamnium calcareum*)	300 mg	30
Iron (ferrous succinate)	20 mg	111
Iodine (potassium iodide)	75 mcg	50
Magnesium (citrate and oxide)	100 mg	25
Zinc (picolinate)	15 mg	100
Selenium (L-selenomethionine)	20 mcg	–
Copper (gluconate)	1 mg	50
Manganese (citrate)	1 mg	–

Herbal Remedies

HERB	FUNCTION	FORM AND DOSAGE
Chamomile	Calms; relieves heartburn	As tea, 1 to 2 cups daily; or add 2–4 drops of essential oil to bath
Horsetail	Contains silica, which supports healthy bones, skin, hair, and nails	250-mg capsule daily
Peppermint	Calms; relieves indigestion	As tea, 2 to 3 cups daily, after meals
Red raspberry leaf	Relieves morning sickness	As tea, 2 cups daily
Slippery elm bark	Relieves heartburn	250-mg capsule, twice daily; or as tea, 2 cups daily; or as Thayer's lozenges, 2–4 daily

Nutritional Supplements

NUTRITIONAL SUPPLEMENT	FUNCTION	FORM AND DOSAGE
Larch arabinogalactan	Relieves constipation	Soluble fiber supplement: 1 tablespoon mixed with water or juice, twice daily
Probiotic	For intestinal health	2 capsules, twice daily*
DHA	Provides essential nutrients for fetal development	300-mg capsule daily

* See appendix B for information on blood type–specific probiotics.

Second Trimester

Vitamins/Minerals

Continue to take your prenatal supplement, preferably one formulated for Type B.

Herbal Remedies

HERB	FUNCTION	FORM AND DOSAGE
Bilberry	Relieves hemorrhoids and varicose veins	25-mg capsule, twice daily
Chamomile	Calms; relieves heartburn; relieves hemorrhoids and varicose veins	As tea, 1 to 2 cups daily; or add 2 to 4 drops of essential oil to bath
Horsetail	Contains silica, which supports healthy bones, skin, hair, and nails	250-mg capsule daily
Peppermint	Calms and relieves indigestion	As tea, 2 to 3 cups daily, after meals
Red raspberry leaf	Treatment for bleeding gums	As tea, 2 cups daily
Rose hips	Treatment for varicose veins, bleeding gums, allergies	One tablespoon concentrate every 30 minutes for allergy attack; as tea, 2 to 3 cups daily
Stinging nettle leaf	Allergy relief	As tea, 2 cups daily for symptoms
Witch hazel	Treatment for hemorrhoids	Use topically as needed

Nutritional Supplements

NUTRITIONAL SUPPLEMENT	FUNCTION	FORM AND DOSAGE
Larch arabinogalactan	Relieves constipation	Soluble fiber supplement: 1 tablespoon mixed with water or juice, twice daily
Probiotic	For intestinal health; prevention of candida infection	2 capsules, twice daily*
DHA	Provides essential nutrients for fetal development	300-mg capsule daily

* See appendix B for information on blood type–specific probiotics.

Third Trimester

Vitamins/Minerals

Continue to take your prenatal supplement, preferably one formulated for Type B.

Herbal Remedies

HERB	FUNCTION	FORM AND DOSAGE
Dandelion leaf/root	Lowers blood pressure; decreases edema	As tea, 2 cups daily; or 250-mg capsule, twice daily
Nettles	Rich in vitamin K, promotes blood clotting	As tea, 2 cups daily; or 250-mg capsule, twice daily
Raspberry leaf	Softens the cervix in preparation for birth; stimulates milk production	As tea, 2 cups daily; as tincture, 15 to 20 drops daily
Squaw vine	Prepares uterus for birth	As tincture, 10 drops in warm water, twice daily

Nutritional Supplements		
NUTRITIONAL SUPPLEMENT	FUNCTION	FORM AND DOSAGE
Larch arabinogalactan	Relieves constipation	Soluble fiber supplement: 1 tablespoon mixed with water or juice, twice daily.
Probiotic	For intestinal health; prevention of candida infection	2 capsules, twice daily*
DHA	Provides essential nutrients for fetal development	300-mg capsule daily

* See appendix B for information on blood type–specific probiotics.

Labor and Delivery

In addition to the general guidelines for labor and delivery (page 32), you have some specific Type B needs.

Labor Preparation

One of the best ways I have found for Type Bs to deal with stress is through organization. When a Type B individual has a clear plan of action, she is more relaxed and confident. This being the case, it makes sense for you to spend time in the days and weeks prior to delivery carefully preparing for the big event. Make a list of questions for your practitioner, pack your bag, create a contingency plan—everything that *can* be controlled.

Type B Blood-Building Needs

To guard against excessive bleeding in the event that a cesarean or other surgical procedure might be required, increase your blood-clotting factors. Follow these guidelines in the final weeks of pregnancy:

- Vitamin K is essential to blood clotting. Eat lots of greens, especially kale, spinach, and collard greens, and supplement your diet with liquid chlorophyll.
- Avoid using aspirin, which has blood-thinning properties and can prolong your bleeding.

Type B Energy Needs

Begin several weeks before your delivery date to prepare yourself for the stress of labor and delivery. Try to get more sleep than usual and eat plenty of nutrient-rich foods. Type Bs have a tendency to let stress levels build, and you don't want to reach the point of labor with all of your energy resources depleted.

The first stage of labor can last many hours. Drink plenty of liquids and keep a light protein snack nearby. Stay hydrated. Be sure to discuss in advance with your doctor or midwife what the policy is about eating light foods or drinking liquids during labor.

Type B Emotional Needs

Type Bs tend to be extraordinarily gifted in their ability to reduce stress and relieve anxiety with mental exercises, such as meditation and visualization.

Breathing is a critical component of meditation. Not surprisingly, a technique called "alternate nostril breathing" is a powerful tool in managing your physiology. Left nostril breathing generates a more relaxing effect, or toning down, of sympathetic activity. Right nostril breathing generates an increase in parasympathetic activity. The alternate nostril breathing technique generates a relative balance between the sympathetic and parasympathetic nervous systems and is a tremendous antistress measure.

CREATIVE VISUALIZATION. This exercise also helps to reduce stress by imagining a very calm and relaxing scene in your mind. Some people picture themselves at the beach feeling the warmth of the sun and the sound of the waves crashing on the shore. Others think of being in the mountains, with eagles soaring overhead, as they breathe in the cool clean air. The goal is to replace negative, stressful thoughts with more relaxing ones. As your mind relaxes, so does your body.

See page 35 for natural childbirth painkillers.

6

The Type AB Pregnancy

TYPE AB IS THE RAREST BLOOD TYPE, comprising less than 5 percent of the population. In some respects, you're more vulnerable to health problems, since your complex immune system shares some aspects of Type A and some aspects of Type B. Similarly, although your digestive profile is A-like, there is a shared Type B preference for meat. So, although Type AB needs a bit more animal protein than Type A, they typically do not do well with a diet centered around animal protein. Similarly, Type AB has difficulty metabolizing combinations of fat and protein, because of low levels of an important enzyme called intestinal alkaline phosphatase. Type ABs should abide by this simple rule of thumb: Most foods that should be avoided by Type A and Type B should also be avoided by Type AB.

Type AB's rather unique immune defenses can hyperfunction, leading to allergies, inflammation, chronic fatigue, and a number of other autoimmune disorders that can sap your vitality and interfere with the ability to conceive. These disorders can also create problems during pregnancy.

Following the blood type diet is an essential foundation, enabling you to optimize your health and prepare for an energetic and enjoyable pregnancy.

The Type AB Diet

The following food lists comprise the Type AB diet. Note that the values for certain foods change in preparation for pregnancy, during pregnancy, and/or while you are breast-feeding. I call these Chameleon Foods, and they are contained in the following table. Use this table for quick reference. Chameleon Foods are also marked with an asterisk (*) in the specific food lists.

Values are calculated for secretors. If you are a non-secretor and want a higher level of compliance, refer to *Live Right 4 Your Type*.

Type AB Chameleon Foods

Chameleons are foods whose values change before pregnancy, during pregnancy, and/or while breast-feeding.

FOOD	PRE-/POST-PREGNANCY	PREGNANCY	FACTORS
SEAFOOD			
Bluefish	Neutral	Avoid	Heightened risk of contamination
Carp	Neutral	Avoid	Heightened risk of contamination
Catfish	Neutral	Avoid	Heightened risk of contamination
Grouper	Beneficial	Avoid	Heightened risk of contamination
Mahimahi	Beneficial	Avoid	Heightened risk of contamination
Salmon	Beneficial	Neutral	Some risk of contamination
Shark	Neutral	Avoid	High mercury content
Swordfish	Neutral	Avoid	High mercury content
Tilapia	Neutral	Avoid	Heightened risk of contamination
Tuna	Beneficial	Avoid	High mercury content
Whitefish	Neutral	Avoid	Heightened risk of contamination
DAIRY/EGGS			
Egg/chicken	Neutral	Beneficial	Good source of DHA
OILS			
Borage	Neutral	Avoid	Uterine stimulant
BEAN/LEGUME			
Soy cheese	Neutral	Beneficial	Good source of calcium/protein
Soy milk	Neutral	Beneficial	Good source of calcium/protein
VEGETABLES			
Parsley	Beneficial	Neutral	Limit intake; can be a uterine stimulant in large amounts
SPICES			
Chocolate	Neutral	Avoid	Contains caffeine
Ginger	Beneficial	Avoid	May cause miscarriage in large amounts
Licorice	Neutral	Avoid	Can influence estrogen levels
Parsley	Beneficial	Neutral	Limit intake; can be a uterine stimulant in large amounts
Turmeric	Neutral	Avoid	Uterine stimulant

FOOD	PRE-/POST-PREGNANCY	PREGNANCY	FACTORS
HERBAL TEAS			
Catnip	Neutral	Avoid	Uterine stimulant
Dandelion	Neutral	Beneficial	Aids digestion
Dong quai	Neutral	Avoid	Can start uterine bleeding
Fenugreek	Neutral	Avoid	Uterine stimulant
Ginger	Beneficial	Avoid	May cause miscarriage in large amounts
Goldenseal	Neutral	Avoid	Potentially harmful to fetus
Licorice	Beneficial	Avoid	Can influence estrogen levels
Parsley	Beneficial	Neutral	Limit intake; can be a uterine stimulant in large amounts
Raspberry leaf	Neutral	Beneficial	Supports the pregnancy
St. John's wort	Neutral	Avoid	Can be harmful to fetus
Vervain	Neutral	Avoid	Uterine stimulant
Yarrow	Neutral	Avoid	Uterine stimulant
BEVERAGES			
Beer	Neutral	Avoid	Alcohol should be completely avoided during pregnancy
Seltzer	Neutral	Avoid	Can cause digestive problems
Tea, green	Beneficial	Avoid	Contains caffeine; start weaning yourself before pregnancy, and avoid during pregnancy
Wine, red	Beneficial	Avoid	Alcohol should be completely avoided during pregnancy
Wine, white	Neutral	Avoid	Alcohol should be completely avoided during pregnancy

Meats and Poultry

Type ABs need to limit the amount of meat you eat, since you do not produce enough stomach acid to effectively digest too much animal protein. The key for you is portion size and frequency. Give preference to lamb, mutton, rabbit, and turkey over beef, and avoid chicken. Choose lean, organic cuts of meat.

HIGHLY BENEFICIAL

Lamb	Rabbit
Mutton	Turkey

NEUTRAL

Goat	Ostrich
Liver	Pheasant

AVOID

All commercially	Ham
processed meats	Heart/sweetbreads
Bacon	Horse
Beef	Partridge
Buffalo	Pork
Chicken	Quail
Cornish hen	Squab
Duck	Squirrel
Goose	Turtle
Grouse	Veal
Guinea hen	Venison

Seafood

Seafood is an excellent source of protein for Type ABs, but pregnant women must use special caution to avoid fish that may contain PCBs or that are otherwise potentially toxic. Check with your local health department about the safety of fish caught in local waters. In addition, avoid certain fish that are especially vulnerable to contamination by environmental pollutants, such as pesticides and PCBs. These include bass, bluefish, flounder, grouper, halibut, mahimahi, fresh salmon, tilapia, and whitefish. Also avoid fish that may contain a high level of mercury—halibut, shark, swordfish, and tuna.

HIGHLY BENEFICIAL

Cod

Grouper*

Mackerel

Mahimahi*

Monkfish

Pickerel

Pike

Porgy

Red snapper

Sailfish

Salmon*

Sardine

Shad

Snail (*Helix pomatia*/escargot)

Sturgeon

Tuna*

NEUTRAL

Abalone

Bluefish*

Bullhead

Butterfish

Carp*

Catfish*

Caviar (sturgeon)

Chub

Croaker

Cusk

Drum

Halfmoon fish

Harvest fish

Herring (fresh)

Mullet

Muskelunge

Mussels

Opaleye fish

Orange roughy

Parrot fish

Perch (all types)

Pollack

Pompano

Rosefish

Scallop

Scrod

Scup

Shark*

Smelt

Snapper

Squid (calamari)

Sucker

Sunfish

Swordfish*

Tilapia*

Tilefish

Weakfish

Whitefish*

AVOID

Anchovy

Barracuda

Bass (all types)

Beluga

Clam

Conch

Crab

Crayfish

Eel

Flounder

Frog

Haddock

Food with different values than the standard Type AB diet are indicated with an asterisk (*).

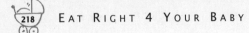

Hake	Shrimp
Halibut	Smoked salmon
Herring (pickled)	Sole (all types)
Lobster	Trout (all types)
Octopus	Whiting
Oysters	Yellowtail
Salmon roe	

Eggs and Dairy

Type ABs benefit from dairy foods, especially cultured and soured products—yogurt, kefir, and sour cream—which are easily digested. If you have respiratory problems, sinus attacks, or ear infections, cut back on dairy foods. Eggs are a very good source of protein for Type ABs, and also contain DHA, which is highly beneficial for pregnant women.

HIGHLY BENEFICIAL

Cottage cheese	Kefir
Egg, chicken	Mozzarella
Farmer cheese	Ricotta
Feta	Sour cream (low-fat)
Goat cheese	Yogurt
Goat's milk	

NEUTRAL

Casein	Jarlsberg
Cheddar	Milk (cow)
Colby	Monterey jack
Cream cheese	Muenster
Edam	Neufchâtel
Egg, chicken*	Paneer
Egg, goose	Quark cheese
Egg, quail	Sherbet
Emmenthal	String cheese
Ghee (clarified butter)	Swiss
Gouda	Whey
Gruyère	

AVOID

American cheese	Brie
Blue cheese	Butter

Buttermilk   Ice cream
Camembert   Parmesan
Egg, duck   Provolone
Half & half

Oils and Fats

When cooking, give preference to the healthful monounsaturated olive oil. Linseed (flaxseed) oil, neutral for Type AB, should be limited during pregnancy, and borage oil should be avoided.

HIGHLY BENEFICIAL

Olive   Walnut

NEUTRAL

Almond   Evening primrose
Black currant seed   Linseed (flaxseed)
Borage*   Peanut
Canola   Soy
Castor   Wheat germ
Cod liver

AVOID

Coconut   Safflower
Corn   Sesame
Cottonseed   Sunflower

Nuts and Seeds

Nuts and seeds present a mixed picture for Type ABs. Eat them in small amounts and with caution. Although they can be a good supplementary protein source, many seeds contain lectins that can induce immune reactions, making them a problem for Type ABs. Others, such as peanuts, are excellent immunity boosters.

HIGHLY BENEFICIAL

Chestnut   Peanut butter
Peanut   Walnut

Food with different values than the standard Type AB diet are indicated with an asterisk (*).

NEUTRAL

Almond	Hickory
Almond butter	Litchi
Almond cheese	Macadamia
Almond milk	Pecan/pecan butter
Beechnut	Pignolia (pine nut)
Brazil nut	Pistachio
Cashew/cashew butter	Safflower seed
Flaxseed (linseed)	

AVOID

Filbert (Hazelnut)	Sesame seed
Poppy seed	Sesame butter (tahini)
Pumpkin seed	Sunflower seed/butter

Beans and Legumes

Beans and legumes are another mixed bag for Type ABs. Lentils are known to contain cancer-fighting antioxidants. On the other hand, kidney and lima beans can cause problems for Type ABs. Soy-based foods are highly beneficial for you during pregnancy, as they are excellent sources of calcium and protein.

HIGHLY BENEFICIAL

Lentil (green)	Soy, miso
Navy bean	Soy, tempeh
Pinto bean	Soy, tofu
Soy bean	

NEUTRAL

Cannellini bean	Pea pod
Copper bean	Snap bean
Green bean	Soy cheese*
Green pea	Soy milk*
Jicama bean	String bean
Lentil (domestic, red)	Tamarind bean
Northern bean	White bean

Food with different values than the standard Type AB diet are indicated with an asterisk (*).

AVOID

Adzuki bean	Garbanzo bean (chickpea)
Black bean	Kidney bean
Black-eyed pea	Lima bean
Fava (broad) bean	Mung bean, sprouts

Grains, Pastas, and Cereals

Generally, Type ABs do well on grains, but you need to limit your wheat consumption, especially if you have a pronounced mucus condition caused by asthma or frequent infections. Oatmeal, soy flakes, millet, farina, rice, and soy granules are good Type AB choices, as are Essene and Ezekiel breads. Avoid buckwheat and corn.

HIGHLY BENEFICIAL

Amaranth	Rice (white, brown, basmati,
Essene bread	wild)
Ezekiel 4:9 bread (100%	Rice (puffed)
sprouted)	Rye bread (100%)
Millet	Rye crisp
Oat bran	Rye flour
Oat flour	Rye vita
Oatmeal	Soy flour bread
Rice bran	Spelt (whole)
Rice bread	Wheat bread (sprouted)
Rice cake	

NEUTRAL

Barley	Seven-grain bread/cereal
Couscous (cracked wheat)	Shredded wheat
Cream of rice	Spelt bread
Cream of wheat	Spinach pasta
Familia	Wheat bran
Farina	Wheat bran muffin
Gluten flour	Wheat (gluten flour products)
Grape-Nuts	Wheat (white flour products)
Quinoa	Wheat (whole-wheat products)
Semolina pasta	Wheat germ

AVOID

Artichoke pasta (pure)   Popcorn
Buckwheat/kasha   Soba noodles (100%
Corn (white, yellow, blue)   buckwheat)
Cornbread or muffin   Sorghum
Cornflakes   Tapioca
Cornmeal   Teff
Grits   Wheat (refined, unbleached)
Kamut

Vegetables

Most vegetables are available to Type ABs, and they are an excellent source of vitamins, minerals, and phytochemicals. Fennel and parsley, normally good for Type AB, should be minimized during pregnancy, as these are uterine stimulants. Also note that although onions and garlic are acceptable for Type AB, you may want to avoid or limit them while you're breast-feeding. Some babies experience colic when moms eat these foods.

Values for whole vegetables apply to their juices, unless otherwise noted.

HIGHLY BENEFICIAL

Alfalfa sprouts   Eggplant
Beet   Garlic
Beet greens   Kale
Broccoli   Mushroom (maitake)
Cabbage juice   Mustard greens
Carrot juice   Parsley*
Cauliflower   Parsnip
Celery   Sweet potato
Collard greens   Yam
Cucumber

NEUTRAL

Arugula   Cabbage (all types)
Asparagus   Carrot
Asparagus pea   Celeriac
Bamboo shoot   Chicory
Bok choy   Coriander leaf (cilantro)
Brussels sprouts   Cucumber juice

Food with different values than the standard Type AB diet are indicated with an asterisk (*).

Daikon
Endive
Escarole
Fennel*
Fiddlehead fern
Horseradish
Kohlrabi
Leek
Lettuce (all types)
Mushroom (silver dollar,
  portabello, tree, oyster,
  enoki)
Okra
Olive (Greek, green, Spanish)
Onion (all types)
Oyster plant
Pea (green, pod)
Poi
Potato (red, white)
Pumpkin

Radicchio
Rappini (broccoli rabe)
Rutabaga
Sauerkraut
Scallion
Seaweeds
Shallot
Snow pea
Spinach
Squash (all types)
String bean
Swiss chard
Taro
Tomato
Turnip
Water chestnut
Watercress
Yucca
Zucchini

AVOID

Aloe
Artichoke (domestic, globe,
  Jerusalem)
Corn
Mushroom (shiitake, abalone)

Olive, black
Peppers (all types)
Pickles (all types)
Radish (red)
Sprouts (mung, radish)

Fruits

Type ABs should emphasize the more alkaline fruits, such as grapes, plums, and berries. Avoid oranges, which are a stomach irritant for Type ABs and also interfere with the absorption of important minerals. Lemons are excellent for Type ABs, helping to aid digestion and clear mucus from the system.

The banana lectin interferes with Type AB digestion. I recommend substituting other high-potassium fruits such as apricots, figs, and certain melons.

Values for whole fruits apply to their juices, unless otherwise noted.

HIGHLY BENEFICIAL

Cherry
Cranberry

Fig (fresh, dried)
Gooseberry

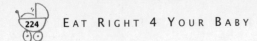

Grape (all types)   Loganberry
Grapefruit   Pineapple
Kiwi   Plum
Lemon   Watermelon

NEUTRAL

Apple   Lime
Apricot   Mulberry
Asian pear   Mush melon
Blackberry   Nectarine
Blueberry   Papaya
Boysenberry   Peach
Breadfruit   Pear
Canang melon   Persian melon
Cantaloupe   Pineapple juice
Casaba melon   Plantain
Christmas melon   Prune
Crenshaw melon   Raisin
Currants (black, red)   Raspberry
Date (all types)   Spanish melon
Elderberry (dark blue, purple) Strawberry
Grapefruit juice   Tangerine
Honeydew   Youngberry
Kumquat

AVOID

Avocado   Orange
Banana   Persimmon
Bitter melon   Pomegranate
Coconut   Prickly pear
Dewberry   Quince
Guava   Sago palm
Mango   Star fruit (carambola)

Spices and Sweeteners

Spices can be either helpful or dangerous, and this is especially true during pregnancy. A number of spices are uterine stimulants and should be avoided—especially if you have a high-risk pregnancy or a history of miscarriage. Ginger can be an excellent remedy for digestive ailments. However, it can cause miscarriage in excessive amounts. Chocolate contains caffeine and should also be avoided. Type ABs should also limit the consumption of sugars.

Certain spices, normally used in small amounts for cooking, should be minimized during pregnancy. These include cinnamon, marjoram, nutmeg, oregano, parsley, rosemary, sage, and thyme.

If you have problems with heartburn, nausea, or morning sickness, which occur mostly in the first trimester, you may find it helpful to eliminate strong spices such as curry and horseradish. However, if you don't suffer digestive problems, go ahead and use these spices.

HIGHLY BENEFICIAL

Blackstrap molasses	Ginger*
Curry	Horseradish
Garlic	Parsley*

NEUTRAL

Agar	Mace
Apple pectin	Maple syrup
Arrowroot	Marjoram
Basil	Molasses
Bay leaf	Mustard (dry)
Bergamot	Nutmeg
Caper	Oregano
Caraway	Paprika
Cardamom	Peppermint
Carob	Rice syrup
Chervil	Rosemary
Chili powder	Saffron
Chive	Sage
Chocolate*	Savory
Cilantro (coriander leaf)	Sea salt
Cinnamon	Senna
Clove	Soy sauce
Coriander	Spearmint
Cream of tartar	Stevia
Cumin	Sugar
Dill	Tamari
Honey	Tamarind
Juniper	Tarragon
Licorice root*	Thyme

Food with different values than the standard Type AB diet are indicated with an asterisk (*).

Turmeric*   Wintergreen
Vanilla   Yeast (baker's, brewer's)

AVOID

Allspice   Fructose
Almond extract   Gelatin, plain
Anise   Guarana
Aspartame   Gum (Arabic, acacia)
Barley malt   Maltodextrin
Carrageenan   Sucanat
Cornstarch   Tapioca
Corn syrup   Vinegar (all types)
Dextrose

Condiments

Avoid all pickled condiments, due to a susceptibility to stomach cancer. Also avoid ketchup, which contains vinegar, and Worcestershire sauce (with its corn syrup).

HIGHLY BENEFICIAL

None

NEUTRAL

Jam (from acceptable fruits)   Mustard
Jelly (from acceptable fruits) Salad dressing (from
Mayonnaise   acceptable ingredients)

AVOID

Ketchup   Pickle relish
Pickles (all types)   Worcestershire sauce

Herbal Teas

Herbal teas can deliver strong doses of herbs, and for this reason many are not advised for pregnant women. However, certain teas are particularly beneficial, especially late in pregnancy. Raspberry leaf is rich in vitamins and nourishes the uterus. Chamomile is excellent as a calming tea and sleep aid. Dandelion tea aids digestion. Rose hip tea is a good source of vitamin C. Slippery elm tea is an excellent remedy for intestinal problems.

HIGHLY BENEFICIAL

Alfalfa

Burdock

Chamomile

Echinacea

Ginger*

Ginseng*

Hawthorn

Licorice root*

Parsley*

Rose hip

Strawberry leaf

NEUTRAL

Catnip*

Cayenne pepper*

Chickweed

Dandelion*

Dong quai*

Elder

Fenugreek*

Goldenseal*

Horehound

Mulberry

Peppermint

Rasberry leaf*

Sage

Sarsaparilla

Slippery elm*

Spearmint

St. John's wort*

Thyme

Valerian

Vervain*

White birch

White oak bark

Yarrow*

Yellow dock

AVOID

Aloe

Coltsfoot

Corn silk

Gentian

Hops

Linden

Mullein

Red clover

Rhubarb

Senna

Shepherd's purse

Skullcap

Miscellaneous Beverage

Start eliminating caffeine and alcohol three to six months before pregnancy and continue until you are no longer breast-feeding. The common caffeine withdrawal symptoms—headache, fatigue, and irritability—won't occur if you wean yourself gradually. Consumption of alcohol during pregnancy can cause miscarriage, lead to birth defects, and cause fetal alcohol syndrome.

Food with different values than the standard Type AB diet are indicated with an asterisk (*).

HIGHLY BENEFICIAL
Tea, green
Wine, red

NEUTRAL
Beer*   Wine, white*
Seltzer water*

AVOID
Coffee (regular, decaf)   Soda (all types)
Liquor   Tea, black (regular, decaf)

Before You Get Pregnant

The best guarantee for a healthy pregnancy is to be in top condition before you get pregnant. Start getting ready at least six months before you conceive.

Pre-pregnancy Diet Strategies

Time and again, we have seen compelling evidence that the blood type diet exerts a powerfully positive influence on fertility and pregnancy. The following strategies provide a blueprint for optimal health.

Get Serious About the Type AB Diet

Begin to increase your compliance to the Type AB diet at least six months prior to attempting to conceive. The most efficient approach is to add to the number of beneficial foods you consume. These beneficial foods exert a powerful medicinal influence on your system, creating the optimal atmosphere for conception. At the same time, make an effort to eliminate those foods that are "avoids" for Type AB. Check the Type AB Chameleon Foods in the table on page 214. Some of these foods show different values for the pre-pregnancy period.

Control Your Weight

For Type AB, weight control relies on a diet that balances digestable proteins and metabolically useful carbohydrates.

Food with different values than the standard Type AB diet are indicated with an asterisk (*).

TYPE AB HEALTHY WEIGHT-LOSS GUIDELINES
1. Minimize your consumption of meat—and eat only those meats that are beneficial.
2. Eat plenty of cultured foods, especially cultured dairy and soy.
3. Include sources of essential fatty acids, especially omega-3 oils found in fish.
4. Eat plenty of fresh vegetables and fruit to provide proper natural fiber. This will aid in the eliminative process.
5. Avoid stimulants found in alcohol, caffeine, and refined sugars. Eliminate carbonated flavored sodas, even diet sodas.
6. Engage in a combination of meditative exercise and rigorous aerobic exercise several times a week.

Type AB

THESE FOODS PROMOTE WEIGHT LOSS	THESE FOODS PROMOTE WEIGHT GAIN
Soy foods	Red meat
Fish and seafood	Chicken
Cultured dairy	Kidney beans
Green vegetables	Lima beans
Kelp (seaweed)	Corn
Pineapple	Wheat
	Buckwheat

Incorporate Detoxifiers into Your Diet

Toxins are the by-products of bacterial activity on unabsorbed foods that grow in your intestinal tract. Most often these toxins are the result of eating foods that are poorly digested by your blood type—including foods that are overly processed and chemically treated.

SIGNS OF TOXICITY IN TYPE AB
- Diminished sex drive
- Circulation problems
- Sensitivity to light
- Bad breath
- Feelings of fullness in lower intestine
- Cystic breasts
- Cold sores

To aid in detoxification before pregnancy, follow this protocol for one week.

TYPE AB DETOXIFICATION PROTOCOL
(Do not use during pregnancy.)

- Burdock root (*Arctium sp.*). As a tea—1 to 3 cups, daily.
- A mixture of fresh red grapes and blueberries. Juice and drink 8 ounces every morning.
- Flaxseeds (*Linum usitatissimum*). Add 1 tablespoon to 8 ounces of water; allow to soak overnight; drink in morning.
- Probiotic supplement (friendly bacteria). Take twice daily (preferably blood type specific).
- Larch arabinogalactan (soluble fiber supplement). Take 1 tablespoon mixed with water or juice, twice daily.
- Dry skin brushing—perform this procedure once a day.

About Dry Skin Brushing

Dry skin brushing is a method of daily hygiene that has many benefits and has been around for a long time. The skin is a major organ of the body that functions as protection and as a means of elimination. Daily skin brushing will:

- Remove dried, dead cells that block the pores of the skin, allowing the skin to breathe easier and increasing its ability to protect and eliminate the waste products of metabolism.
- Increase circulation of the blood and lymph vessels that lie close to the surface just under the skin. The blood, fluid, and its contents are returned to the heart for redistribution and/or elimination.
- Increase the nutrients to the skin. By clearing out stagnant materials, there is an increased oxygen/carbon dioxide exchange, and other nutrients, vitamins, minerals, enzymes, etc., are also brought to the area.
- Remove waste products of cellular metabolism through the blood vessels and sweating.
- Decrease the workload on the rest of the body with regard to circulation and elimination.
- Warm the skin.

PROCEDURE

Skin brushing should be done with a natural or nylon bristle body brush before the bath or shower. It is suggested the brushing be done toward the heart; start with the lower limbs, arms, and back, and then the front of the body, using a moderate pressure with short strokes upward and inward. If you have a soft complexion brush, the face can be done as well using more circular motions. Strokes should bring a slight pink color or slight tingling sensation to the skin—never bruising, scraping, bleeding, or painful. One time through for each body area is sufficient.

AVOID SKIN BRUSHING IF:

- You have delicate skin.
- You have easily damaged skin.
- You have an open wound.
- You have known malignancies of the skin or lymph system.

Detoxifying foods that are especially effective for Type AB include cultured dairy foods, such as yogurt and kefir, and soy products, such as miso, natto, okara, soy sauce, and tempeh.

Pre-pregnancy Supplement Guidelines

VITAMINS	MINERALS	HERBS
Vitamin C from rose hip or acerola cherry—250 mg daily	Zinc—25 mg daily	Dandelion—250-mg capsule daily; also use fresh in salads or as tea
		Green tea—1 to 3 cups daily *before* pregnancy

The Type AB diet offers abundant quantities of important nutrients and it's important to get as many of those nutrients as possible from fresh foods. Only use supplements to fill in the minor blanks in your diet. In addition to vitamins, minerals, protein, carbohydrates, and fats, many grains, beans, vegetables, and fruits are excellent sources of fiber, which are necessary for proper digestion. In addition, fresh vegetables are an important source of phytochemicals, the substances in foods that strengthen the immune system and support pregnancy.

VITAMINS

VITAMIN C. Type AB can benefit from an extra dose (250 to 500 milligrams) of vitamin C every day to strengthen your immune system and improve your ability to digest food. Look for food-derived vitamin C preparations, such as those found from rose hip or acerola cherry.

MINERALS

ZINC. A small amount of zinc supplementation can help protect Type AB against infection. However, zinc in high doses can be teratogenic and upset the balance of other minerals, such as copper. Consume less than 25 milligrams per day.

HERBS

GREEN TEA (*Camellia sinensis*). Regular consumption of green tea appears to enhance chances of conception. Green tea does contain small amounts of caffeine, so if you are sensitive, refrain from drinking it after 6 P.M. (Do not drink green tea during pregnancy.)

DANDELION (*Taraxacum officinale*). This is very effective for mild water retention. It can be used in salads or as a tea. It is also a good source of potassium.

Improve Your Emotional Health

Your emotional well-being—especially your ability to adapt to stress—is every bit as important to your overall health as is your physical well-being. Indeed, the two are inextricably linked. As a Type AB you share Type O's susceptibility to an imbalance of the stress hormones called catecholamines. Yet you have the additional complexity of Type B's rapid clearing of nitrous oxide, which can spark high emotions.

It is crucial that you take steps to regulate your stress levels before you become pregnant, since pregnancy requires optimal health and energy. The key to Type AB stress regulation is the Type AB diet and exercise program.

Pre-pregnancy Exercise Guidelines

Type AB requires both calming activities and more intense physical exercise. Vary your routine to include a mix of the following—two days calming, three days aerobic.

CALMING

HATHA YOGA. Hatha yoga has become increasingly popular in Western countries as a method for coping with stress, and in my experience it is an excellent form of exercise for Type ABs. Make sure that you spend plenty of time outdoors. The effects of sunlight and fresh air work marvels at tempering the Type AB immune system, in particular the function of the body's natural killer (NK) cells, which can influence conception and fertility.

AEROBIC/WEIGHT-BEARING
Any of the following are useful to round out your fitness regimen.

EXERCISE	DURATION	FREQUENCY
Aerobics	45–60 minutes	2–3 × week
Martial arts	30–60 minutes	3 × week
Cycling	45–60 minutes	3 × week
Hiking	30–60 minutes	3 × week
Weight lifting	30 minutes	2 × week

Your Pregnancy:
Type AB Three-Trimester Plan

Diet Strategies

First Trimester

Choose Type AB Beneficial Foods

Continue your compliance with the Type AB diet, paying special attention to the Type AB Chameleon Foods in the table on page 214. These are foods whose normal values are different during pregnancy. If you are new to the Type AB diet, your most important first steps are inclusion of high-quality protein found in soy foods, fish, and cultured dairy, and the avoidance of red meat, chicken, wheat, buckwheat, and corn.

The first trimester is such a critical time that you should emphasize your beneficial foods whenever possible. These foods act as medicine for Type AB. While many foods are good choices of important nutrients, your power foods offer an extra benefit. For example:

Choose turkey over lamb.
Choose goat cheese and kefir over gouda and cheddar.
Choose oat flour over wheat flour.
Choose collard greens and alfalfa sprouts over carrots and leeks.
Choose cherries and figs over melons and peaches.

Emphasize Pregnancy Power Foods

There are some nutrients that have special importance. These include protein, calcium, iron, and folic acid.

Blood Type AB Pregnancy Power Foods			
PROTEIN	**CALCIUM**	**IRON**	**FOLIC ACID**
Lean, organic venison	Cultured dairy	Beef liver*	Beef liver*
Fish	Soy milk	Eggs	Fish
Cultured dairy and soy	Sardines (unboned)		Dark green leafy vegetables
	Canned salmon (with bones)		
	Tofu		

* Although red meat is discouraged for Type AB, you may have occasional small amounts of beef liver (3 to 5 ounces), which is an excellent source of iron. Avoid chicken liver: It has a deleterious protein (galectin) that can adversely effect your immune function.

Enhance Digestive Enzymes

Type ABs can have lower levels of stomach acid, pepsin, and gastrin, which may contribute to digestive problems common early in pregnancy. By improving digestive efficiency, you'll experience far less heartburn, nausea, and morning sickness.

- Limit meat, which requires high levels of digestive enzymes, to small portions—3 to 5 ounces.
- If you experience morning sickness, chamomile is a good replacement for ginger. A cup of chamomile tea will soothe your stomach.
- Avoid carbonated beverages, such as mineral water, seltzer, and soda. The carbonation can influence gastrin production, which decreases stomach acidity.

Balance Your Moods

Mood swings are common in the first months of pregnancy, triggered by the many hormonal changes that are occurring, as well as the extra stress that comes with a major life change. Recognize your tendencies and work to avoid stresses that might increase your emotional distress. Here are some suggestions for reducing mood swings:

- Find a support group or friend you can share your anxieties with. Better still, volunteer to help others. Type ABs reduce stress and elevate moods when they are focused outside themselves.
- Keep a journal detailing what you are experiencing.
- Break up your workday with physical activity, especially if your job is sedentary. You'll feel more energized, and exercise serves as a natural mood elevator.
- Plan ahead to have foods on hand for a quick energy snack when you're feeling tired or moody. Mood changes can be triggered by a decrease in blood sugar.
- Type ABs who suffer from mood swings should always supplement with extra folic acid, along with other B-complex vitamins. Folic acid has the additional benefit of being essential for fetal development. (See Supplement Guidelines, page 264).

Fight Fatigue

It is common for women to feel especially fatigued during the first trimester of pregnancy, as your body adapts to the tremendous changes taking place. You need to get at least 1 to 2 hours of additional sleep every night. Establish a regular sleep schedule and adhere to it as closely as possible. During the day, schedule at least two breaks of 20 minutes each for complete relaxation. Combat sleep disturbances with regular exercise and a relaxing pre-bedtime routine. A light snack before bedtime will help raise your blood sugar levels. Your menu plans offer many suggestions for evening snacks. In addition, a neutral (room temperature) bath before bedtime will help you sleep.

Type ABs may also benefit from the daily consumption of what I call the Membrane Fluidizer Cocktail, which improves the health of your immune and nervous systems:

MEMBRANE FLUIDIZER COCKTAIL

1 tablespoon flaxseed oil
1 tablespoon high-quality lecithin granules
6 to 8 ounces fruit juice

Shake well and drink.

A contributing factor to Type AB fatigue is a susceptibility to iron deficiency anemia. Ask your doctor about taking an iron supplement and increase your consumption of foods high in folic acid, vitamin C, iron, selenium, and zinc. These include: cold water fish (salmon, mackerel, herring, and sardines), eggs, lentils, beets, green vegetables, green beans, spinach, parsley, mustard greens, yams, apricots, blackberries, apples, currants, kelp, lettuce, peaches, molasses, mustard greens, and mulberries.

Handle Your Cravings and Aversions

If you crave foods that are not beneficial for your blood type, find healthy, blood type–friendly substitutes. For example:

WHEN YOU CRAVE . . .	EAT . . .
Sugar	Raisins or a plum; any suitable fruit
Salty foods	Nori (seaweed) snack; miso soup
Ice cream	Frozen yogurt; soy-based ice cream
Fatty foods	Peanuts; walnuts
Creamy foods	Vegetable puree—sweet potato, onion, pumpkin, or turnip; yogurt; soy smoothie

First Trimester Menu Plans

The following menus offer a guide to healthy eating during the first trimester of your pregnancy. They are designed to offer well-balanced, delicious meals that include the primary values critical for Type AB:

- They emphasize a variety of delicious meat, fish, soy, dairy, beans, fresh fruits, and vegetables.
- They provide an extra boost of calcium and protein with Type AB–specific smoothies.
- They provide many foods to help overcome first trimester problems, such as constipation, fatigue, and morning sickness.

They break the daily diet into six meals/snacks a day—aiding digestion and reducing fatigue by avoiding an empty stomach. The menus are flexible and can be mixed and reorganized according to your personal needs. I have purposely not included portion sizes for most dishes, since caloric needs vary depending on your height and weight. However, try to eat about 300 calories a day more than normal during the first trimester.

Although beverages are listed with some meals, I suggest you drink them half an hour before or after eating. Liquids consumed with solid foods dilute the digestive juices. Don't forget to keep drinking water throughout the day.

Menus

DAY 1

BREAKFAST
One-Egg Omelet* with mozzarella and
  broccoli
Ezekiel toast
Pineapple juice

MID-MORNING SNACK
Silken Smoothie*

LUNCH
Lentil Soup*
Tossed salad
Crackers

MID-AFTERNOON SNACK
Beneficial fruit

DINNER
Spicy Stir-fried Tofu with Apricots
  and Almonds*
Braised shiitake mushrooms
Braised greens with garlic
Raw Enzyme Relish*

EVENING SNACK
Super Baby Smoothie*

DAY 2

BREAKFAST
Poached egg
Spelt flakes with raisins and soy milk
Mixed berries

MID-MORNING SNACK
Beneficial fruit or protein

LUNCH
Farmer's Vegetable Soup*
Mesclun Salad*

MID-AFTERNOON SNACK
Type AB Trail Mix-2*

DINNER
Broiled Salmon Steak*
Wild rice
Braised leeks

EVENING SNACK
Super Baby Smoothie*

DAY 3

BREAKFAST
Cottage cheese with fresh pineapple
    and kiwi
Ezekiel toast with cherry preserves
Slippery elm tea

MID-MORNING SNACK
High-Energy Protein Shake*

LUNCH
Sardine Salad* on rye bread
Apple

MID-AFTERNOON SNACK
Toasted Tamari Pumpkin Seeds*
Glass of soy milk

DINNER
Roasted Turkey*
Vegetable Fritters*
Green Bean Salad with Walnuts and
    Goat Cheese*

EVENING SNACK
Super Baby Smoothie*

DAY 4

BREAKFAST
Brown Rice–Spelt Pancakes*
Sautéed Apples*
Cranberry juice
Strawberry leaf tea

MID-MORNING SNACK
Beneficial fruit or protein

LUNCH
Salmon with Wakame Seaweed*
Turkey Soup*

MID-AFTERNOON SNACK
Type AB Trail Mix-2*

DINNER
Indian Lamb Stew with Spinach*
Sweet Potato Pancakes*
Braised greens with garlic

EVENING SNACK
Super Baby Smoothie*

DAY 5

BREAKFAST
Date-Prune Smoothie*
Pumpkin-Almond Bread*
Burdock-rose hip tea

MID-MORNING SNACK
Apricot Yogurt Drink*

LUNCH
Turkey sandwich on spelt bread, with
    Romaine lettuce and tomato
Grapes

MID-AFTERNOON SNACK
Beneficial fruit or protein

DINNER
Broiled cod
Steamed spinach
Turnip puree

EVENING SNACK
Peanut Butter Cookies*
Chamomile tea

DAY 6

BREAKFAST
2 scrambled eggs
½ grapefruit
Essene toast with peanut butter

MID-MORNING SNACK
Super Baby Smoothie*

LUNCH
Mixed Roots Soup*
Mesclun Salad*

MID-AFTERNOON SNACK
Beneficial fruit or protein

DINNER
Roast Turkey*
Braised greens with garlic
Raw Enzyme Relish*

EVENING SNACK
Rice pudding with Soy Milk*
Chamomile tea

DAY 7

BREAKFAST
Wheat-free Waffles*
Mixed berries
Vegetable juice
Burdock-rose hip tea

MID-MORNING SNACK
High-Energy Protein Shake*

LUNCH
Sardine Salad*
Rye vita crackers
Mixed greens

MID-AFTERNOON SNACK
Rice cakes with prune butter
Glass of soy milk

DINNER
Lasagna with Portabello Mushrooms
    and Pesto*
Tossed salad with lemon vinaigrette

EVENING SNACK
Super Baby Smoothie*

DAY 8

BREAKFAST
Vegetable Frittata*
Ezekiel toast
Mixed berries

MID-MORNING SNACK
Pineapple Yogurt Drink*

LUNCH
White Bean and Wilted Greens Soup*
Spinach Salad*
Crackers

MID-AFTERNOON SNACK
Beneficial fruit or protein

DINNER
Tofu Vegetable Stir-fry*
Steamed cauliflower
Wild rice

EVENING SNACK
Super Baby Smoothie*

DAY 9

BREAKFAST
Poached egg on toasted Ezekiel bread
Pineapple slices
Rose hip tea

MID-MORNING SNACK
Beneficial fruit or protein

LUNCH
Speltberry and Rice Salad*
Carrot and celery sticks
Yogurt

MID-AFTERNOON SNACK
Type AB Trail Mix-1*

DINNER
Broiled cod*
Braised greens
Lentil Salad*

EVENING SNACK
Super Baby Smoothie*

DAY 10

BREAKFAST
Oatmeal with raisins and soy milk
Mixed fruit
Raspberry leaf tea

MID-MORNING SNACK
Slice of spelt bread with apple butter
Glass of soy-rice milk

LUNCH
Grilled portabello mushroom burger
    on a spelt bun with Romaine
Mixed green salad

MID-AFTERNOON SNACK
Raisins and chopped walnuts

DINNER
Tempeh Kabobs*
Steamed brown rice
Sesame Broccoli*
Herbal ice tea

EVENING SNACK
Super Baby Smoothie*

DAY 11

BREAKFAST
Poached egg
Spelt flakes with fresh berries and soy
    milk
Rose hip tea

MID-MORNING SNACK
Apricot Yogurt Drink*

LUNCH
Cucumber Yogurt Soup*
Mesclun Salad*

MID-AFTERNOON SNACK
Beneficial fruit or protein

DINNER
Fried Monkfish*
Green beans
Wild rice

EVENING SNACK
Super Baby Smoothie*

DAY 12

BREAKFAST
Tropical Salad*
Ezekiel toast with cherry preserves
Slippery elm tea

MID-MORNING SNACK
Beneficial fruit or protein

LUNCH
Miso Soup with tofu*
Brown rice
Carrot Raisin Salad*

MID-AFTERNOON SNACK
Type AB Trail Mix-2*

DINNER
Broiled Salmon, Marinated in Tamari
    Dipping Sauce*
2 beneficial vegetables

EVENING SNACK
Super Baby Smoothie*

DAY 13

BREAKFAST
Omelet* with fresh spinach and feta
Essene toast with cherry preserves

MID-MORNING SNACK
Fresh figs with yogurt

LUNCH
Super Broccoli Salad*
Sliced turkey on a bed of Romaine

MID-AFTERNOON SNACK
Beneficial fruit

DINNER
Steamed Whole Red Snapper*
Glazed Turnips and Onions*
Braised mustard greens with garlic

EVENING SNACK
Super Baby Smoothie*

DAY 14

BREAKFAST
Blueberry Muffin*
Mixed fruit
Glass of soy milk
Strawberry leaf tea

MID-MORNING SNACK
Rice cakes with apple butter

LUNCH
Sliced tomato, fresh mozzarella, and
    basil on spelt bread
Berries with yogurt

MID-AFTERNOON SNACK
Type AB Trail Mix-1*

DINNER
Grilled Loin of Lamb Chops*
Sautéed greens
Romaine-feta salad

EVENING SNACK
Super Baby Smoothie*

Second Trimester

Adjust to an Increased Appetite

Fetal growth is rapid during the second trimester, and you may experience a greater appetite, especially if you no longer suffer from the nausea that may have plagued you during the first three months. Use your extra calories to maximum benefit.

---

* You can find recipes for asterisk-marked items in appendix A.

EMPHASIS FOR EXTRA CALORIES

- High-quality protein—fish and soy foods
- Calcium-rich foods—cultured dairy, sardines, canned salmon with bones, soy milk, tofu
- Vitamin C–rich foods—dark green leafy vegetables, plums, pineapple

Keep Your Blood Sugar in Check

For Type AB, blood sugar irregularities are usually the result of carbohydrate intolerance—especially if you're eating too many grains, beans, and potatoes. While some increase in blood sugar is normal during pregnancy, be aware that severely elevated blood sugar leads to a dangerous condition called gestational diabetes, which can cause premature birth and even birth defects. The following symptoms should alert you to blood sugar imbalances:

> Fatigue
> Extreme hunger
> Dry skin
> Anxiety
> Dizziness and light-headedness

To restore a proper balance:

- Increase the protein and decrease the carbohydrates in your diet.
- Eliminate refined sugars and starches.
- Eat fiber-rich foods every day.
- Never skip meals, especially breakfast. Preferably, eat six small meals a day.

Avoid Urinary Tract Infections

Many women are susceptible to urinary tract infections during the second trimester. As a Type AB, you need to be aware of this tendency, because Type ABs typically have an extremely high risk factor for UTIs. In addition to following the Type AB diet, you can guard against UTIs with the following:

- Eat plenty of cultured dairy foods, such as yogurt and kefir.
- Eat cranberries or blueberries—effective UTI fighters.
- Urinate frequently to avoid buildup of urine in the bladder.
- Continue taking your probiotic supplement. It will help keep the colon flora, vaginal flora, and urinary tract healthy.

Build Your Immunity

Type AB often struggles with compromised immune function, which can make you more vulnerable to colds and flus. Your overall immune health is critical to your ability to carry a fetus to term, since your immune system is suppressed during pregnancy to accept the fetus. If you have a history of miscarriages, immune health should be your top priority. Many dietary factors have been linked to immune function. Failure to eat breakfast, irregular eating habits, low vegetable intake, inadequate protein, excessive wheat intake, and high-fat diets (especially those with excessive amounts of polyunsaturated fatty acids) have all been associated with lowered immune function.

Deficiencies in a range of nutrients can result in decreased immune function, so keep your nutrient levels high. In particular, selenium, zinc, vitamin C, beta-carotene, vitamin A, vitamin E, and vitamin D deficiencies should be addressed.

Check the nutrient chart below to be sure your diet contains plenty of these nutrient-rich foods.

SELENIUM	ZINC	VITAMIN C	BETA-CAROTENE
Whole grains	Turkey	Citrus fruit	Dark green
Seafood	Dried beans	Strawberries	vegetables
	and peas	Brussels sprouts	Carrots
		Dark green	Pumpkin
		vegetables	Peaches
VITAMIN A	**VITAMIN E**	**VITAMIN D**	
Chicken liver	Spinach	Fatty fish	
Eggs	Safflower oil	Egg yolk	

Eliminate Excess Mucus Production

Type AB has a tendency to suffer from excessive mucus production, which can cause a stuffy nose, respiratory problems, and ear infections. I recommend that all Type ABs begin the day with a glass of room temperature water mixed with the juice of one quarter to one half a lemon. This will reduce mucus.

Second Trimester Menu Plans

The following menus offer a guide to healthy eating during the second trimester of your pregnancy. They include some adjustments from the first trimester, taking into account the special emphasis on this period in your pregnancy.

- The menu suggestions place an even greater emphasis on meat, soy, fish, grains, and fresh fruits and vegetables—all foods that help regulate Type AB blood sugar.
- They include more calories than the first trimester menus, to accommodate the growing nutritional needs of your fetus.
- They provide an extra boost of calcium and protein with Type AB–specific smoothies.
- They provide additional foods that will help to overcome second trimester problems, such as hemorrhoids, varicose veins, and mucus production.

The menus are flexible and can be mixed and reorganized according to your personal needs. I have purposely not included portion sizes for most dishes, since caloric needs vary depending upon your height and weight. However, these menus do offer more foods than the first trimester—and you should try to increase your intake by 100 to 300 calories per day.

Note that although beverages are listed with some meals, I suggest you drink them half an hour before or after eating. Liquids consumed with solid foods dilute the digestive juices. Don't forget to keep drinking water throughout the day.

Menus

DAY 1

BREAKFAST
Fruit Silken Scramble*
Fresh vegetable juice
Ezekiel bread

MID-MORNING SNACK
Beneficial fruit or protein

LUNCH
Salmon with Wakame Seaweed*
Rice crackers
Raisins and walnuts with yogurt

MID-AFTERNOON SNACK
Type AB Trail Mix-1*

DINNER
Peter's Escargot*
Steamed broccoli
Pureed root vegetables
Wild rice

EVENING SNACK
Super Baby Smoothie*

DAY 2

BREAKFAST
Omelet* with fresh spinach and feta
Tropical Salad*
Essene toast

MID-MORNING SNACK
Pineapple Yogurt Drink*

LUNCH
Miso Soup*
Mesclun Salad*
Rye crisps

MID-AFTERNOON SNACK
Beneficial fruit or protein

DINNER
Grilled red snapper
Braised Collards*
Wild and Basmati Rice Pilaf*

EVENING SNACK
Rice Pudding*
Chamomile tea

DAY 3

BREAKFAST
Wheat-free Waffles*
Cherry preserves
Cranberry juice
Rose hip tea

MID-MORNING SNACK
Beneficial fruit or protein

LUNCH
Grilled eggplant and feta on Ezekiel
    bread
Mixed green salad
Grape Ice*

MID-AFTERNOON SNACK
Type AB Trail Mix-2*

DINNER
Tofu Vegetable Stir-fry*
Steamed broccoli
Lentil Salad*
Raw Enzyme Relish*

EVENING SNACK
Super Baby Smoothie*

DAY 4

BREAKFAST
Scrambled eggs
Poached Fruit*
Essene toast with peanut butter
Strawberry leaf tea

MID-MORNING SNACK
Date-Prune Smoothie*

LUNCH
Broiled lean ground turkey patty with
    melted goat cheese, lettuce,
    tomato, and onion
Yogurt with fruit

MID-AFTERNOON SNACK
Beneficial fruit

DINNER
Broiled Salmon with Lemongrass*
Baked sweet potato
Steamed spinach

EVENING SNACK
Super Baby Smoothie*

DAY 5

BREAKFAST
Pineapple Yogurt Drink*
Pumpkin Almond Bread*

MID-MORNING SNACK
Beneficial fruit or protein

LUNCH
Farmer's Vegetable Soup*
Super Broccoli Salad*
Crackers

MID-AFTERNOON SNACK
Peanut Butter Cookies*
Soy milk

DINNER
Soba Noodles with Pumpkin
    and Tofu*
Broccoli Rabe*
Mixed Roots Puree*

EVENING SNACK
Super Baby Smoothie*

DAY 6

BREAKFAST
Poached egg on toasted spelt bread
Fresh pineapple slices
Slippery elm tea

MID-MORNING SNACK
Date-Prune Smoothie*

LUNCH
Grilled Goat Cheddar on Ezekiel
Miso Soup*

MID-AFTERNOON SNACK
Beneficial fruit or protein

DINNER
Green Leafy Pasta*
Romaine salad with Olive Oil and
    Lemon Dressing*

EVENING SNACK
Super Baby Smoothie*

DAY 7

BREAKFAST
Silken Scramble*
Sautéed Pears*
Spelt toast with berry preserves
Strawberry leaf tea

MID-MORNING SNACK
Beneficial fruit or protein

LUNCH
Farmer's Vegetable Soup*
Mesclun Salad*
Crackers

MID-AFTERNOON SNACK
Cottage cheese and fresh fruit

DINNER
Indian Lamb Stew with Spinach*
Braised greens with garlic
Pureed root vegetables

EVENING SNACK
Super Baby Smoothie*

DAY 8

BREAKFAST
Quinoa Almond Muffin*
Stewed plums
Pineapple juice

MID-MORNING SNACK
Beneficial fruit or protein

LUNCH
Sardine Salad*
Rice crackers
Fruit and yogurt

MID-AFTERNOON SNACK
Super Baby Smoothie*

DINNER
Steamed Whole Red Snapper*
Grilled Sweet Potato Salad*
Steamed broccoli

EVENING SNACK
Wild or Basmati Rice Pudding*
Mint-chamomile tea

DAY 9

BREAKFAST
Heidi's Early Morning Shake*
Mixed berries
Strawberry leaf tea

MID-MORNING SNACK
Beneficial fruit or protein

LUNCH
Greek Salad*
Spelt pita bread
Yogurt

MID-AFTERNOON SNACK
Type AB Bar
Bunch of grapes

DINNER
Tasty Tofu Pumpkin Stir-fry*
Basmati rice
Beneficial vegetable

EVENING SNACK
Super Baby Smoothie*

DAY 10

BREAKFAST
Poached eggs
Mixed fruit
Vegetable juice
Burdock tea

MID-MORNING SNACK
Silken Smoothie*

LUNCH
Peanut butter, raisins, and honey on
    spelt toast
Yogurt and fruit

MID-AFTERNOON SNACK
Beneficial fruit or protein

DINNER
Tofu Vegetable Stir-fry*
Brown rice
Beneficial vegetable

EVENING SNACK
Super Baby Smoothie*

DAY 11

BREAKFAST
Wheat-free Waffles*
Yogurt
Mixed berries
Rose hip tea

MID-MORNING SNACK
Super Baby Smoothie*

LUNCH
Salmon with Wakame Seaweed*
Rice cakes
Vegetable consommé

MID-AFTERNOON SNACK
Papaya-Kiwi Drink*

DINNER
Fried Monkfish*
Pureed root vegetables
Braised Collards*

EVENING SNACK
Glass of soy milk
Chamomile tea

DAY 12

BREAKFAST
Poached egg
Tropical Salad*
Ezekiel toast with blackberry
    preserves
Type AB Tea

MID-MORNING SNACK
Pineapple Yogurt Drink*

LUNCH
Sardines on spelt bread with
    horseradish
Spinach Salad*

MID-AFTERNOON SNACK
Beneficial fruit or protein

DINNER
Braised Rabbit*
Braised greens
Grilled Sweet Potato Salad*

EVENING SNACK
Super Baby Smoothie*

DAY 13

BREAKFAST
Silken Scramble* with parsley-alfalfa
    sprouts
Sautéed Pears*
Ezekiel toast

MID-MORNING SNACK
High-Energy Protein Shake*

LUNCH
White Bean and Wilted Greens Soup*
Mixed green salad with Olive Oil and
    Lemon Dressing*

MID-AFTERNOON SNACK
Beneficial fruit

DINNER
Tofu Vegetable Stir-fry*
Faro Pilaf*
Glass of soy milk

EVENING SNACK
Super Baby Smoothie*

DAY 14

BREAKFAST
Wheat-free Pancakes* with blackberry
   preserves
Cranberry juice
Dandelion tea

MID-MORNING SNACK
Super Baby Smoothie*

LUNCH
Simple Fish Soup*
Green Bean Salad with Walnuts and
   Goat Cheese*

MID-AFTERNOON SNACK
Beneficial fruit or protein

DINNER
Green Leafy Pasta*
Romaine salad with Olive Oil and
   Lemon Dressing*

EVENING SNACK
Peanut Butter Cookies*
Glass of soy-rice milk

Third Trimester

Increase Healthy Blood Flow

Pregnancy places extra stress on your blood vessels as your blood volume increases to support your fetus. Type AB has naturally "thicker" blood, making you more susceptible to pulmonary embolisms and clots. To keep your blood flowing efficiently:

- Drink a glass of water with the juice of half a fresh lemon every morning upon rising.
- Get serious about reducing stress. There is good evidence that Type ABs react to stress by increasing the viscosity (thickness) of your blood. Get out into the garden; pull a few weeds! Reduce clutter. Take long walks.
- Continue to take a DHA supplement, 300 milligrams daily.

Control Your Blood Pressure

Type ABs need to be particularly careful to keep blood pressure under control during pregnancy. Preeclampsia, or pregnancy-induced hypertension, is a very serious condition that afflicts some women in the late stages of pregnancy.

Maintaining your blood type diet is essential.

NATURAL BLOOD PRESSURE REDUCTION TONIC. One excellent method for ensuring healthy blood pressure is to juice several stalks of celery, taking 6 to 8 ounces as fresh juice daily.

---

* You can find recipes for asterisk-marked items in appendix A.

Third Trimester Menu Plans

During the third trimester you may feel full after eating very little. Smaller meals, eaten at regular intervals of 3 to 4 hours may be required to get all the nutrients you need. The following menus offer a guide to healthy eating during the third trimester of your pregnancy. They include some adjustments to account for the special emphasis of this period in your pregnancy.

- They place even greater emphasis on soy foods, fish, and fresh fruits and vegetables—all foods that help maintain metabolic balance.
- They provide an extra boost of calcium and protein with Type AB–specific smoothies. This will help you prepare for the rigors of labor and delivery.
- Vitamin A– and C–rich foods are abundant, also in preparation for delivery.

The menus are flexible and can be mixed and reorganized according to your personal needs. I have purposely not included portion sizes for most dishes, since caloric needs vary depending upon your height and weight. You may need to divide up the meals and snacks further if you don't think you can finish them at one sitting. However, it's vital that you maintain your overall caloric level.

Note that although beverages are listed with some meals, I suggest you drink them half an hour before or after eating. Liquids consumed with solid foods dilute the digestive juices and fill you up faster. Don't forget to keep drinking water throughout the day.

Menus

DAY 1

BREAKFAST
Omelet* with fresh spinach and feta
Essene toast with peanut butter
Cranberry juice
Strawberry leaf tea

MID-MORNING SNACK
Papaya-Kiwi Drink*

LUNCH
Simple Fish Soup*
Carrot Raisin Salad*

MID-AFTERNOON SNACK
Beneficial fruit or protein

DINNER
Pasta with Rappini*
Mixed steamed vegetables

EVENING SNACK
Super Baby Smoothie*

DAY 2

BREAKFAST
Spelt flakes with raisins and soy milk
½ grapefruit
Ezekiel toast

MID-MORNING SNACK
Yogurt with sliced kiwi
Strawberry leaf tea

LUNCH
Wild Rice Salad*
Sliced tomatoes and cucumbers
Glass of soy milk

MID-AFTERNOON SNACK
Beneficial fruit or protein
Rose hip tea

DINNER
Roast Turkey*
Mashed Plantains*
Steamed broccoli

EVENING SNACK
Super Baby Smoothie*

DAY 3

BREAKFAST
Scrambled eggs
Ezekiel toast with black cherry
    preserves
Mixed fruit salad
Raspberry leaf tea

MID-MORNING SNACK
Beneficial fruit or protein

LUNCH
Turkey Soup*
Super Broccoli Salad*

MID-AFTERNOON SNACK
Type AB Trail Mix-2*

DINNER
Broiled Salmon with Lemongrass*
Carrots and Parsnips with Garlic and
    Cilantro*
Faro Pilaf*

EVENING SNACK
Super Baby Smoothie*

DAY 4

BREAKFAST
Poached eggs
2 plums
Glass of goat's milk
Rose hip tea

MID-MORNING SNACK
Cherry-Peach Smoothie*

LUNCH
Grilled Goat Cheddar on Ezekiel
    or Spelt*
Mesclun Salad*

MID-AFTERNOON SNACK
Beneficial fruit or protein

DINNER
Broiled Salmon Steak* with cherry
    tomatoes
Brown basmati rice
Steamed cauliflower

EVENING SNACK
Super Baby Smoothie*

DAY 5

BREAKFAST
Oatmeal with dried cranberries, maple
    syrup; and goat's milk
Pineapple slices

MID-MORNING SNACK
Beneficial fruit or protein

LUNCH
Salmon with Wakame Seaweed* on a
    bed of Romaine lettuce
Farmer's Vegetable Soup*

MID-AFTERNOON SNACK
Rice cakes with prune butter

DINNER
Green Leafy Pasta*
Endive salad

EVENING SNACK
Super Baby Smoothie*

DAY 6

BREAKFAST
Spinach Frittata*
2 plums
Rose hip tea

MID-MORNING SNACK
Papaya-Kiwi Drink*

LUNCH
Greek Salad*
Yogurt with fruit
Lemon-chamomile tea

MID-AFTERNOON SNACK
Sliced apple, raisins, and walnuts
Glass of soy milk

DINNER
Broiled Lamb Chops*
Speltberry Salad*
Steamed carrots

EVENING SNACK
Super Baby Smoothie*

DAY 7

BREAKFAST
Wheat-free Waffles* with plum
    preserves
Mixed fruit

MID-MORNING SNACK
Beneficial fruit or protein

LUNCH
Waldorf Salad*
Grilled eggplant and feta on spelt
    bread

MID-AFTERNOON SNACK
Rye crisp snack with prune butter

DINNER
Turkey Burger*
Mesclun Salad*

EVENING SNACK
Super Baby Smoothie*

DAY 8

BREAKFAST
Puffed rice cereal with dried cherries
    and goat's milk
Sliced honeydew melon
Essene bread with peanut butter
Strawberry leaf tea

MID-MORNING SNACK
Beneficial fruit or protein

LUNCH
White Bean and Wilted Greens Soup*
Mixed Mushroom Salad*
Crackers

MID-AFTERNOON SNACK
Rice cakes with peanut butter and
    prune butter

DINNER
Steamed Whole Red Snapper* with
    Seaweed Dressing*
Steamed broccoli
Grilled Sweet Potato Salad*

EVENING SNACK
Super Baby Smoothie*

DAY 9

BREAKFAST
High-Energy Protein Shake*
Essene bread with plum preserves

MID-MORNING SNACK
Beneficial fruit or protein

LUNCH
Broiled lean ground turkey patty with
    melted goat cheese and raw
    spinach leaves
Mixed green salad

MID-AFTERNOON SNACK
Type AB Trail Mix-1*
Carrot juice

DINNER
Tempeh Kabobs*
Brown rice
2 Beneficial vegetables

EVENING SNACK
Super Baby Smoothie*

DAY 10

BREAKFAST
Poached egg on toasted Ezekiel bread
Pineapple slices

MID-MORNING SNACK
Cherry-Peach Smoothie*

LUNCH
Sardine Salad*
Rye vita crackers
Cream of broccoli soup

MID-AFTERNOON SNACK
Beneficial fruit or protein

DINNER
Fried Monkfish*
Brown rice
Beneficial vegetable
Mixed green salad

EVENING SNACK
Super Baby Smoothie*

DAY 11

BREAKFAST
Spelt flakes with raisins and soy milk
Pineapple slices
Ezekiel toast

MID-MORNING SNACK
Apricot Yogurt Drink*

LUNCH
Smoked Mackerel Salad*
Mixed green salad
Yogurt with sliced peaches
Rose hip tea

MID-AFTERNOON SNACK
Beneficial fruit

DINNER
Roast Chicken with Garlic and Herbs*
Broccoli Rabe*
Baked sweet potato

EVENING SNACK
Super Baby Smoothie*

DAY 12

BREAKFAST
Scrambled eggs
Ezekiel toast with plum preserves
Beneficial fruit

MID-MORNING SNACK
Beneficial fruit or protein

LUNCH
Turkey Burger*
Mesclun Salad*

MID-AFTERNOON SNACK
Type AB Trail Mix-2*

DINNER
Tasty Tofu Pumpkin Stir-fry*
Basmati rice
Beneficial vegetable

EVENING SNACK
Super Baby Smoothie*

DAY 13

BREAKFAST
Oatmeal with raisins and soy milk
Beneficial fruit
Raspberry leaf tea

MID-MORNING SNACK
Papaya-Kiwi Drink*

LUNCH
Grilled portabello mushroom burger
   on a spelt bun with Romaine
Mesclun Salad*

MID-AFTERNOON SNACK
Beneficial fruit or protein

DINNER
Eggplant Casserole*
Brown rice
Beneficial vegetable

EVENING SNACK
Super Baby Smoothie*

DAY 14

BREAKFAST
Blueberry Muffin*
Glass of soy-rice milk
Mixed fruit
Dandelion tea

MID-MORNING SNACK
Tofu Carob Protein Drink*

LUNCH
Greek Salad*
Yogurt
Spelt pita

MID-AFTERNOON SNACK
Super Baby Smoothie*

DINNER
Steamed Whole Red Snapper*
Brown rice
Braised Collards*

EVENING SNACK
Tofu Pumpkin Pudding*
Strawberry leaf tea

Exercise Guidelines

First Trimester

Maintenance for Healthy Type ABs

If you are healthy, continue to combine moderate aerobic exercise with relaxation and calming exercises on a normal schedule during the first trimester (page 232).

Choose from among the following Type AB exercises for a minimum regimen of 45 minutes, three to four times a week.

EXERCISE	DURATION
Tennis	45–60 minutes
Cycling	25–30 minutes
Hiking	30–60 minutes
Treadmill	30–40 minutes
Golf (no cart)	60 minutes
Swimming	30–45 minutes

* You can find recipes for asterisk-marked items in appendix A.

CAUTIONS FOR HIGH-RISK PREGNANCIES

Consult with your doctor before continuing your exercise regimen if you are in a high-risk pregnancy. Most doctors will discourage exercise if you:

- Have a history of miscarriages, or have had even one miscarriage, if it is recent.
- Have a history of recurrent pelvic or abdominal infections.
- Have an incompetent cervix. This condition causes the cervix to open early, usually in the second trimester, leading to miscarriage.
- Have had toxemia in a previous pregnancy.
- Have a history of premature deliveries.
- Have or have had a serious medical condition, such as cancer, heart disease, asthma, or kidney disease.

Second Trimester

Adaptations for Advancing Pregnancy

Continue your regular program of exercise during the second trimester, with an additional emphasis on gentle stretching and calming exercises. An ideal second trimester regimen for Type AB includes:

THREE TIMES A WEEK, CHOOSE ONE:

EXERCISE	DURATION
Water aerobics	40–50 minutes
Treadmill	30 minutes
Cycling (recumbent bike)	30 minutes
Swimming	30 minutes
Brisk walking	45 minutes

TWO TIMES A WEEK, CHOOSE ONE:

EXERCISE	DURATION
Light yoga	40–50 minutes
T'ai Chi	30 minutes
Labor preparation class	40–50 minutes

DAILY:

EXERCISE	DURATION
Kegel exercises	2 minutes, 10–20 times

- Join a yoga class specifically designed for pregnant women.
- Spend more time on your warm-up and cooldown to fully warm and stretch your muscles. This will minimize the muscle cramps that are common as your pregnancy progresses.
- Look for opportunities to incorporate fitness into your daily routine. If feasible, walk to work instead of driving. Take the stairs instead of the elevator.
- Swimming is an excellent exercise for the second and third trimesters. It places minimum stress on your joints and heart rate. A water aerobics class is an ideal substitution for more strenuous aerobics.
- If you haven't already started your Kegel exercises (see page 28), do so now.

PREGNANCY-SAFE EXERCISE SUBSTITUTIONS

INSTEAD OF . . .	TRY . . .
Bicycling	Indoor stationary bike (recumbent)
Tennis	Brisk walking/treadmill
Aerobics	Water aerobics

Third Trimester

Adaptations for Late Pregnancy

Exercise is essential during the third trimester. It can help keep your blood pressure in check, combat fatigue, regulate your blood sugar, and reduce the effects of stress. It can also keep you limber and reduce some of the aches and pains you're probably experiencing. However, even if you have been exercising vigorously for years, you need to pay close attention to the signs that you may be pushing yourself too hard. If you feel light-headed or crampy during your workout routine, stop exercising. Avoid any exercises that place pressure on your abdominal area.

Sign up for a prenatal yoga class. Also begin your daily perineal massage to tone the vaginal canal (page 31).

An excellent third trimester exercise regimen for Type AB would be the following.

TWO TIMES A WEEK, CHOOSE ONE:

EXERCISE	DURATION
Water aerobics	40–50 minutes
Treadmill	30 minutes
Cycling (recumbent bike)	30 minutes
Swimming	30 minutes
Brisk walking	45 minutes

THREE TIMES A WEEK, CHOOSE ONE:

EXERCISE	DURATION
Light yoga	40–50 minutes
Relaxation, stretching	30 minutes
Labor preparation class	40–50 minutes

DAILY, PERFORM BOTH:

EXERCISE	DURATION
Kegel exercises	2 minutes, 10–20 times
Perineal massage	5 minutes, 1–2 times

Supplement Guidelines

First Trimester

Vitamins/Minerals

Take a standard prenatal vitamin supplement, choosing one made from whole food, not synthetic ingredients. Powder-in-capsule forms dissolve most efficiently. If you would like to use a prenatal supplement specifically formulated for Type AB, see appendix B for information about Healthy Start ABO Prenatal. The following nutrient breakdown is the optimal formula for Type AB.

PRENATAL SUPPLEMENT—TYPE AB		% DAILY VALUE
Vitamin A (100% as natural beta-carotene from *Dunaliella salina*)	3,000 iu	60
Vitamin C (100% from acerola berry, *Malpighia puncifolia*)	75 mg	125
Vitamin D (cholecalciferol)	125 iu	31
Vitamin K (phytonadione)	20 mcg	–
Vitamin E (Natural d,alpha-tocopheryl succinate)	125 iu	416
Thiamin (from Thiamin HCl)	20 mg	1,333
Riboflavin	10 mg	588
Niacin and niacinamide (vitamin B_3)	15 mg	75
Vitamin B_6 (from pyridoxine HCl)	10 mg	500
Folic acid	800 mcg	200
Vitamin B_{12} (methylcobalamin)	15 mcg	250
Biotin	400 mcg	133
Pantothenic Acid (from D-calcium pantothenate)	15 mg	150
Calcium (seaweed base, derived from *Lithothamnium corralliodes* and *Lithothamnium calcareum*)	300 mg	30
Iron (ferrous succinate)	22 mg	122
Iodine (potassium iodide)	100 mcg	66
Magnesium (citrate and oxide)	100 mg	25
Zinc (picolinate)	27 mg	180
Selenium (L-selenomethionine)	25 mcg	–
Copper (gluconate)	1 mg	50
Magnesium (citrate)	1 mg	–

Herbal Remedies

HERB	FUNCTION	FORM AND DOSAGE
Chamomile	Calms; relieves heartburn	As tea, 1 to 2 cups daily; or add 2–4 drops of essential oil to bath
Horsetail	Contains silica, which supports healthy bones, skin, hair, and nails	250-mg capsule daily
Peppermint	Calms; relieves indigestion	As tea, 2 to 3 cups daily, after meals
Red raspberry leaf	Relieves morning sickness	As tea, 2 cups daily

HERB	FUNCTION	FORM AND DOSAGE
Slippery elm bark	Relieves heartburn	250-mg capsule, twice daily; or as tea, 2 cups daily; or as Thayer's lozenges, 2–4 daily

Nutritional Supplements

NUTRITIONAL SUPPLEMENT	FUNCTION	FORM AND DOSAGE
Larch arabinogalactan	Relieves constipation	Soluble fiber supplement: 1 tablespoon mixed with water or juice, twice daily
Probiotic	For intestinal health	2 capsules, twice daily*
DHA	Provides essential nutrients for fetal development	300-mg capsule daily

* See appendix B for information on blood type–specific probiotics.

Second Trimester

Vitamins/Minerals

Continue to take your prenatal supplement, preferably one formulated for Type AB.

Herbal Remedies

HERB	FUNCTION	FORM AND DOSAGE
Bilberry	Relieves hemorrhoids and varicose veins	25-mg capsule, twice daily
Chamomile	Calms; relieves heartburn; relieves hemorrhoids and varicose veins	As tea, 1 to 2 cups daily; or add 2–4 drops of essential oil to bath
Horsetail	Contains silica, which supports healthy bones, skin, hair, and nails	250-mg capsule daily
Peppermint	Calms; relieves indigestion	As tea, 2 to 3 cups daily, after meals
Red raspberry leaf	Treatment for bleeding gums	As tea, 2 cups daily
Rose hips	Treatment for varicose veins, bleeding gums, and allergies	1 tablespoon concentrate every 30 minutes for allergy attack; as tea, 2 to 3 cups daily

HERB	FUNCTION	FORM AND DOSAGE
Stinging nettle leaf	Allergy relief	As tea, 2 cups daily for symptoms
Witch hazel	Treatment for hemorrhoids	Use topically as needed

Nutritional Supplements

NUTRITIONAL SUPPLEMENT	FUNCTION	FORM AND DOSAGE
Larch arabinogalactan	Relieves constipation	Soluble fiber supplement: 1 tablespoon mixed with water or juice, twice daily
Probiotic	For intestinal health; prevention of candida infection	2 capsules, twice daily*
DHA	Provides essential nutrients for fetal development	300-mg capsule daily

* See appendix B for information on blood type–specific probiotics.

Third Trimester

Vitamins/Minerals

Continue to take your prenatal supplement, preferably one formulated for Type AB.

Herbal Remedies

HERB	FUNCTION	FORM AND DOSAGE
Astragalus	Prevents edema; lessens abdominal achiness	500 mg daily
Dandelion leaf/root	Lowers blood pressure; decreases edema	As tea, 2 cups daily; or 250-mg capsule, twice daily
Nettles	Rich in vitamin K, promotes blood clotting	As tea, 2 cups daily; or 250-mg capsule, twice daily
Raspberry leaf	Softens the cervix in preparation for birth; stimulates milk production	As tea, 2 cups daily; as tincture, 15–20 drops daily
Squaw vine	Prepares uterus for birth	As tincture, 10 drops in warm water, twice daily

Nutritional Supplements		
NUTRITIONAL SUPPLEMENT	FUNCTION	FORM AND DOSAGE
Larch arabinogalactan	Relieves constipation	Soluble fiber supplement: 1 tablespoon mixed with water or juice, twice daily
Probiotic	For intestinal health; prevention of candida infection	2 capsules, twice daily*
DHA	Provides essential nutrients for fetal development	300-mg capsule daily

* See appendix B for information on blood type–specific probiotics.

Labor and Delivery

In addition to the general guidelines for labor and delivery (page 32), you have some specific Type AB needs.

Type AB Energy Needs

Begin several weeks before your delivery date to prepare yourself for the stress of labor and delivery. Try to get more sleep than usual and eat plenty of nutrient-rich foods.

The first stage of labor can last many hours. Drink plenty of liquids and keep a light protein snack nearby. Stay hydrated. Be sure to discuss in advance with your doctor or midwife what the policy is about eating light foods or drinking liquids during labor.

Type AB Emotional Needs

Type AB shows major physiological benefits from positive social interaction and support. You might consider engaging a doula to assist in labor, since you feel stronger and more emotionally stable when you are working with others to achieve a common purpose. (See page 32 for a discussion of the role of a doula.)

Anxiety is enhanced by fear of the unknown. Arrange in advance for your doctor, nurse, midwife, and other providers to keep you informed about the process and apprised of any problems or complications.

See page 35 for natural childbirth painkillers.

The "Fourth" Trimester
(After the Birth)

THE THREE-MONTH PERIOD following your child's birth is sometimes referred to as the fourth trimester, as all of you—mother, baby, father, and other siblings—begin your new life together. This is an extraordinary period of time in which so many elements must be coordinated and taken into account that the stress factors can threaten to overwhelm all involved.

The fourth trimester is a time of adaptation to the new demands of motherhood, biological repair, and reintegration into the flow of life.

Whatever you may have imagined was going to happen in terms of your thoughts and emotions, give yourself an opportunity to relax and let go now. Don't push yourself to maintain your normal standards. This is a time to "go with the flow." Permit yourself to get plenty of rest. If your home is messier than you'd like, let it be so. Don't force yourself to do more than you may be capable of doing. Concentrate on your baby's needs, and your own needs. Those are the paramount concerns at this time.

Easing Postpartum Discomfort

Vaginal discharge after birth is called lochia. It is a combination of the sluffed uterine lining and blood. The lochia usually changes from bright red, to pink, to whitish over the course of several weeks.

It is very common for the bleeding to stop and start intermittently as well as contain clots. Decrease your activity if you notice an increase in the amount of bleeding, as this is a signal for you to slow down and rest more. Special care in cleansing the perineum should be taken as long as postpartum bleeding continues. If you are comfortable, you will be better able to care for your baby during the first days after birth.

Your perineum may be sore and slightly swollen after birth. If you have had an episiotomy, your stitches will be tender. The puffiness decreases in a few days. Any increased pain or swelling should be reported to your health-care provider.

Advice from the Naturopath Midwife
Cathy Rogers, N.D.

SITZ BATHS FOR POSTPARTUM DISCOMFORT

Fill a tub with water so that it covers the hip and reaches up to mid-abdomen. If possible, immerse the pelvic and abdominal regions in the sitz bath water with your feet immersed in a separate basin with water, which is a few degrees warmer.

When using hot sitz bath, the tub should be filled with water about 110 degrees F. Stay in the bath for 20 to 40 minutes and then take a quick cold shower or bath. For cold sitz bath, fill the tub with ice water and stay in the cold bath for 30 to 60 seconds. Then towel yourself dry.

For alternating hot and cold baths, fill one tub with hot water and a second with ice water. Stay in the hot sitz bath first for 3 to 4 minutes and then shift to the cold sitz bath for 30 to 60 seconds; repeat this three to four times.

Handling Postpartum "Blues" and Depression

Many women I've treated in my clinic suffer from some form of "baby blues" in the weeks following delivery. These mood swings, triggered by hormonal changes, are usually short-lived. The best remedy is to engage in stress-reduction practice, exercise, and get enough rest.

New research indicates that pregnant or nursing women could reduce their chances of developing postpartum depression and improve the neurological development of their babies by increasing the amount of the essential fatty acid DHA they consume. DHA (docosahexaenoic acid) is an omega-3 fatty acid mostly found in eggs and salmon. The standard dosage is 300 milligrams daily.

If fatigue is a factor, and it often is in the early days, the remedy is rest, your blood type diet, and moderate energizing exercise, such as gentle stretching or walking. Refer to your blood type section below.

Postpartum depression is a different matter. Between 10 and 15 percent of new mothers experience a more severe form of depression and need professional help. The symptoms include:

- Anxiety or panic attacks
- Feelings of hopelessness or guilt
- Insomnia
- Lack of interest in your baby
- Thoughts about harming your baby

If your depression is severe and is not eased by stress reduction, exercise, diet, and rest, seek professional help.

Getting Back into Shape

Most women I've treated are extremely anxious to get back into shape as soon as possible after the birth of their babies. Your blood type guidelines offer strategies for doing this. However, I urge you to take it slow and not rush into a weight-loss program. Place your focus on health and fitness rather than weight loss, and don't use any extreme measures. It is not safe or healthy to lose weight rapidly, especially while nursing. You do not want to risk a reduced milk production or a depletion of your bone and muscle tissue for the sake of getting back to your pre-pregnancy weight. As a general rule, the breastfeeding mother should be carrying an extra 10 pounds of weight.

In order to lose weight while nursing, and, in particular, fat weight, a combination of diet and exercise is best. Maintain a calorie level of 1,800 to 2,000 calories a day. While you maintain a relatively high calorie level to provide your baby with the proper nutrients, also increase the intensity of your exercise routine. For example, try running instead of walking, or walk at a brisker pace for a longer time. Also, add weight lifting two times a week to your routine. Muscles burn more calories than fat, plus a muscular body has a higher metabolism. The increase in caloric intake along with the exercise will raise your metabolism and therefore help you to lose weight.

It may take you as long as a year to return to your pre-pregnancy condition. That's okay. Your best approach to the first year is to focus on nurturing your baby—and nurturing yourself.

The Type O Mother

Personal Recovery Guidelines

The Type O new mother will benefit enormously from talking about your birth experience—both the positive experience and the painful elements. If you have a doula, she can help you process your experience and provide guidance and support for the early weeks. Also be sure to share your feelings and experiences with your mate. When you meet the new challenges as a team, there will be less stress and anxiety.

Be aware of your own tendencies and work to overcome those that will add to your stress. In particular, be aware of your tendency to exhibit "type A personality" characteristics.

To reduce stress:

- Express yourself in writing. Keep a journal and write down what you are experiencing during the early weeks after the birth of your baby.
- Learn problem-solving techniques. Frustration and anger are most often the result of feeling a loss of control. When you are intent on solving a problem, rather than exploding in a helpless rage, your stress hormones will remain steady.
- Make sure to have a person or persons you can talk to when you're frustrated or angry. The extroverted Type O releases stress by engaging in a supportive conversation. The Internet provides many supportive Web communities that can help you build confidence and security in your parenting.

TYPE O POSTPARTUM RECOVERY PROTOCOL

Use this protocol for four weeks:

- General multivitamin—preferably Type O specific (see appendix B)
- L-Carnitine—50 mg. Take 1 to 2 capsules, twice daily
- Extra vitamin C, from acerola cherry or rose hip—250 mg, twice daily
- DHA—300-mg capsule, once daily
- L-tyrosine—500 mg, two times a day

Postpartum Exercise Guidelines

If your delivery was routine, you can begin exercising again soon after your baby's birth, and I encourage you to do so. Exercise is such an essential part of Type O's well-being, both mind and body. Take it slow, though. Your sessions should be shorter and less vigorous than normal, with plenty of attention to stretching. If you're able, sign up for a new mothers' exercise class.

You'll benefit physically and emotionally if you can get away on your own for exercise—even for half an hour. Take a walk or attend a class while someone watches your baby.

Eight Type O Strategies for Getting Back in Shape

1. KNOW YOUR METABOLIC PROFILE

Your body weight alone is not a reliable indicator of your fitness. Your goal is not just to lose pounds but to build muscle and to burn calories efficiently. In addition to weight in pounds, it is important to know your metabolic rate (how efficiently you burn calories) and your body mass index (the ration of muscle to fat).

BASAL METABOLIC RATE. This is the rate at which you burn calories at rest. That is, how many calories you need to sustain basic functions. You can estimate your average basal metabolic rate by multiplying your weight by 10 calories. If you engage in moderate activity (the level recommended in the average Type O exercise plan), multiply that number by 1.6 to estimate the number of calories you burn in a day.

> *Example:*
> 150 pounds × 10 calories = 1,500 (at rest)
> 1,500 × 1.6 = 2,400
> Total calorie expenditure: 2,400

BODY MASS INDEX. This is a measurement of body fat, based on your height and weight. A body mass index above 25 is considered overweight. To calculate your body mass index, multiply your weight by 704.5. Then multiply your height (in inches) by your height (in inches). Divide the first result by the second.

> *Example:*
> An individual who is 5'5" and weighs 140 pounds
> 140 pounds × 704.5 = 98,630
> 65 × 65 = 4,225
> 98,630 ÷ 4,225 = 23

You can find more information about body mass index by going to the website of the National Heart, Lung, and Blood Institute—www.nhlbi.nih.gov.

2. RESOLVE ANY MEDICAL CONDITIONS

Get a thorough checkup to determine whether you have any metabolic impediments to fitness. In particular, thyroid irregularities and insulin resistance syndrome can impede fitness and weight loss.

3. CHOOSE FOODS THAT ARE METABOLICALLY EFFICIENT

Many common grain lectins have the effect of inhibiting the breakdown of fats through their effects on insulin. When Type Os adopt low-fat diets rich in metabolically inactivating lectins, you gain weight. Let the Type O diet be your guide. To jump-start your program, adhere to the following plan.

SEVEN-DAY SUPER O DIET
- Lean, organic meat—4 to 6 servings weekly
- Fish rich in omega-3 fatty acids—3 to 4 servings weekly
- Eggs—2 to 3 eggs weekly
- Soy milk, tofu—5 to 7 servings weekly (while breast-feeding)
- Olive or flaxseed oil—1 serving daily
- Green vegetables—2 to 3 servings daily
- Other beneficial vegetables—5 to 7 servings weekly
- Fruit—2 to 3 servings daily
- Grains (allowed)—3 to 4 servings weekly

4. ELIMINATE ARTIFICIAL STIMULANTS

Many people use stimulants as a weight-loss method, but this approach is counterproductive for Type Os. Often, stimulants contain some form of caffeine. There is strong evidence that even moderate amounts of caffeine can activate the Type O sympathetic nervous system, resulting in a higher adrenaline release. This adrenaline release mimics hypoglycemia, even when your blood sugar levels are not actually low.

5. TRICK YOUR CARBOHYDRATE CRAVING

When you crave carbohydrates, especially sugars, your serotonin levels are low, and your brain is demanding stimulants to raise the levels. As a rule, when you crave sugar, eat some protein.

6. GET AEROBIC

Aerobic exercise, at least four times a week, for 30 to 45 minutes, is a necessity for Type Os. In fact, it constitutes 50 percent of your health plan. Watch for signs of boredom or strain and adjust your routine accordingly. Choose from among the following exercises:

EXERCISE	DURATION	FREQUENCY
Aerobics	40–50 minutes	3–4 × week
Running	40–45 minutes	3–4 × week
Calisthenics	30–45 minutes	3 × week
Treadmill	30 minutes	3 × week
Cycling	30 minutes	3 × week
Swimming	30 minutes	2–3 × week

7. LIFT WEIGHTS TO BUILD MUSCLE MASS

Lift weights at least twice a week to build muscle mass. Muscles burn more calories than fat, plus a muscular body has a higher metabolism. The increase in calorie intake along with the exercise will raise your metabolism and therefore help you to lose weight. Lifting weights will also train you to lift and carry your growing child with ease.

8. DON'T RUSH IT

Place your focus on health and fitness rather than weight loss, and don't use any extreme measures, especially while you're breast-feeding. It is not safe or healthy to lose weight rapidly, especially while nursing.

The Type A Mother

Personal Recovery Guidelines

The new Type A mother faces one of the great stressful moments of her life—and we know that Type As are extremely vulnerable to the effects of stress.

Ease some of your stress by making decisions. This is very important. When a matter remains unresolved, it acts as a chronic stressor. Unresolved issues are like a virus on your computer's hard drive. They eat up all the available memory and make it impossible to run "programs" like good health and peace of mind. Suppressed emotions compromise the quality of your life and your health. They limit mental clarity, productivity, and your ability to adapt to stress. Allow your feelings. Acknowledge that life includes both positive and negative emotions.

TYPE A POSTPARTUM RECOVERY PROTOCOL

Use this protocol for four weeks:

- General multivitamin—preferably Type A specific (see appendix B)
- DHA—300 mg, twice daily

- Liquid chlorophyll supplement—1 teaspoon daily (can be added to a clear glass of spring water and placed by a window for a few minutes; it will absorb light energy and supercharge the molecules)
- Pantothenic acid—250 mg, 1 to 2 capsules daily
- Potassium citrate—100 mg, twice daily
- Extra vitamin C, from acerola cherry or rose hip—250 mg, twice daily
- Chamomile (*Matricaria chamomilla*)—herbal tincture; 25 drops in warm water, two to three times daily
- Holy Basil (*Ocinum sanctum*)—leaf extract, take 250-mg capsule, twice daily

Postpartum Exercise Guidelines

If your delivery was routine, you can begin exercising again soon after your baby's birth, and I encourage you to do so. Take it slow, though. Your sessions should focus on gentle, calming exercises, with plenty of attention to stretching. If you're able, sign up for a new mothers' exercise class.

Eight Type A Strategies for Getting Back in Shape

1. KNOW YOUR METABOLIC PROFILE

Your body weight alone is not a reliable indicator of your fitness. Your goal is not just to lose pounds but to build muscle and to burn calories efficiently. In addition to weight in pounds, it is important to know your metabolic rate (how efficiently you burn calories) and your body mass index (the ration of muscle to fat).

BASAL METABOLIC RATE. This is the rate at which you burn calories at rest. That is, how many calories you need to sustain basic functions. You can estimate your average basal metabolic rate by multiplying your weight by 10 calories. If you engage in moderate activity (the level recommended in the average Type A exercise plan), multiply that number by 1.6 to estimate the number of calories you burn in a day.

> *Example:*
> 150 pounds × 10 calories = 1,500 (at rest)
> 1,500 × 1.6 = 2,400
> Total calorie expenditure: 2,400

BODY MASS INDEX. This is a measurement of body fat, based on your height and weight. A body mass index above 25 is considered overweight. To calculate your body mass index, multiply your weight by 704.5. Then multiply your height (in inches) by your height (in inches). Divide the first result by the second.

> *Example:*
> An individual who is 5′5″ and weighs 140 pounds
> 140 pounds × 704.5 = 98,630
> 65 × 65 = 4,225
> 98,630 ÷ by 4,225 = 23

You can find more information about body mass index by going to the website of the National Heart, Lung, and Blood Institute—www.nhlbi.nih.gov.

2. RESOLVE ANY MEDICAL CONDITIONS

Get a thorough checkup to determine whether you have any metabolic impediments to fitness. In particular, make sure that your cardiovascular and digestive systems are all in good working order, so that you can exercise safely and eliminate toxins efficiently.

3. CHOOSE FOODS THAT ARE METABOLICALLY EFFICIENT

Let the Type A diet be your guide. To jump-start your program, adhere to the following plan.

SEVEN-DAY SUPER A DIET
- Soy foods (tofu, tempeh, soy milk, etc.)—1 to 2 servings daily
- Lean, organic poultry—1 to 3 servings weekly
- Fish rich in omega-3 fatty acids—3 to 5 servings weekly
- Eggs—2 to 3 eggs weekly
- Olive or flaxseed oil—1 serving daily
- Beans and legumes
- Grains
- Green vegetables—2 to 3 servings daily
- Other beneficial vegetables—5 to 7 servings weekly
- Fruit—2 to 3 servings daily

4. EAT ENOUGH FOOD

Don't undereat or skip meals. Use appropriate blood type snacks between meals if you get hungry. Avoid low-calorie diets. Remember, food deprivation is a huge stress. It raises cortisol levels, lowers metabolism, encourages fat storage, and depletes healthy muscle mass.

5. BOOST YOUR METABOLISM

Many meat-eating Type As report feeling fatigued and lacking energy, especially when they engage in aerobic exercise and restrict complex carbohydrates. Another common Type A problem with excessive meat consumption is fluid retention, the result of the inability to properly digest high-protein foods. While Type Os have the capacity to break down the complex proteins in meat, most Type As lack this ability.

6. REDUCE STRESS

Type As who struggle with low metabolism and weight gain have another challenge—the effects of high cortisol. Being under constant stress causes weight gain for Type A. That's because high levels of the stress hormone cortisol promote insulin resistance and catabolize (burn) muscle tissue instead of fat. Obesity itself leads to cortisol resistance; it becomes a dangerously vicious circle for Type As. High cortisol is also associated with leptin, a hormone related to the obesity gene, which increases your appetite.

7. REGULATE YOUR MEALS

Often, how much you eat is less important than when you eat it. Eat the same amount of calories early in the day and most people lose weight; eat them at night and most people gain weight. Skipping breakfast or eating only a small amount of food for breakfast will have detrimental effects on your slow Type A metabolism. Cortisol and thyroid hormones will both be impacted. The same applies to skipping lunch. If you are serious about losing weight, a critical strategy is to eat a well-balanced breakfast, well-balanced lunch, and an adequate dinner—early in the evening. Resist the late-night munchies.

8. EXERCISE FOR YOUR TYPE

The following comprises the ideal exercise regimen for Type A.

THREE TO FOUR TIMES A WEEK, CHOOSE ONE:

EXERCISE	DURATION
Hatha yoga	40–50 minutes
T'ai Chi	40–50 minutes

TWO TO THREE TIMES A WEEK, CHOOSE ONE:

EXERCISE	DURATION
Aerobics (low impact)	40–50 minutes
Treadmill	30 minutes
Weight training (5–10 lb free weights)	15 minutes
Cycling (recumbent bike)	30 minutes
Swimming	30 minutes
Brisk walking	45 minutes

The Type B Mother

Personal Recovery Guidelines

The new Type B mother faces one of the great stressful moments of her life—and we know that Type Bs are vulnerable to the effects of stress when they are overwhelmed or overtired.

Be aware of your own tendencies and work to overcome those that will add to your stress. The collective research that has been done on the Type B personality seems to confirm these neurochemical attributes. When you are in a state of balance, you can be flexible, creative, sensitive, and mentally agile, with a strong intuitive sense. Out of balance, you can suffer from the effects of high stress hormones, such as cortisol, and a susceptibility to viral infections, chronic fatigue, mental fogginess, and autoimmune diseases. Your focus in achieving mind-body integrity needs to be on lowering your cortisol levels and increasing your mental acuity.

According to Japanese pop psychology (and my own clinical experience), individuals with Type B blood tend to exhibit so-called "Type B personality" patterns. People who exhibit these patterns tend to be easygoing. They're able to take upsets in stride, keep their priorities in perspective, and understand their limitations. They are less driven and perhaps less obsessive than other blood types. These qualities can be extremely helpful to a new mother. You'll be happier and healthier (and so will your baby) if you can maintain a balanced perspective and not try to strive for perfection.

TYPE B POSTPARTUM RECOVERY PROTOCOL
Use this protocol for four weeks:

- General multivitamin, preferably Type B specific
- Phosphatidyl choline. Take 1 gram, 2 capsules daily

- Siberian ginseng. Take 200 mg, 1 capsule, twice daily
- Magnesium. Take 350 mg, 1 capsule, twice daily
- Extra vitamin C, from acerola cherry or rose hip. Take 250 mg, twice daily
- DHA. Take 300 mg, twice daily
- Cordyceps (*Cordyceps sinensi*). Take 500 mg, 1 to 2 capsules, twice daily
- Inositol. Take 500 mg, 1 to 2 capsules, twice daily

Postpartum Exercise Guidelines

If your delivery was routine, you can begin exercising again within a few days. Take it slow. Your sessions should be shorter and less vigorous than normal, with plenty of attention to stretching. If you're able, join an exercise class for new mothers.

Eight Type B Strategies for Getting Back in Shape

1. KNOW YOUR METABOLIC PROFILE

Your body weight alone is not a reliable indicator of your fitness. Your goal is not just to lose pounds but to build muscle and burn calories efficiently. In addition to weight in pounds, it is important to know your metabolic rate (how efficiently you burn calories) and your body mass index (the ratio of muscle to fat).

BASAL METABOLIC RATE. This is the rate at which you burn calories at rest. That is, how many calories you need to sustain basic functions. You can estimate your average basal metabolic rate by multiplying your weight by 10 calories. If you engage in moderate activity (the level recommended in the average Type B exercise plan), multiply that number by 1.6 to estimate the number of calories you burn in a day.

> *Example:*
> 150 pounds × 10 calories = 1,500 (at rest)
> 1,500 × 1.6 = 2,400
> Total calorie expenditure: 2,400

BODY MASS INDEX. This is a measurement of body fat, based on your height and weight. A body mass index above 25 is considered overweight. To calculate your body mass index, multiply your weight by 704.5. Then multiply your height (in inches) by your height (in inches). Divide the first result by the second.

> *Example:*
> An individual who is 5'5" and weighs 140 pounds
> 140 pounds × 704.5 = 98,630
> 65 × 65 = 4,225
> 98,630 ÷ by 4,225 = 23

You can find more information about body mass index by going to the website of the National Heart, Lung, and Blood Institute—www.nhlbi.nih.gov.

2. RESOLVE ANY MEDICAL CONDITIONS

Get a thorough checkup to determine whether you have any metabolic impediments to fitness. In particular, chronic viral infections and autoimmune conditions, such as chronic fatigue syndrome, can impede fitness and slow weight loss.

3. CHOOSE FOODS THAT ARE METABOLICALLY EFFICIENT

SEVEN-DAY SUPER B DIET

- Lean, organic venison or lamb—4 to 6 servings weekly
- Fish rich in omega-3 fatty acids—3 to 4 servings weekly
- Cultured dairy foods—1 to 2 servings daily
- Noncultured dairy foods—4 to 7 servings weekly
- Eggs—2 to 3 eggs weekly
- Olive or flaxseed oil—1 serving daily
- Green vegetables—2 to 3 servings daily
- Other beneficial vegetables—5 to 7 servings weekly
- Fruit—2 to 3 servings daily
- Grains (allowed)—3 to 4 servings weekly

4. REDUCE STRESS

Type Bs who struggle with low metabolism and weight gain have another challenge—the effects of high cortisol. For Type B, being in a condition of stress equals weight gain. That's because the stress hormone cortisol promotes insulin resistance. Obesity itself leads to cortisol resistance; it becomes a dangerously vicious cycle for Type Bs. High cortisol is also associated with leptin, a hormone related to the obesity gene, which increases your appetite.

5. REGULATE YOUR MEALS

Often, how much you eat is less important than when you eat it. Eat the same amount of calories early in the day and most people lose weight; eat them at night and most people gain weight. Skipping breakfast or eating only a small amount of food for breakfast will have detrimental effects on your slow Type B metabolism. Cortisol and thyroid hormones will both be impacted. The same applies to skipping lunch. If you are serious about losing weight, a critical strategy is to eat a well-balanced breakfast, well-balanced lunch, and an adequate dinner—early in the evening. Resist the late-night munchies.

6. ENGAGE IN MODERATE AEROBIC EXERCISE

Stay active by participating in moderate aerobic exercise at least four times a week, for 30 to 45 minutes each session. Choose from among the following exercises:

EXERCISE	DURATION	FREQUENCY
Tennis	45–60 minutes	2–3 × week
Cycling	45–60 minutes	3 × week
Hiking	30–60 minutes	3 × week
Golf (no cart!)	60–90 minutes	2 × week

7. BALANCE AEROBIC EXERCISE WITH MENTALLY CHALLENGING DISCIPLINES

For Type Bs, overall fitness is achieved with a balance of moderate aerobic activity and mentally soothing exercise. At least twice a week, participate in a stress-reducing activity, such as T'ai Chi or Hatha yoga.

8. DON'T RUSH IT

Place your focus on health and fitness rather than weight loss, and don't use any extreme measures, especially while you're breast-feeding. It is not safe or healthy to lose weight rapidly, especially while nursing.

The Type AB Mother

Personal Recovery Guidelines

Since many Type ABs have a tendency to internalize their emotions, the new Type AB mother will benefit enormously from resisting that impulse and talking openly about your feelings and experiences. You may want to join a support group for new mothers, where you can not only work on your own emotions but also enjoy the benefits derived from reaching out to others.

Be aware of your own tendencies, and work to overcome those that will add to your stress. Type ABs are extremely sensitive to criticism, so try to be easy on yourself and stay away from people who are overly judgmental. Being a new mother—especially if this is your first time—is full of ups and downs. No one is perfect. In time you'll adjust to your new role.

TYPE AB POSTPARTUM RECOVERY PROTOCOL
Use this protocol for four weeks:

- General multivitamin—preferably Type AB specific
- DHA—300 mg daily
- Vitamin B$_6$ (pyridoxal phosphate)—25 mg, daily
- Pantothenic acid—250 mg, 1 to 2 capsules, twice daily
- Zinc—25 mg, 1 capsule daily
- Extra vitamin C, from acerola cherry or rose hip—250 mg, twice daily
- Chamomile (*Matricaria chamomilla*)—herbal tincture, 25 drops in warm water, two to three times daily
- Holy basil (*Ocinum sanctum*)—leaf extract, 250-mg capsule, twice daily

Postpartum Exercise Guidelines

If your delivery was routine, you can begin exercising again soon after your baby's birth, and I encourage you to do so. Take it easy, though. Your sessions should focus on gentle, calming exercises, with plenty of attention to stretching. If you're able, sign up for a new mothers' exercise class.

Eight Type AB Strategies for Getting Back in Shape

1. KNOW YOUR METABOLIC PROFILE
Your body weight alone is not a reliable indicator of your fitness. Your goal is not just to lose pounds but to build muscle and burn calories efficiently. In addition to weight in pounds, it is important to know your metabolic rate (how efficiently you burn calories) and your body mass index (the ratio of muscle to fat).

BASAL METABOLIC RATE. This is the rate at which you burn calories at rest. That is, how many calories you need to sustain basic functions. You can estimate your average basal metabolic rate by multiplying your weight by 10 calories. If you engage in moderate activity (the level recommended in the average Type AB exercise plan), multiply that number by 1.6 to estimate the number of calories you burn in a day.

Example:
150 pounds × 10 calories = 1,500 (at rest)
1,500 × 1.6 = 2,400
Total calorie expenditure: 2,400

BODY MASS INDEX. This is a measurement of body fat, based on your height and weight. A body mass index above 25 is considered overweight. To calculate your body mass index, multiply your weight by 704.5. Then multiply your height (in inches) by your height (in inches). Divide the first result by the second.

Example:
An individual who is 5′5″ and weighs 140 pounds
140 pounds × 704.5 = 98,630
65 × 65 = 4,225
98,630 ÷ 4,225 = 23

You can find more information about body mass index by going to the website of the National Heart, Lung, and Blood Institute—www.nhlbi.nih.gov.

2. RESOLVE ANY MEDICAL CONDITIONS
Get a thorough checkup to determine whether you have any metabolic impediments to fitness. In particular, make sure that your cardiovascular and digestive systems are all in good working order, so that you can exercise safely and eliminate toxins efficiently.

3. CHOOSE FOODS THAT ARE METABOLICALLY EFFICIENT
Let the Type AB diet be your guide. To jump-start your program, adhere to the following plan.

SEVEN-DAY SUPER AB DIET
- Soy foods (tofu, tempeh, soy milk, etc.)—1 to 2 servings daily
- Lean, organic turkey—1 to 2 servings weekly
- Fish rich in omega-3 fatty acids—5 to 7 servings weekly
- Cultured dairy foods—4 to 5 servings weekly
- Eggs—2 to 3 eggs weekly
- Olive or flaxseed oil—1 serving daily
- Green vegetables—2 to 3 servings daily
- Other beneficial vegetables—5 to 7 servings weekly
- Fruit—2 to 3 servings daily
- Grains (allowed)—3 to 4 servings weekly

4. EAT ENOUGH FOOD

Don't undereat or skip meals. Use appropriate blood type snacks between meals if you get hungry. Avoid low-calorie diets. Remember, food deprivation is a huge stress. It raises cortisol levels, lowers metabolism, encourages fat storage, and depletes healthy muscle mass.

5. REGULATE YOUR MEALS

Often, how much you eat is less important than when you eat it. Eat the same amount of calories early in the day and most people lose weight; eat them at night and most people gain weight. Skipping breakfast or eating only a small amount of food for breakfast will have detrimental effects on your slow Type AB metabolism. Cortisol and thyroid hormones will both be impacted. The same applies to skipping lunch. If you are serious about losing weight, a critical strategy is to eat a well-balanced breakfast, well-balanced lunch, and an adequate dinner—early in the evening. Resist the late-night munchies.

6. ENGAGE IN MODERATE AEROBIC EXERCISE

Stay active by participating in moderate aerobic exercise at least four times a week, for 35 to 45 minutes each session. At least three times a week, engage in one of the following aerobic activities:

EXERCISE	DURATION	FREQUENCY
Aerobics	45–60 minutes	2–3 × week
Martial arts	30–60 minutes	3 × week
Cycling	45–60 minutes	3 × week
Hiking	30–60 minutes	3 × week
Weight lifting	30 minutes	2 × week

7. BALANCE AEROBIC EXERCISE WITH CALMING EXERCISES

For Type ABs, overall fitness is achieved with a balance of moderate aerobic activity and calming exercises. At least twice a week, participate in a stress-reducing activity, such as T'ai Chi or Hatha yoga.

8. DON'T OBSESS

It can take time to get back into the shape that you enjoyed prior to conception and pregnancy. Don't push yourself. Let the changes happen at their own pace. Place your focus on health and fitness rather than weight loss, and don't use any extreme measures. It is not safe or healthy to lose weight rapidly, especially while you're nursing.

8

A Healthy Start for Baby

YOUR BABY IS AN INDIVIDUAL from the moment of birth. Most parents say they are immediately aware of their child's unique qualities. Martha and I certainly found this to be true with each of our daughters. It's important to keep this in mind as you begin to develop your infant's patterns and schedules.

A key aspect of your baby's individuality is his or her blood type. It may be the same as yours, or different. Although every newborn has a blood type, infants are not born with functioning antibodies to opposing blood types. However, within two weeks of exposure to the outside world, those antibodies are activated and in play.

Breast-feeding Diet Strategies

Many parents get especially anxious about feeding schedules—how often, how much. Allow your baby to develop his or her own patterns. Babies will want to feed between eight and eighteen times every day. Some learn the skill of suckling more quickly than others. Be patient, relax, and let your child find his or her own rhythm.

Now, more than ever, you will be focused on eating right for your baby. If you are wondering whether or not to breast-feed, consider the following benefits for you and your baby.

All Blood Types

BENEFITS OF BREAST-FEEDING FOR YOUR BABY

- The nutrients in breast milk change according to the needs of the baby. For example, if your baby is born prematurely, the nutrient ratio in your milk will increase to aid in accelerating your newborn's neurodevelopment.
- Antibodies are passed through the breast milk, providing a great deal of immunity to your baby during a time when his or her immune system is still developing. This can result in fewer allergies, colds, and ear infections later in the child's life.
- Breast-feeding is particularly protective against some common childhood conditions, including eczema, otitis media, and iron-deficiency anemia.

BENEFITS OF BREAST-FEEDING FOR MOM

- Nursing contracts your uterus, which helps to prevent postpartum bleeding.
- Breast-feeding appears to provide substantial protection against breast cancer and osteoporosis later in life.
- Breast-feeding creates a deep bond between you and your baby.

GENERAL BREAST-FEEDING TIPS

- Type O, Type A, and Type AB should avoid cow's milk and cheese, which can cause infant colic and other digestive disorders. For Type B, cultured dairy foods, such as yogurt and kefir, are preferable to noncultured dairy. (See blood type breast-feeding power foods later in this chapter.)
- Increase your intake of omega-3 fatty acids (DHA) found in fish oils.
- Continue to abstain from alcohol, which can get into your breast milk. Also be aware that caffeine and chocolate often cause colic in babies.
- Stay away from potential toxins. It's especially important to eat organic foods, clear of pesticides and antibiotics. These can get into your milk supply.
- Be aware that extreme and rapid weight loss can lead to toxicity in your milk supply. When you lose excessive amounts of weight, there is a breakdown of fat tissue. If PCBs are stored in this tissue, they could be released into the bloodstream and contaminate your milk supply.
- Avoid broccoli, cabbage, cauliflower, and Brussels sprouts. They may cause colic in some babies.
- Avoid onions and garlic, as well as hot or sweet peppers, as they also affect the quality of the milk supply and may cause your baby to refuse your breast.
- Drink plenty of fluids. Have a glass of water or juice with every feeding.
- Exercise to increase your fitness and the quality of your milk supply. While extreme weight loss can be hazardous, regular exercise promotes overall fitness and a healthy, gradual weight loss.

- Don't undereat or skip meals. You need to eat 300 to 500 calories a day more than normal while you are breast-feeding. About half the extra calories your baby needs will come from your fat stores and the other half from the food you eat. If you cut back on calories, you're shortchanging your baby's nutritional needs.

Advice from the Naturopath Midwife
Cathy Rogers, N.D.

RELIEVING BREAST-FEEDING ANXIETIES

It's normal to be a little anxious when you start breast-feeding for the first time. The most common worries are: Is the baby getting enough milk? Will breast-feeding hurt? Will it feel too sensual? (The action of breast-feeding contracts the uterus.) Some mothers feel anxious about the claim a breast-feeding baby places on their body, fearing they'll never be "themselves" again.

Whatever your anxieties, the best way to alleviate them is to press forward into the breast-feeding process and ride out the adjustment period. You and your baby will adjust. And the payoff is enormous. Now your baby, who lived in your womb, has full access to your touch, smell, and heartbeat. Relax and enjoy the intimacy as your baby bonds with you out in the world.

FOUR HERBS THAT IMPROVE MILK PRODUCTION

Each of these herbs can be made into a tea infusion. Drink as often as needed if you are having problems with milk production.

1. Borage (*Borago officinalis*): infusion of flowers and leaves; drink freely to promote nursing.
2. Hops (*Humulus lupulus*): infusions, promote lactation—especially for women whose milk production is impaired by tension or anxiety.
3. Motherwort (*Leonurus cardiaca*): a general women's herb; promotes milk production.
4. Anise (*Pimpinella anisum*): contains phytosterols that promote lactation. Bruise or crush the whole seeds to make a tea.

GETTING COMFORTABLE WITH BREAST-FEEDING

It's normal to feel some nipple soreness when you start breast-feeding. Give yourself a week or so to get comfortable with the experience. You can alleviate your temporary soreness by trying the following:

- Apply warm black teabags to your nipples between feedings, using a Band-Aid or surgical tape to keep them in place.
- Apply lanolin cream to your nipples after feeding—unless you are allergic to wool. Don't use soap on your nipples for a month or two before giving birth and while you're breast-feeding. It is drying.
- Go braless for periods of time, if you can, to expose your breasts to the air.
- Express a little milk and rub it around your aerola and allow to air-dry.
- Apply vitamin E oil directly to your sore nipple.
- When your baby is done feeding, break the suction by gently placing a finger in your baby's mouth before removing him or her from your breast.
- Try holding your baby in a position that will help him or her grasp the aereola and nipple, not just the nipple itself. This provides better stimulus for milk production.

Advice from the Naturopath Midwife Cathy Rogers, N.D.

TURN OFF THE PHONE AND CONNECT WITH YOUR BABY

When you have a new baby in the house, relatives, friends, and neighbors are eager to pay their respects, meet the baby, and shower you with food, gifts, and advice. You in turn feel obligated to be the perfect host. This is *not* a good use of the postpartum period, which should be devoted to bonding with your baby.

Leave a message on your machine and pin a note on your door, politely discouraging visitors. If a relative or friend plans to come and help, ask her to delay her visit for a week.

Make your time all about connecting. Mom, dad, and baby should snuggle together and get to know each other.

Your privacy is paramount. And it's so important for a mother to learn to trust her own instincts, without feeling pressured to fulfill others' expectations.

If you experience clogged ducts or mastitis, continue nursing on the affected breast. Cessation of nursing can impair milk flow, increase discomfort, and even endanger your milk supply. Nurse frequently, but just enough to empty your breast of milk. To relieve discomfort:

- Gently massage your breast inward toward the nipple to encourage drainage of lymphatic tissue.
- Use a castor oil pack: soak a washcloth in castor oil and apply it to your breast. Cover the cloth with plastic wrap, then hot wet towels, and leave it on for 20 minutes. Wash the oil off with baking soda and water.

WHAT TO DO IF YOU CAN'T BREAST-FEED

There will be some mothers who are unable to nurse their babies for a variety of reasons, or will not be able to produce enough milk to meet their baby's needs. If the issue is related to feeding (latch-on problems, prematurity, etc.) and not to milk production, you can still pump your breast milk to give your baby the benefits. If you need to use a commercial formula, there are many available, including:

1. Dairy-based—SMA, Similac, Enfamil, Follow-Up formula, Good Start, Alimentum
2. Soy-based—Isomil, Nursoy, Prosobee
3. Predigested protein—Nutramigen, Pregestimil

Talk to your pediatrician about the best formula for your baby. Increasingly, the soy formulas are gaining in popularity, since so many infants develop colic and digestive problems from cow's milk.

If you are bottle-feeding, you need not give up the special bonding with your baby. Hold him close as you feed him, establish skin-to-skin contact, and look into his eyes, establishing the connection that is so vital in early life.

EAT RIGHT FOR *YOUR* TYPE, NOT YOUR BABY'S

New mothers always ask me: Should they eat for their own blood type or their baby's blood type when they're breast-feeding? The answer is that you eat what's right for *your* blood type, which constitutes the healthiest formula for your baby. If you and your baby have different blood types, there's no reason to be concerned about your breast milk. Breast milk is, to a degree, immunologically privileged. Human breast milk is inordinately high in the sugar fucose, which is the staple sugar of the O antigen. This is not normally a problem, as the O factor is considered universal. None of the other blood types will react negatively to it.

Type O Mother—Breast-feeding Power Foods

PROTEIN	CALCIUM	IRON	ZINC
• Lean, organic meats, especially beef, beef liver, and venison • Fish and seafood	• Sardines with bone • Canned salmon with bone • Soy milk • Tofu	• Lean, organic meat • Calf's liver, heart, sweetbreads • Dried apricots • Dark green leafy vegetables	• Oysters • Black-eyed peas • Lima beans
VITAMIN B_6	VITAMIN C	VITAMIN D	VITAMIN K
• Chicken • Fish • Bananas • Black-eyed peas	• Strawberries • Grapefruit • Pineapple	• Fortified juice and soy milk • Fatty fish	• Calf's liver • Egg yolks • Green, leafy vegetables

Type A Mother—Breast-feeding Power Foods

PROTEIN	CALCIUM	IRON	ZINC
• Soy foods, fish, organic poultry, beans	• Sardines with bone • Canned salmon with bone • Soy milk • Tofu • Cultured dairy • Seaweed • Spinach	• Molasses • Egg yolks • Dried apricots • Dark green leafy vegetables	• Snails • Black-eyed peas • Adzuki beans
VITAMIN B_6	VITAMIN C	VITAMIN D	VITAMIN K
• Chicken • Fish • Apricots, figs • Black-eyed peas	• Cherries • Grapefruit • Pineapple	• Fortified juice and soy milk • Fatty fish	• Fatty fish • Egg yolks • Green, leafy vegetables

Type B Mother—Breast-feeding Power Foods

PROTEIN	CALCIUM	IRON	ZINC
• Lean, organic meats, especially lamb, mutton, liver, and venison • Fish and seafood	• Cow's milk • Goat's milk • Yogurt • Canned sardines with bone • Seaweed	• Lean, organic meat • Calf's liver, heart, sweetbreads • Dried apricots • Dark green leafy vegetables	• Black-eyed peas • Lima beans
VITAMIN B$_6$	VITAMIN C	VITAMIN D	VITAMIN K
• Turkey • Fish • Bananas • Black-eyed peas	• Strawberries • Watermelon • Pineapple	• Fortified juice and milk • Fatty fish	• Egg yolks • Green, leafy vegetables

Type AB Mother—Breast-feeding Power Foods

PROTEIN	CALCIUM	IRON	ZINC
• Fish and seafood • Soy foods • Cultured dairy • Small amounts of lean, organic venison	• Cow's milk • Soy milk • Tofu • Sardines with bone • Canned salmon with bone	• Lean, organic calf's liver • Dried apricots • Dark green leafy vegetables	• Oysters • Black-eyed peas • Lima beans
VITAMIN B$_6$	VITAMIN C	VITAMIN D	VITAMIN K
• Turkey • Fish • Black-eyed peas	• Strawberries • Grapefruit • Pineapple	• Fortified cow's milk • Fortified juice and soy milk • Fatty fish	• Calf's liver • Egg yolks • Green, leafy vegetables

Starting Solids—All Blood Types

Your breast milk is the best food for your baby. Don't rush the introduction of solid foods. Begin to introduce solids between four and six months, depending on your baby's readiness. Before four months, your baby lacks the digestive enzymes necessary to handle solid foods. Furthermore, the swallowing and tongue reflexes are not yet developed. However, don't delay the introduction of solid foods beyond six months. (See appendix A for recipes.)

When you do begin to introduce strained or pureed foods, go very slowly, beginning with a rice cereal of a semiliquid consistency. If you have a food processor, blender, or grinder, you can make your own strained fruits and vegetables, selected from organic whole foods. Introduce meat last—between nine months and a year. Your baby is already receiving its best protein source from your milk.

Even when you do introduce solids, continue breast-feeding for at least nine months to a year, if possible. Don't be too rigid, though. Infants really do have minds of their own when it comes to eating. Our first daughter, Claudia, was comfortable breast-feeding for a year. Emily, however, was eager to get off the breast after six months and eat like her big sister, a response that is probably more common when there are older children in the house.

Just Say No to Commercial Baby Foods

In spite of the hype, commercial baby foods are not a healthy choice for your child. Most of them include fillers, such as tapioca, rice flour, and modified cornstarch. Many contain sugar, salt, and corn syrup. Look for organic baby foods in your market or health-food stores, or, better still, make your own baby food. It doesn't have to be a big production. Once your baby has been introduced to foods beyond breast milk, you can even puree your own organic food, and your baby can eat what you're eating. There are some helpful recipes for homemade baby food in appendix A.

Safety Rules for Homemade Baby Food

1. Wash your hands thoroughly before you begin preparing food.
2. Wash utensils and cutting board between preparing different foods, and use different cutting boards for raw and cooked foods.
3. Only store prepared foods in the refrigerator or freezer for the recommended times: Refrigerate pureed meats and eggs for one day; refrigerate pureed fruit and vegetables for three days; freeze prepared foods in airtight containers for up to two months.
4. Refrigerate or freeze unused foods immediately.

5. Wash fresh fruits and vegetables thoroughly to remove any chemical residue. Use an organic vegetable wash, available in health-food markets.

Avoid These Foods in the First Year

- Honey is dangerous to children under age one because of the possible contraction of botulism.
- Nuts, raisins, popcorn, raw vegetables, and peanut butter can cause choking.
- Salt, sugar, or strong spices should not be added to homemade baby food.
- Canned vegetables are usually loaded with sodium and additives.
- Highly acidic fruits, such as oranges, tangerines, and pineapples, are not suitable for an immature digestive system.
- Egg whites can cause allergic reactions (yolks are okay).

Your Baby's First Blood Type Diet

Babies are marvelous creatures, full of curiosity about themselves and the vast world that surrounds them. As your infant begins to explore the world of food beyond your breast milk, it's your job to respect his individuality. That means beginning to introduce him to the foods that are right for his blood type. Begin with the basics of the blood type diet. Choose as many highly beneficial foods and juices as you possibly can and make them the centerpiece of your child's diet. There are plenty of wonderful choices for all of the blood types, and they ensure optimum health and vitality for your growing child.

The following chapters provide individual guidelines for your baby's first year, according to blood type.

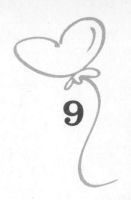

9

The Type O Baby

Type O Baby Health Issues

AS YOUR BABY GROWS, his or her blood type will provide protection against some health conditions and increase susceptibility to others. In particular, watch for:

- A tendency to develop colic or gastric problems.
- A susceptibility to food and environmental allergies.
- Bacterial infections—in particular, those causing digestive distress and ulcerative conditions (such as infection with *H. pylori*).
- Skin rashes, including diaper rash.
- Restlessness, inability to be comforted.

Type O Remedies for Common Conditions

FOOD ALLERGIES

Almost all food allergies your Type O baby experiences will be related to the introduction of wheat or dairy into the diet. Avoid these foods altogether. If you are breast-feeding during the first year, your baby is getting plenty of nutrients. Otherwise, you can substitute soy or rice milk and choose from the allowable grains on your baby's Type O diet (below).

GASTRIC DISTRESS

Type Os have high levels of stomach acid, which can sometimes contribute to acid reflux and gastric distress. I believe digestive discomfort is the most common cause of colic. Prevent gastric distress this way:

- While you are breast-feeding, avoid milk, sugars, coffee, hot and spicy foods, onions, and garlic.
- While you are breast-feeding, drink fennel, lemon, ginger, and chamomile teas. Choose those you prefer and drink 1 cup, two to three times a day.
- Rub a calming mixture of 3 drops of lavender oil and 3 drops of almond oil over your baby's abdomen.

Advice from the Naturopath Midwife Cathy Rogers, N.D.

SOOTHING CHAMOMILE TREATMENTS FOR THE COLICKY BABY

- Make chamomile tea, using 1 tablespoon tea to 1 quart water. Steep 5 to 10 minutes. Cool. Using a teaspoon, dribble the liquid into your baby's mouth.
- Add 3 to 4 drops of chamomile oil to baby's bath.
- Warm 1 tablespoon olive oil and mix with 2 drops of chamomile oil. Gently massage oil over baby's belly.

DIARRHEA

Type O children often experience mild to moderate diarrhea in reaction to eating dairy products. If your baby is eating some solids and drinking liquids, avoid giving him or her fruit juice. Instead, replenish fluids with vegetable or meat broths.

Advice from the Naturopath Midwife Cathy Rogers, N.D.

A GENTLE REMEDY FOR MILD INFANT DIARRHEA

Occasional mild diarrhea is normal. If the diarrhea is severe or continues, see your doctor immediately to rule out a bacterial infection.

To prevent dehydration, try the following with a very small infant. Cook carrots (well washed and peeled) in boiling water for 20 minutes or longer, until the water has become a carrot broth. Cool the broth and dribble a teaspoon into your baby's mouth several times a day.

If your child is eating solids, limit fruit. Too much fruit can stimulate diarrhea. Rice cereal is binding.

EAR INFECTIONS

Although Type O babies are less susceptible to ear infections than others, I've found that any child can contract chronic ear infections if she eats foods that react poorly in her system. My personal feeling is that ear infections can be prevented in Type O children simply by breast-feeding instead of bottle-feeding. Breast-feeding for a period of a year or so allows a child's immune system and digestive tract time to develop. When your child begins to eat solid foods, avoid wheat and dairy.

DIAPER RASH

Type O babies are more susceptible to inflammations and rashes. If your baby has diaper rash, try the following remedies:

- Avoid rubber pants and change your baby's diaper often. Leave the diaper off whenever possible.
- Use cloth diapers and change them often.
- Treat the area with goldenseal (*Hydrastis canadensis*) powder and marigold (*Calendula off.*) cream.

Advice from the Naturopath Midwife Cathy Rogers, N.D.

AN EASY REMEDY FOR DIAPER RASH

At the changing table, mix 1 tablespoon baking soda with 4 ounces spring water and rub on rash, then pat dry. Gently rub area with a small amount of calendula cream.

RESTLESSNESS/HYPERACTIVITY

Research shows that many hyperactive children also suffer from hypersensitivity and allergies. Typically, I find that Type Os with allergies are eating wheat-based foods. Do not give your baby wheat—be it cream of wheat cereal, teething biscuits, or prepared foods with wheat-starch fillers. See the diet below for alternatives.

The Type O Baby Diet

When you begin to introduce solid foods and liquids other than breast milk, follow these guidelines for your Type O baby:

- Limit sugars and artificial sweeteners. This will help your baby avoid infections and strengthen his immune system.
- Avoid any wheat-based foods or wheat-based fillers in seemingly innocuous foods. Wheat flour and wheat gluten are in a wide variety of

foods, so read the ingredient labels before allowing your child to eat an unfamiliar food product.
- Avoid foods made with cow's milk.
- Avoid acidic fruits, such as oranges and kiwi.
- Choose organic foods only.
- Pay attention to the recommended "start date" for different foods (see below).

Type O Beneficial Baby Foods—First Year

NOTE: Most foods in the first year are strained, mashed, or pureed.

CEREALS
Cream of rice—6 months
Kasha—9 to 12 months

VEGETABLES
Beets—12 months
Broccoli—12 months
Carrots—6 months
Collard greens—12 months
Pumpkin—6 months
Spinach—12 months
Squash—6 months
Sweet potato—6 months

FRUITS
Apple—7 to 9 months
Apricot—6 months
Banana—6 months
Blueberries—6 months
Grapes—9 to 12 months
Mango—9 to 12 months
Papaya—12 months
Pear—6 months
Pineapple—12 months
Plum—7 to 9 months
Strawberries—12 months

BEANS/LEGUMES
  Black-eyed peas—9 to 12 months
  Green beans and peas—6 months
  Lima beans—7 to 9 months
  Miso—7 to 9 months
  Soy milk—6 to 9 months
  Tofu—9 to 12 months

GRAINS/RICE/PASTA
  Quinoa pasta—12 months
  Rice—12 months
  Rice cakes—9 to 12 months
  Rice milk—12 months
  Rolled oats—6 to 9 months
  Soba noodles—12 months

MEAT
  Beef—9 to 12 months
  Chicken—9 to 12 months
  Turkey—9 to 12 months

Type O Avoid Baby Foods—First Year

CEREALS
  Cornflakes
  Cream of wheat
  Oatmeal
  Wheat flakes

VEGETABLES
  Corn
  Potato

FRUITS
  Avocado
  Kiwi
  Orange
  Tangerine

BEANS/LEGUMES
  Kidney beans

Lima beans
Navy beans

GRAINS/RICE/PASTA
Semolina pasta
All wheat-based grains

DAIRY
Cheese
Cottage cheese
Cow's milk
Yogurt

MEAT
All pork-based foods

See appendix A for nutritious, delicious recipes for Type O homemade baby food.

10

The Type A Baby

Type A Baby Health Issues

AS YOUR BABY GROWS, his or her blood type will provide protection against some health conditions and increase susceptibility to others. In particular, watch for:

- Overproduction of mucus.
- Throat and respiratory problems.
- Eczema-like skin rashes.
- Increased ear infections.
- Frequent colds and viruses.
- Restlessness and sleep problems.

Type A Remedies for Common Conditions

EAR INFECTIONS/OVERPRODUCTION OF MUCUS
Avoid dairy foods and sugar. In addition to diet, treating Type A children with ear infections almost always involves enhancing their immunity. The simplest way to enhance the immunity of any child is to cut down on his or her intake of sugar. Also note that longer breast-feeding (nine months to one year) is associated with stronger immune system protection.

COLDS AND CONGESTION
The Type A immune system is highly sensitive, and your baby may be more prone to colds and respiratory infections. While you are breast-feeding, keep your

own immune system in healthy shape and take extra precautions with hygiene around the baby.

ECZEMA-LIKE SKIN RASHES

Type A children often have scaly, itchy skin patches on the legs, stomach, and arms. If your child displays these symptoms, it is a sure sign that he or she is consuming too much dairy or that the diet is deficient in essential fatty acids. If you're still breast-feeding, you may want to increase your own intake of fatty acids either by taking a black currant seed oil supplement or by increasing your intake of olive oil. If your child is on solids already, try to wiggle a little of these products into his or her diet. For example, black currant seed oil capsules can be opened and added to fruit purees.

COLIC

I believe digestive discomfort is the most common cause of colic. Prevent gastric distress this way:

- While you are breast-feeding, avoid milk, sugars, coffee, hot and spicy foods, onions, and garlic.
- While you are breast-feeding, drink these teas: fennel, dill, lemon balm, chamomile, and ginger. Choose those you prefer and drink 1 cup, two to three times a day.
- Rub a calming mixture of 3 drops of lavender oil and 3 drops of almond oil over your baby's abdomen.

See box on page 298 for naturopath Cathy Rogers' Soothing Chamomile Treatments for the Colicky Baby.

DIARRHEA

Type A children often experience mild to moderate diarrhea in reaction to eating dairy products. If your baby is eating some solids and drinking liquids, avoid giving him or her fruit juice. Instead, replenish fluids with vegetable or meat broths. Also, see box on page 298 for naturopath Cathy Rogers' Gentle Remedy for Mild Infant Diarrhea.

DIAPER RASH

Any baby can develop diaper rash, but diarrhea and infections can make your Type A baby more vulnerable. To prevent diaper rash:

- Avoid rubber pants and change your baby's diaper often. Leave the diaper off whenever possible.
- Use cloth diapers and change them often.

- Treat the area with goldenseal (*Hydrastis canadensis*) powder and marigold (*Calendula off.*) cream.

See the box on page 299 for naturopath Cathy Rogers' Easy Remedy for Diaper Rash.

RESTLESSNESS/SLEEP PROBLEMS

Type A babies show special sensitivity to their environments, so don't rule out environmental factors if your infant is restless or has trouble sleeping. Keep baby's sleep area away from the noise of the household. Dim the lights, play soft music, or sing softly.

The Type A Baby Diet

When you begin to introduce solid foods and liquids other than breast milk, follow these guidelines for your Type A baby:

- Limit sugars and artificial sweeteners. This will help your baby avoid infections and strengthen his or her immune system.
- When your baby begins to eat more complex solid foods (after nine months), avoid beef and favor soy foods such as tofu over chicken and turkey.
- Avoid noncultured dairy foods. Small amounts of cultured dairy, such as yogurt and kefir, are allowed.
- Choose organic foods only.
- Pay attention to the recommended "start date" for different foods (see below).

Type A Beneficial Baby Foods—First Year

NOTE: Most foods in the first year are strained, mashed, or pureed.

CEREALS
Cream of rice—6 months
Oatmeal—9 to 12 months

VEGETABLES
Beets—12 months
Broccoli—12 months
Carrots—6 months

Collard greens—12 months
Corn—9 to 12 months
Pumpkin—6 months
Spinach—7 to 9 months
Squash—6 months

FRUITS
Apple—7 to 9 months
Apricot—6 months
Avocado—7 to 9 months
Blueberries—6 months
Kiwi—9 to 12 months
Pear—6 months
Plum—7 to 9 months
Strawberries—12 months

BEANS/LEGUMES
Black-eyed peas—9 to 12 months
Green beans and peas—6 months
Lentil beans—9 to 12 months
Miso—9 months
Soy milk—6 to 9 months
Tofu—9 months

GRAINS/RICE/PASTA
Cornbread—12 months
Quinoa pasta—12 months
Rice—12 months
Rice cake—12 months
Rice milk—12 months
Rolled oats—6 to 9 months
Soba noodles—12 months

DAIRY
Goat cheese—9 to 12 months
Goat's milk—9 to 12 months
Yogurt—7 to 9 months

MEAT
Chicken—9 to 12 months
Turkey—9 to 12 months

Type A Avoid Baby Foods—First Year

CEREALS
Cream of wheat
Farina

VEGETABLES
Cabbage
Potato
Sweet potato
Tomato

FRUITS
Banana
Orange
Papaya
Tangerine

BEANS/LEGUMES
Chickpeas
Kidney beans
Lima beans
Navy beans

GRAINS/RICE/PASTA
Wheat bran
Wheat germ

DAIRY
Cheese
Cottage cheese
Cow's milk

MEAT
Beef
Pork and pork-based foods

See appendix A for nutritious, delicious recipes for Type A homemade baby food.

11

The Type B Baby

Type B Baby Health Issues

AS YOUR BABY GROWS, his or her blood type will provide protection against some health conditions and increase susceptibility to others. In particular, you may observe:

- A tendency to develop strep infections.
- A tendency to develop chronic ear infections.
- A tendency to develop respiratory problems, which may become chronic.
- A susceptibility to food allergies.

Type B Remedies for Common Conditions

RESPIRATORY/EAR INFECTIONS

In Type B children, ear infections are usually the result of an underlying infection with a bacteria called *Hemophilus*, to which Type B is unusually susceptible. The dietary fix involves restricting tomatoes, corn, and chicken. The lectins in these foods react with the surface of the digestive tract, causing swelling and mucus secretion, which usually carry over to the ears and throat.

Here's an interesting note for Type B babies who may have asthmatic tendencies. Studies show that babies who are breast-fed at least nine months to one year have fewer incidences of asthma, thanks to the immune system protection of mother's milk.

FOOD ALLERGIES

Type B children are extremely sensitive to foods containing reactive lectins. While you are breast-feeding, the foods you eat can cause allergic reactions in your baby. These reactions can include a rash or cramping, nausea, vomiting, or diarrhea. Other common symptoms are hives, wheezing, sneezing, runny nose, unusual crying, and shortness of breath. In extreme cases, a child may develop a life-threatening condition called anaphylactic shock. Severe symptoms or reactions to any allergen require immediate medical attention.

Foods a mother eats that are the most likely to cause an allergy for a Type B infant are wheat, shellfish, peanuts, corn, buckwheat, and chicken.

DIARRHEA

Type B children will contract diarrhea if they overindulge in wheat products, or in reaction to eating chicken and corn. If the diarrhea is caused by a food-related intolerance or allergy, your child will often exhibit other symptoms, such as dark, puffy circles under the eyes, rash, or wheezy breathing. Also, see box on page 298 for naturopath Cathy Rogers' Gentle Remedy for Mild Infant Diarrhea.

DIAPER RASH

Allergies and diarrhea can be factors in skin inflammation and diaper rash. In particular, food allergies are known to cause eczema. If your infant has diaper rash, see the box on page 299 for naturopath Cathy Rogers' Easy Remedy for Diaper Rash.

RESTLESSNESS/HYPERACTIVITY

Research shows that many hyperactive children also suffer from hypersensitivity and allergies. Typically, I find that Type Bs with allergies are eating foods with reactive lectins, the worst offenders being corn, buckwheat, lentils, peanuts, and tomatoes. See the diet below for the appropriate foods to give your Type B baby when he or she starts eating solids.

The Type B Baby Diet

When you begin to introduce solid foods and liquids other than breast milk, follow these guidelines for your Type B baby:

- Limit sugars and artificial sweeteners. This will help prevent infections and strengthen your baby's immune system.
- When your baby begins to eat more complex solid foods (after nine months), avoid chicken, which causes allergic reactions.
- Gradually introduce dairy foods, starting with cultured dairy such as sugar-free yogurt made from organic milk.

- Choose organic foods only.
- Pay attention to the recommended "start date" for different foods listed below.

Type B Beneficial Baby Foods—First Year

NOTE: Most foods in the first year are strained, mashed, or pureed.

CEREALS
Cream of rice—6 months
Oatmeal—9 months

VEGETABLES
Beets—12 months
Broccoli—12 months
Cabbage—12 months
Carrots—6 months
Potato—9 months
Seaweed—9 to 12 months
Spinach—12 months
Squash—6 months
Sweet potato—6 months

FRUITS
Apple—7 to 9 months
Apricot—6 months
Banana—6 months
Blueberries—6 months
Papaya—12 months
Pear—6 months
Pineapple—12 months
Plum—7 to 9 months
Strawberries—12 months

BEANS/LEGUMES
Green beans and peas—6 months
Kidney beans—9 to 12 months
Lima beans—9 to 12 months
Navy beans—9 to 12 months

GRAINS/RICE/PASTA
Rice—9 to 12 months
Rice cake—9 to 12 months
Rice milk—9 to 12 months
Rolled oats—6 to 9 months
Spelt flour—9 to 12 months

DAIRY
Butter—12 months
Cottage cheese—9 to 12 months
Goat cheese—12 months
Kefir—9 to 12 months
Ricotta—12 months
Yogurt—7 to 9 months

MEAT
Beef—9 to 12 months
Lamb—9 to 12 months
Turkey—9 to 12 months
Venison—12 months

Type B Avoid Baby Foods—First Year

CEREALS
Cream of wheat
Kasha

VEGETABLES
Corn
Pumpkin
Tomato

FRUITS
Avocado
Star fruit (carambola)

BEANS/LEGUMES
Black-eyed peas
Chickpeas
Lentils

Miso
Pinto beans
Soy milk
Tofu

GRAINS/RICE/PASTA
Buckwheat
Cornmeal
Soba noodles
Wheat bran
Wheat germ

DAIRY
American cheese
Ice cream

MEAT
Chicken
Pork and pork-based foods

See appendix A for nutritious, delicious recipes for Type B homemade baby food.

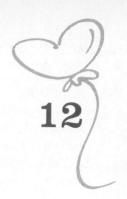

12

The Type AB Baby

Type AB Baby Health Issues

AS YOUR BABY GROWS, his or her blood type will provide protection against some health conditions and increase susceptibility to others. In particular, watch for:

- Overproduction of mucus.
- Throat and respiratory problems.
- Increased risk of ear infections.
- Susceptibility to frequent colds and viruses.

Type AB Remedies for Common Conditions

EAR INFECTIONS/OVERPRODUCTION OF MUCUS

Avoid dairy foods and sugar. In addition to diet, treating Type AB children with ear infections almost always involves enhancing their immunity. The simplest way to enhance the immunity of any child is to cut down on his or her intake of sugar, so keep that in mind when your baby begins eating solid foods. Many commercial brands contain sugar. Also note that longer breast-feeding (nine months to one year) is associated with stronger immune system protection.

COLDS AND CONGESTION

The Type AB immune system is highly sensitive, and your baby may be more prone to colds and respiratory infections. While you are breast-feeding, keep your own immune system in healthy shape and take extra precautions with hygiene around the baby.

DIARRHEA

Type AB children can suffer from digestive upset if they overindulge in wheat products or in reaction to eating chicken and corn. If the diarrhea is caused by a food-related intolerance or allergy, your child will often exhibit other symptoms, such as puffy circles under the eyes, rashes, and wheezy breathing. Also, see box on page 298 for naturopath Cathy Rogers' Gentle Remedy for Mild Infant Diarrhea.

DIAPER RASH

Any baby can develop diaper rash, but diarrhea and infections can make your Type AB baby more vulnerable. To prevent diaper rash:

- Avoid rubber pants and change your baby's diaper often. Leave the diaper off whenever possible.
- Use cloth diapers and change them often.
- Treat the area with goldenseal (*Hydrastis canadensis*) powder and marigold (*Calendula off.*) cream.

See box on page 299 for naturopath Cathy Rogers' Easy Remedy for Diaper Rash.

The Type AB Baby Diet

When you begin to introduce solid foods and liquids other than breast milk, follow these guidelines for your Type AB baby:

- Limit sugars and artificial sweeteners. Type AB babies are highly sensitive to the effects.
- When your baby begins to eat more complex solid foods (after nine months), avoid chicken, which causes allergic reactions.
- Go easy on meats, such as turkey and lamb. Start with very small quantities—two to three spoonfuls.
- Choose organic foods only.
- Pay attention to the recommended "start date" for different foods listed below.

Type AB Beneficial Baby Foods—First Year

NOTE: Most foods in the first year are strained, mashed, or pureed.

CEREALS
Cream of rice—6 months
Oatmeal—9 to 12 months

VEGETABLES

Beets—12 months

Broccoli—12 months

Cabbage—12 months

Carrots—6 months

Collard greens—9 to 12 months

Potato—9 months

Pumpkin—6 months

Spinach—9 to 12 months

Sweet potato—6 months

Tomato—12 months

FRUITS

Apple—7 to 9 months

Apricot—6 months

Blueberries—6 months

Cranberries—7 to 9 months

Grapes—9 to 12 months

Kiwi—9 to 12 months

Pineapple—12 months

Plum—9 to 12 months

Strawberries—9 to 12 months

BEANS/LEGUMES

Green beans and peas—6 months

Lentil beans—7 to 9 months

Miso—7 to 9 months

Pinto beans—9 to 12 months

Soy milk—7 to 9 months

Tofu—9 to 12 months

GRAINS/RICE/PASTA

Rice—9 to 12 months

Rice cake—9 to 12 months

Rice milk—9 to 12 months

Rolled oats—6 to 9 months

Spelt flour—9 to 12 months

DAIRY

Cottage cheese—9 to 12 months

Goat cheese—12 months

Kefir—9 to 12 months
Ricotta—12 months
Yogurt—6 months

MEAT
Lamb—9 to 12 months
Turkey—9 to 12 months
Venison—12 months

Type AB Avoid Baby Foods—First Year

CEREALS
Grits
Kasha

VEGETABLES
Artichoke
Corn
Sprouts

FRUITS
Avocado
Banana
Mango
Orange

BEANS/LEGUMES
Black-eyed peas
Kidney beans
Lima beans

GRAINS/RICE/PASTA
Buckwheat
Cornbread
Soba noodles

DAIRY
American cheese
Cow's milk
Ice cream

MEAT
Beef
Chicken
All pork products

See appendix A for nutritious, delicious recipes for Type AB homemade baby food.

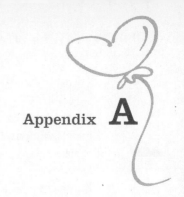

Blood Type Friendly Recipes for Mom and Baby

THE FOLLOWING RECIPES provide a wide variety of healthy choices for every blood type. They are adapted from *Cook Right for Your Type* and from the personal recipes of visitors to Dr. D'Adamo's blood type website. Use them according to the suggested meal plans in your blood type sections or create your own menus. Just be sure to include a variety of nutritious foods that provide the necessary nutrients—and stay with those foods that are approved for your blood type.

There is also a section of homemade baby foods, according to blood type. Try them when your baby starts on solid foods.

See appendix B for more information about cooking for your blood type, including where to find blood type–specific recipes and how to order *Cook Right 4 (for) Your Type*.

For Mom

Contents

Meat and Poultry
Seafood
Tofu and Tempeh
Pasta and Noodles
Legumes and Grains
Soups and Stews

Salads
Vegetables
Sandwiches, Eggs, Tarts, and Frittatas
Breads, Muffins, Pancakes, and Batters
Snacks
Desserts
Beverages
Dressings and Relishes

Meat and Poultry

BRAISED RABBIT

(O, B, AB)

2 tablespoons olive oil
1 rabbit, cut into about 12 pieces
2 tablespoons butter
1 large carrot, diced
4 cloves garlic, chopped
1 stalk celery, finely sliced
1 medium onion, diced
1-plus cup water

Heat the oil in heavy skillet and add the rabbit, cooking over a low flame until nicely browned. Remove the rabbit to a platter, add the butter to the pan. When melted, add the carrot, garlic, celery, and onion, turning until golden. Pushing aside the vegetables, put the rabbit back into skillet, spoon the vegetables over the rabbit pieces and add 1 cup of water, or enough to braise the rabbit. Bring to a boil, cover, reduce heat, and take care that there is always enough braising liquid in the pan. Cook the rabbit 1½ hours, or until very tender. Spoon the "sauce" over rice. *Serves 3 to 4.*

SESAME CHICKEN

(O, A)

8 chicken pieces or breasts on bone
2 tablespoons soy sauce or tamari
3 to 5 cloves garlic, crushed
¼ cup black sesame seeds

Preheat the oven to 375 degrees. Put the chicken pieces in a baking dish. Sprinkle each piece with the soy sauce. Rub with the crushed garlic. Sprinkle the black sesame seeds over the top and bake for 50 minutes or until done. *Serves 4 to 8.*

BROILED LAMB CHOPS

(O, B, AB)

Allow 2 to 3 rib lamb chops per person
1 large clove garlic, peeled and cut
1 tablespoon dry rub of salt and pepper
Olive oil

Preheat the broiler and adjust the shelf so that chops are 3 to 4 inches from the flame. Remove excess fat from the chops and place in a flame-proof pan. Rub the meat with the cut garlic clove, then the salt and pepper rub. Pour a few teaspoons of olive oil over the chops and turn them once to coat both sides with oil. Place under the broiler and cook 5 to 7 minutes, or until the meat is well browned. Turn the chops and replace under broiler, browning other side as well. Serve with mashed sweet potatoes and braised greens.

PEANUT CHICKEN

(A)

2 pounds boneless chicken breasts
2 cups peanuts

Poach, cool, and drain the chicken breasts. Cut into finger-length pieces. Toast the nuts by placing in a skillet and flipping them around for a few minutes. Watch carefully so they do not scorch. When cooled, place them in the bowl of a food processor or into a blender and pulse until the nuts are finely chopped. Dip the chicken in the Chutney-Yogurt Sauce (recipe below), then roll each piece in the nuts. Carefully arrange on a serving tray or on a bed of lettuce.

CHUTNEY-YOGURT SAUCE

1 cup of pineapple chutney
2 tablespoons plain yogurt
2 tablespoons Egg-Free Mayonnaise (page 406)

In the bowl of a food processor, blend all ingredients.

TURKEY BURGERS

(O, A, B, AB)

1 pound ground turkey
2 slices spelt or Ezekiel bread
1 tablespoon olive oil
1 medium onion, finely chopped
2 eggs
Handful of tarragon, chopped
Pinch salt
Olive oil for frying

Place the ground turkey in a large bowl and shred the bread over the meat. In a skillet, heat the oil and sauté the onion over medium heat until soft and golden. Add to the bowl. Beat the eggs in a small bowl, then combine with other ingredients. Add the chopped tarragon and salt. With your hands, mix the ingredients gently but completely, using a very light touch. Do not condense the mixture; keep it fluffy. When the ingredients are well mixed, shape them into 5 or 6 patties and fry in olive oil over medium heat until brown. Turn and continue to fry. Cover the pan after a few minutes, reduce heat, and let them "steam" just a little until the juices run clear. This also keeps them moist.

GRILLED LOIN OF LAMB CHOPS

(O, B, AB)

6 to 8 double loin chops or 1 leg of lamb
Tamari-Mustard Marinade (see below)

Marinate the lamb in the marinade for 1 to 2 hours. Grill over medium heat 15 minutes on each side for chops or 30 to 35 minutes on each side for boneless leg. Let sit for 10 minutes before serving.

TAMARI-MUSTARD MARINADE

¼ cup tamari
2 tablespoons Dijon or dry mustard
1 tablespoon honey
2 cloves garlic, minced
1 lemon, zest and juice
1 tablespoon ground ginger

1 tablespoon ground cumin
2 tablespoons sesame oil

Mix all the ingredients together and store in the refrigerator. *Makes ¾ cup.*

OLD-FASHIONED YANKEE POT ROAST

(O, B)

¼ cup olive oil
3 to 4 pounds chuck roast
4 cups Vegetable Stock (page 354)
¼ cup chopped sweet basil
1 bay leaf
2 large carrots
2 stalks of celery
1 large onion
1 sweet potato
Salt to taste

In a large pot, heat the oil and brown the meat on both sides. Add the stock and herbs, bring to a boil, reduce heat to simmer, and cook 1½ hours. Add all the vegetables and cook another 45 to 60 minutes. Check the meat for tenderness. If it is not easy to pierce with a fork, then continue to cook another 20 to 30 minutes, or until done.

GRILLED CURRIED LEG OF LAMB

(O, B, AB)

2 tablespoons curry powder
2 tablespoons cumin
1 tablespoon iodized salt
2 tablespoons kelp powder
1 tablespoon 5-spice powder
1 leg of lamb, boned and butterflied

Combine spices and dry rub each side of the leg of lamb. Let sit for 1 hour. Grill 20 minutes on each side for medium; 25 minutes for well done. Remove lamb from the grill, and let stand for 10 minutes, then slice thin. *Serves 4.*

GREAT MEATLOAF

(O)

1 egg
1 cup rice, soy, or almond milk, or Chicken Stock (page 353)
3 slices stale bread (Ezekiel, spelt, or rice/almond)
1 pound ground organic beef
1 pound free-range turkey, ground
2 tablespoons kelp powder
1 tablespoon ground cumin
2 tablespoons tamari
3 tablespoons ketchup or tomato paste

In a large bowl, beat the egg and mix in the milk or chicken stock. Cut the stale bread into cubes and soak in egg and milk mixture until soggy. Mix the rest of the ingredients together in the bowl. Preheat the oven to 375 degrees. Form meat into a 10- by 5- by 5-inch loaf and bake on a sheet pan for 1 hour and 15 minutes or until juices run clear. Let sit for 10 minutes before serving.

TURKEY CUTLETS

(O, A, B, AB)

2 tablespoons canola or olive oil
1 package turkey cutlets, about 1 pound
¼ cup spelt breadcrumbs
Squeeze of lemon
Salt to taste

In a large skillet, heat oil until very hot, but not smoking. Roll each cutlet in bread-crumbs and slip into pan, being careful not to overcrowd. Make two batches if necessary. Cook each side for 4 to 5 minutes or until nicely browned. Turn once only. Serve with a squeeze of lemon and add salt to taste. *Serves 2.*

PAN-FRIED LIVER AND ONIONS

(O, B, AB)

2 tablespoons olive oil
1 large onion, peeled and sliced thin
¼ cup butter or light olive oil
1 pound sliced calves or beef liver

½ cup spelt flour (¼ white and ¼ whole is fine)
Salt to taste

In a medium skillet, heat the olive oil and cook onions until wilted and slightly browned. In a large skillet, heat the butter or oil until almost smoking. Dredge the liver in the flour one piece at a time, shake off any excess flour, and cook each side for 4 to 5 minutes. Be careful not to overcrowd the pan. Turn once only. Salt to taste. Serve the liver smothered with onions. *Serves 4 to 5.*

FLANK STEAK

(O, B)

2 tablespoons minced garlic
2 tablespoons ground cumin
1 tablespoon ground chili powder
1 tablespoon ground coriander
½ teaspoon ground cloves
½ teaspoon red pepper flakes
1 tablespoon salt
1 16-ounce flank steak

Mix the garlic and spices together and rub generously over the flank steak. Grill over medium fire for 8 to 10 minutes per side. Allow to rest 5 minutes before slicing. Serve with Fresh Mint Sauce (page 408) as a refreshing contrast to the spicy rub.

ROAST TURKEY

(O, A, B, AB)

1 8- to 10-pound turkey or turkey breast
Summer savory herbs
1 tablespoon salt

There are no secrets to roasting a great turkey. The rule is 15 to 18 minutes per pound or until the juices run clear if poked in the thigh. A 10-pound turkey will roast for a good 2½ hours. Always allow it to rest 10 minutes before carving.

Preheat the oven to 375 degrees. Remove all innards from the turkey, front and back. Save them for future stock by freezing in a Ziploc bag. Rinse the cavity and rub the bird with the herbs and salt. If that is unappealing to you, then stick the herbs in the cavity and sprinkle with salt. Roast until done. If the bird is large, you can make a tent out of foil to cover the breast for the first 1½ hours, but don't forget to remove for the last hour of cooking. Crispy skin is part of the whole appeal. When done, please be careful removing the hot roasting pan from the oven. Make sure the surface on which you place the turkey is close-by.

ROAST CHICKEN WITH GARLIC AND HERBS

(O, A)

1 large chicken
10 cloves garlic, peeled and smashed
2 tablespoons Herbs de Provence
1 teaspoon salt

Preheat the oven to 375 degrees. Prepare the chicken for baking and rub well with a little of the garlic. Put the rest of the cloves in the cavity and season the chicken with the Herbs de Provence and salt. Bake 1 hour and 15 minutes or until the juices run clear. Allow to rest 5 minutes before carving.

Seafood

BROILED SALMON WITH LEMONGRASS

(O, A, B, AB)

3 stalks of lemongrass, bottom ⅓ only, chopped fine
3 tablespoons soy sauce
2 plum tomatoes (Types A and B omit)
2 tablespoons finely chopped fresh coriander
Juice of one lemon
2 scallions, sliced fine
1 small side of salmon, 1 to 1½ pounds, filleted

Combine all the ingredients except the salmon. Put the salmon on a large platter and pour the marinade over the whole fillet. Let marinate for approximately 2 hours. Remove the salmon from the marinade and broil 15 minutes for medium, 20 minutes for well done. *Serves 4.*

PETER'S ESCARGOT

(A, AB)

¼ cup olive oil
2 tablespoons chopped and pressed garlic
12 escargots
Fresh savory flakes

Preheat the broiler. Combine the oil and garlic in a small bowl and mash into a paste using the back of a spoon. Arrange the escargots on a broiling sheet and brush them with the garlic paste. Broil about 10 minutes. When almost done, sprinkle with savory flakes and broil another 30 seconds. *Serves 2.*

BROILED SALMON STEAKS

(O, A, B, AB)

4 salmon steaks
1 tablespoon Garlic-Shallot Mixture (page 409)
2 tablespoons olive oil
1 lemon
3 tablespoons chopped fresh dill
Salt to taste

Rub the steaks with the Garlic-Shallot Mixture, oil, and lemon. Preheat the broiler and cook the fish as close to the heat as possible, about 4 minutes on each side. Test for doneness by poking with a finger and seeing if the flesh separates. Serve hot or cold with chopped fresh dill, salt, and an additional squeeze of lemon.

FRIED MONKFISH

(O, A, B, AB)

1 pound monkfish
1 teaspoon dried basil
Brown rice or spelt flour
1 to 2 eggs

2 tablespoons olive oil
Salt
Pepper

Cut the monkfish into 1-inch cubes. Add the basil to the flour. Beat the eggs well and dip the monkfish in, a few pieces at a time. Heat the olive oil in a heavy skillet. Roll the pieces of monkfish in the seasoned flour. Put the floured fish into the skillet, but do not overcrowd the pan. Fry gently, several minutes on each side, until the batter is crisp and the fish is done. Season with salt and pepper. *Serves 4.*

SHRIMP KABOBS

(O)

1 lemon, juiced
¼ cup olive oil
3 cloves garlic, peeled and smashed
2 tablespoons chopped sweet basil
1 stalk lemongrass, bottom third removed, peeled and chopped
1-inch piece of ginger, peeled and chopped or grated
1 pound large shrimp, cleaned and deveined

Combine the lemon juice, olive oil, garlic, sweet basil, lemongrass, and ginger. Place the shrimp in the marinade and marinate for at least 4 hours. The longer marinating time the better. Overnight is just about right. Skewer 4 to 6 on each rod and grill over high heat 3 minutes on a side. *Serves 2.*

STEAMED WHOLE RED SNAPPER

(O, A, B, AB)

Any small, whole, white-fleshed fish can be steamed by this method. Varying the sauce permits you a wide range of delicious possibilities (see Dressings and Relishes on page 405). Steam the fish on a heavy, restaurant-style platter that fits inside the top of a steaming utensil. A large wok, bamboo steamer, or a traditional fish poacher with removable "tray" modified to lift fish above the boiling water are all suitable. It is worth working out some kind of system for this recipe because not only is it easy, it is a way to serve mixed blood types the same meal using personalized sauces.

1½ pounds red snapper, head and tail on; washed, cleaned, scaled, and trimmed
3 tablespoons olive oil
3 cloves garlic, peeled and smashed
5 scallions, sliced small

2 tablespoons tamari
1 to 2 tablespoons sesame oil (Type O only)
1 scallion, slivered lengthwise
Handful cilantro, chopped

Steam the fish for 10 to 15 minutes. To prepare the sauce, heat the oil in a heavy skillet and gently sauté garlic and scallions until just soft but not brown. Remove from the heat and add the tamari. Type O can add 1 to 2 teaspoons sesame oil. When the fish is done, drain accumulated juices and pour the sauce over fish. Garnish with slivered scallion and cilantro. *Serves 3 to 4.*

Tofu and Tempeh

TOFU VEGETABLE STIR-FRY

(O, A, AB)

2 to 3 tablespoons olive oil
1 medium onion, diced
1 head broccoli, cut into flowers, stems sliced
1 small bunch bok choy, sliced into 1-inch pieces
6 cloves garlic, crushed
½ cup Vegetable Stock (page 354) or water
½ pound snow peas
1 cake tofu, cut into ½-inch cubes
1 tablespoon tamari
¼ teaspoons arrowroot (optional)

In a wok or large heavy skillet, heat the olive oil and add the onion, stirring constantly over a fairly high heat. Add the broccoli, stirring a moment or two. Add the bok choy, stirring again. Add the garlic. Add the vegetable stock or water, let it come to a boil, and then cover, steaming vegetables for several minutes until the broccoli is tender but still crisp. Add the snow peas, and a minute or two later, the tofu. Reduce the heat and let it steam a few more minutes. Add tamari, stir well, and serve. If you prefer a thick sauce, push the vegetables to one side, add 1¼ teaspoons arrowroot, stirring until thickened. Remix the contents of the wok before serving. *Serves 4 to 6.*

RICE STICKS AND TOFU WITH VEGETABLES

(O, A, AB)

These rice sticks are not the same as the rice spaghetti you find in the stores. They are, instead, similar in texture to bean threads.

½ cup tamari sauce
¼ cup water
1 tablespoon sugar
5 cloves garlic, peeled and mashed or put through a press
5 scallions, sliced thin
1-inch piece of ginger, grated
2 tablespoons canola oil
2 containers firm tofu, drained
1 package rice sticks
1 package fresh spinach, washed and stems removed
1 pound green beans or sugar snap peas, washed, stems removed
¼ cup chopped fresh cilantro

Combine the tamari, water, sugar, garlic, scallions, ginger, and canola oil. Marinate the tofu in this mixture for at least 1 hour. Grill or broil the tofu for 5 minutes on each side. Set aside.

Cook the noodles according to the package. Drain and rinse again in warm water; drain well. Remove to a platter. Steam the vegetables and arrange around the noodles. Slice the tofu and place on top of the noodles. Pour the marinade over the tofu and top with chopped cilantro. *Serves 4.*

TEMPEH KABOBS

(O, A, AB)

1 package tempeh, any flavor
6 ounces plum jam
2 ounces pineapple juice (from the pineapple)
3 tablespoons tamari sauce
2 cloves garlic, through a press
2 scallions, sliced thin
1 large onion, quartered and separated into layers, two layers per piece
2 portabello mushrooms, cut into 1- by 1-inch pieces

2 medium zucchini, cut into 1-inch slices
1 pound pineapple chunks, about 1- by 1-inch pieces

Steam the tempeh for 10 to 15 minutes. Meanwhile, combine the plum jam, pineapple juice, tamari, garlic, and scallions to make the barbecue sauce. When the tempeh is cool enough to handle, slice into same-sized pieces as the vegetables. Skewer the pieces by alternating vegetables with the tempeh and pineapple. Brush with the marinade and grill over medium heat until nicely browned. Note: When skewering the zucchini, do so through the green, since the inside is pulpy and will not hold on well. Serve on a bed of rice. *Serves 4.*

BUTTERNUT SQUASH AND TOFU WITH MIXED VEGETABLES

(A, AB)

1 butternut squash
1 package of tofu (fresh and soft is best)
½ cup of soy or other nut milk
¾ cup low-salt soy sauce
½ cup raw honey
2 tablespoons ground mace
2 tablespoons ground ginger
1 teaspoon ground nutmeg
1 pressed clove of garlic
Pinch of curry powder (optional)
1 head of organic broccoli
½ head of organic cauliflower
1 pound green beans
6 large carrots, julienned
Garnish: shelled sunflower or pumpkin seeds, and fresh cilantro

Remove the seeds and clean the center of the squash. Slice lengthwise and steam for 15 to 20 minutes or until soft. Remove the skin and cut into small pieces. Add the squash and all of the other ingredients (except vegetables) to a large mixing bowl. Whip with an electric mixer until smooth and fluffy. Transfer to a large skillet and simmer on low for 15 to 20 minutes. Steam the broccoli, cauliflower, beans, and carrots until al dente, about 10 to 15 minutes, or until brightly colored and moist. To serve, place 2 ladles of mashed squash in the center of a dinner plate. Arrange the steamed veggies around the squash. Garnish with nuts or seeds and cilantro. *Serves 6.*

TOFU AND BLACK BEAN CHILI

(O, A)

¼ cup canola oil
2 onions, diced
1 red pepper, diced (Type O only)
½ tablespoon ground chili
½ tablespoon ground cumin
1 tablespoon ground coriander
1 tablespoon fresh thyme
1 teaspoon ground cloves
2 tablespoons spelt flour
2 cans black beans, drained and rinsed or 1 cup dry black beans,
soaked overnight and cooked al dente
1 to 1½ cups Chicken Stock (page 353)
1 bay leaf
6 cloves garlic, peeled and chopped
1 container firm tofu, drained and cubed

In a large pot heat the oil and add the onions and red pepper. Cook 2 minutes, until wilted, and add all of the spices, stirring and toasting well to release the flavors. Add the flour and cook 2 more minutes. Be sure this spice paste does not burn. Add the black beans, stirring well to coat with the spices. Add 1 cup of the chicken stock, bay leaf, and garlic. Stir to incorporate and simmer for 30 minutes, adding additional chicken stock as needed. For the last 10 minutes of cooking, add the tofu. Since tofu can be rather fragile, handle it gently, using a wooden spoon. Be sure to remove the bay leaf before serving. Serve with rice or homemade tortillas. *Serves 4 to 6.*

KUNG PAO TOFU AND CHICKEN

(A)

½ pound extra-firm tofu, cubed
4 tablespoons water
1 tablespoon cornstarch
4 tablespoons soy sauce
1 teaspoon sugar
Canola oil for frying

2 to 10 dried red chilies (the ones that look like trumpets)
⅓ cup unskinned, unsalted peanuts
½ pound boneless, skinless chicken breast, cubed
1 bunch scallions, cut into 1-inch pieces (white and green parts)

Put a medium pot of salted water to boil; place the tofu into the rapidly boiling salted water. Let the tofu remain in the water until it returns to a boil and the tofu cubes rise to the top. Drain.

To make the sauce: In a bowl, mix the cornstarch into the water. Add the soy sauce and sugar. Stir to blend.

To cook the dish: (A flat-bottomed Teflon skillet works well; keep the flame/temperature on medium high throughout the approximately 10 minutes it takes to complete the dish.) Heat the skillet and pour enough oil to coat the bottom of the skillet. Fry chilies until they begin to turn brown. Remove with a slotted spoon to a plate. In the same oil, fry the peanuts until they begin to turn brown and remove them with a slotted spoon to a plate. In same oil, fry the tofu and chicken cubes. Let the chicken and tofu cook until brown (the tofu will be crispy-looking), turning to brown all sides, about 5 to 7 minutes. Pour the sauce over all. The sauce will thicken very quickly—30 to 60 seconds. (This is not a runny-sauce dish.) Add the green onions and cook together less than a minute. Add the chilies and peanuts back to re-warm for a few seconds and serve! Serve with a nice Asian rice.

TOFU-SESAME FRY

(O, A, AB)

2 tablespoons olive oil
1 cake tofu
1 to 2 tablespoons white sesame seeds
1 to 2 tablespoons black sesame seeds
Salt
Lemon juice
3 to 4 tablespoons tahini
Juice of ½ lemon
1 teaspoon tamari

Heat olive oil in a heavy skillet. Slice tofu about ½ inch thick. Coat half the slices with the white seeds, the other half with the black. Carefully fry in the oil, a few minutes on each side. Serve with a sprinkle of salt and a squeeze of lemon. Or drizzle a little tahini, thinned with a little lemon juice and 1 teaspoon tamari, over the tofu. *Allow 2 slices per serving.*

SILKEN SCRAMBLE

(O, A, AB)

Silken is the softest tofu available and makes a wonderful substitute for eggs, ricotta, or yogurt.

> *1 tablespoon olive oil*
> *1 teaspoon Garlic-Shallot Mixture (page 409)*
> *1 small carrot, grated*
> *1 small zucchini, grated*
> *5 ounces silken tofu*
> *Salt to taste*
> *1 tablespoon chopped fresh basil*

In a small skillet, heat the oil and sauté the Shallot-Garlic Mixture on low for 2 minutes. Add the grated carrot and cook another 3 to 4 minutes. Add the zucchini and silken tofu. With a spoon, chop the silken tofu as it warms and stir the whole mix until warmed. Season with salt and basil.

FRUIT SILKEN SCRAMBLE

(O, A, B, AB)

TYPE O	TYPES A, B, AB
2 tablespoons unsalted butter	*2 tablespoons canola margarine*
1 banana, sliced	*1 peach, sliced with pit removed*
¼ cup blueberries	*¼ cup blueberries*
8 ounces silken tofu, drained	*8 ounces silken tofu, drained*
Salt to taste	*Salt to taste*

In a medium skillet, melt the shortening and gently cook the fruit for 2 to 3 minutes. Bananas are always extra delicious if they can caramelize a bit. Push the fruit to one side and add the silken to the other side, chopping and warming it. The fruit and silken tofu are kept separate so that the silken doesn't get too discolored by the berries. At the final minute of cooking, toss together, add the salt, and serve in a fruit bowl.

GRILLED WILD RICE TEMPEH

(O, A, AB)

1 package wild rice tempeh
3 tablespoons olive oil
2 tablespoons tamari
2 tablespoons Garlic-Shallot Mixture (page 409)
2 tablespoons chopped fresh cilantro
2 tablespoons lemon juice

Remove the tempeh from the wrapper and place in a shallow bowl. In a small bowl, mix together the remaining ingredients and pour this marinade over the tempeh, turning once. Refrigerate for several hours. For a quick marinade, first steam tempeh loaf for 20 minutes then marinate for 1 hour. Grill over medium flame, turning and basting with the marinade until nicely browned, about 15 minutes. Let it sit a few minutes before slicing. Serve with brown rice pilaf and a crisp romaine salad for a delightfully light but satisfying meal. *Serves 4.*

SPICY STIR-FRIED TOFU WITH APRICOTS AND ALMONDS

(O, A, AB)

SPICY CURRY MARINADE

2 tablespoons tamari
1 tablespoon fresh lemon or lime juice (about ½ lemon)
1 tablespoon chopped cilantro
1 tablespoon chopped chives
1 tablespoon sugar
2 teaspoons curry powder
1 teaspoon chili powder
1 teaspoon black sesame seeds
1 cake firm tofu, drained and cut into cubes

Combine the tamari, lemon or lime juice, cilantro, chives, sugar, curry powder, chili powder, and black sesame seeds to make the marinade. Add the tofu cubes, tossing lightly once to cover. Let marinate for 1 hour or longer. Prepare the rest of the stir-fry.

3 tablespoons olive oil
1 small onion or 3 scallions, sliced

3 carrots, sliced on an angle
2 cloves garlic, crushed
½ cup sliced apricots (dried or fresh)
⅓ cup sliced almonds

Heat the oil in a wok or large skillet. Quickly cook the onion or scallions, add the carrots and the garlic, and cook 2 minutes on a medium-high flame, watching that the garlic doesn't burn. Add the tofu all at once and reserve whatever marinade is leftover, adding 2 tablespoons of water. Set the diluted marinade aside. Cook the tofu until heated through, and then add the apricots and almonds. Cook 3 more minutes and serve over white basmati rice with the remainder of the marinade.

TASTY TOFU-PUMPKIN STIR-FRY

(A, AB)

One small sugar pie pumpkin, diced (raw)
One package of honey-sesame flavored (or other flavor) baked tofu, diced
2 tablespoons vegetable oil
½ teaspoon mace
⅛ teaspoon cloves
Salt to taste

Stir-fry the diced pumpkin in oil. When the pumpkin begins to soften, add spices and toss for a minute or two. Add diced tofu and stir-fry until tofu is heated through. Serve the stir-fried mixture over steamed rice (optional) and salt to taste, if desired. *Makes 2 to 3 servings.*

TERIYAKI TOFU STEAK

(A, AB)

1 pound extra-firm tofu, well drained
2 medium cloves garlic, crushed
2 scallions, chopped
2 tablespoons honey
6 tablespoons soy sauce
4 tablespoons olive oil
1 tablespoon arrowroot powder

Cut the tofu into six equal ½-inch strips. Marinate the tofu in garlic, scallions, honey, soy sauce, and 2 tablespoons oil for 20 minutes. Heat the remaining oil in wok over medium heat. Grill the tofu in the wok until brown on both sides. Place on a serving platter. Bring the leftover marinade sauce to a boil and simmer for 2 minutes. Thicken the sauce with the arrowroot. Pour over the tofu before serving. *Makes 5 servings.*

Pasta and Noodles

SOBA NOODLES WITH PUMPKIN AND TOFU

(O, A, AB)

2 tablespoons olive oil
6 cloves garlic, crushed
1 medium leek, thinly sliced (Type O use onion)
Small fresh sugar pumpkin
1 pound tofu
1 pound soba noodles

Put a pot of water on to boil. In a large, heavy skillet, heat the olive oil and add the crushed garlic and the leek, stirring for a few moments. Add ½ cup of water, cover, and let steam over low heat until the leeks are tender, 10 to 15 minutes. Add more water if necessary. Meanwhile, cut the pumpkin in half, remove the seeds (save for toasting later) and carefully peel. Cut into manageable pieces for eating (½ to 1 inch) and add to the skillet with the garlic and leek. Add another ½ cup of water again and steam the pumpkin until tender, about 10 to 15 minutes. The water for the soba should be boiling. Add the noodles and cook according to the package directions. When all the vegetables are done, cut the tofu into ½-inch pieces, add to the skillet, and heat thoroughly. Put the pumpkin mixture on top of the hot soba noodles. *Serves 4 to 6.*

STUFFED SHELLS WITH PESTO

(B, AB)

1 pound shell pasta (either spelt, semolina, or rice flour)
1 pound ricotta cheese
½ pound mozzarella cheese
½ cup Vegetable Stock (page 354)
Pesto (page 409)

Boil the pasta until done, undercooking by a minute or two. In a bowl, combine the ricotta and mozzarella. Put about 1 tablespoon inside each shell, then place shells into a buttered glass baking dish, lining them up in neat little rows. When all the shells are filled, pour in the vegetable stock, cover dish with aluminum foil, and bake in 300-degree oven for about 20 minutes. Remove from oven and serve, spooning pesto over the shells. *Serves 4.*

GREEN LEAFY PASTA

(A, B, AB)

1 pound spinach pasta (Types B and AB) or 1 pound artichoke pasta (Type A)
¼ cup olive oil
2 leeks, washed and sliced
3 cloves garlic, chopped
1 bunch spinach, washed and rinsed
1 bunch Swiss chard, washed and trimmed
Salt and pepper to taste
Romano cheese to taste

Bring a large pot of water to a boil, cook the pasta, drain, and dress with a little oil. Keep covered. Meanwhile, in a large skillet, heat the olive oil and add the leeks, turning to coat with the oil. Over a medium heat, cook them gently for several minutes, until they begin to soften and wilt. Add the garlic and stir, and a few moments later add the spinach and Swiss chard and turn to coat with oil and garlic. The greens will begin to wilt. Steam, uncovered, so the water evaporates for several more minutes, or until the greens are fully cooked. Season to taste and grate on some Romano. *Serves 4.*

LASAGNA WITH PORTABELLO MUSHROOMS AND PESTO

(AB)

One box of lasagna noodles
1 32-ounce container part-skim ricotta
6 to 8 cups organic tomato sauce
4 firm portabello mushrooms, sliced ¼-inch thick
½ pound part-skim mozzarella
½ cup Pesto (page 409)

Preheat oven to 375. In an 8- by 13-inch Pyrex pan, assemble the ingredients as follows:

A quarter of the tomato sauce on the bottom
A third of the uncooked noodles to cover the sauce
Half the ricotta, spread evenly
Paint on half of the pesto
Half of the sliced portabelli over the pesto
Another quarter of the tomato sauce
Another third of the noodles
The rest of the ricotta
The rest of the pesto
The rest of the portabelli
The last of the noodles
The rest of the tomato sauce (about half)
All the mozzarella

Bake 1 hour and 15 minutes, remove from oven, and let sit 15 minutes.

CELLOPHANE NOODLES WITH GRILLED SIRLOIN AND GREEN VEGETABLES

(O, B)

MARINADE

⅔ cup tamari (wheat-free—check the labels)
4 tablespoons water
5 cloves garlic, minced or through a press
1 tablespoon sugar
2 scallions, sliced thin
2 tablespoons canola oil
2 pounds lean sirloin steak

Combine the tamari, water, garlic, sugar, scallions, and canola oil and pour over the steak, turning at least once. Marinate for at least 1 hour, but the longer the better.

NOODLES

Cellophane noodles (made from beans)
2 cloves garlic, peeled
1 pound sugar snap peas or haricot verte or delicate string beans, stems removed
1 package of fresh spinach
¼ cup chopped fresh cilantro

After marinating the steak, grill it to medium rare and set aside. Bring a pot of water to a boil for the noodles and a small pot of water to a boil to steam the vegetables. Soften the noodles in hot water and then boil according to directions, or until tender. Rinse in warm water and drain thoroughly. Pile high on a platter. Quickly steam the garlic and peas for a minute or so, then add the spinach on top, and steam for 2 more minutes. Arrange the vegetables around the noodles. Slice the steak, place it on top of noodles, and drizzle with the dipping sauce. Top with fresh cilantro. *Serves 4.*

TAMARI DIPPING SAUCE

¼ cup tamari
1 lime, juiced
1 tablespoon olive oil
2 tablespoons chopped cilantro
1 tablespoon sugar
2 tablespoons brown rice vinegar
1 clove garlic, mashed

Combine all ingredients.

FETTUCCINE WITH GRILLED LAMB SAUSAGES AND VEGETABLES

(O, B, AB)

2 red peppers
2 yellow peppers
2 portabello mushrooms
2 cloves mashed garlic (for rubbing vegetables and to toss with pasta)
¼ cup olive oil (for brushing on vegetables and on pasta)
1 pound lamb sausages
1 pound rice fettuccine (any shape rice pasta is fine)
Salt to taste
¼ cup chopped fresh basil
Romano cheese

Prepare a medium-hot fire on the grill. Prepare the vegetables by slicing the peppers in half lengthwise and removing the seeds and stems. Remove the stems from the mushrooms so they lay flat on the grill. Rub all vegetables with garlic and brush with oil. Grill sausages until nicely browned and juices run clear. Hold the sausages on the side of the grill to keep them warm while the vegetables are cooking. Meanwhile, cook the fettuccine in plenty of boiling water, drain, and rinse with warm water when done. Pour remaining olive oil over pasta and season with salt. When all the vegetables are nicely grilled (they should be soft but not burned), slice into long strips and toss with garlic. Serve atop the fettuccine along with a couple of sausages. Sprinkle with fresh basil and grated Romano cheese. *Serves 4.*

COLD BUCKWHEAT NOODLES WITH PEANUT SAUCE

(A)

1 package buckwheat (soba) noodles
2 cups shredded Romaine, washed and dried
1 cup grated carrots
2 scallions, sliced thin
chopped fresh cilantro

Cook the noodles in plenty of water, according to the package. Drain and rinse in tepid water. Toss with the Peanut Sauce. On a platter or 2 serving plates spread the lettuce and then the grated carrots and roll the noodles on top. Sprinkle with chopped scallions and fresh cilantro and serve. *Serves 2.*

PEANUT SAUCE

1 clove garlic, peeled and crushed
2 scallions
¼ cup fresh coriander, washed and coarsely chopped
½ cup peanut butter
¼ cup tamari
1 tablespoon brown rice vinegar
½ cup water
Juice of 1 lemon

In a food processor, chop the garlic, scallions, and coriander on high speed. Add peanut butter, tamari, lemon juice, and vinegar. The mixture will be very thick. Slowly add water until the sauce reaches the desired consistency.

PASTA (RICE OR SPELT) WITH RAPPINI (BROCCOLI RABE)

(O, A, B, AB)

1 package pasta of choice
2 tablespoons olive oil
2 tablespoons Garlic-Shallot Mixture (page 409)

1 bunch rappini (broccoli rabe), washed and trimmed
2 to 3 tablespoons water
2 tablespoons tamari
1 tablespoon olive oil
Salt to taste
Freshly shaved Pecorino Romano

Prepare to cook the pasta by bringing a pot to boil with plenty of water. Heat the oil in a large skillet. Add the Garlic-Shallot Mixture and cook for 1 minute. Meanwhile, cut the tip off the stems of the broccoli rabe and discard. Cut the remaining greens into thirds. Put in the skillet and cook a few minutes, turn once, add 2 tablespoons water, cover, and cook another few minutes. "Throw" the pasta in boiling water and stir well, return to a boil, and stir again. The pasta will cook in about 5 to 7 minutes. At this point, check the broccoli rabe. If it is tender, remove from the skillet and dress with 2 tablespoons tamari and set aside. Drain the pasta and toss with a tablespoon of oil and salt to taste. Serve pasta topped with the rabe and freshly shaved Pecorino Romano cheese. *Serves 4.*

QUINOA FLOUR TORTILLAS WITH PUREED PINTO BEANS

(O, A, AB)

TORTILLAS

2½ cups quinoa flour
1½ cups white spelt flour
1 teaspoon salt
1½ teaspoons baking powder
4 tablespoons canola oil (for Type B, substitute olive oil)
1½ cups warm water

In a large mixing bowl, stir together the dry ingredients. Add the oil and water. Using a wooden spoon, mix until the dough forms a ball. Turn onto a well-floured surface and knead for 10 minutes. Cover loosely with plastic wrap and let the dough "rest" for another 10 minutes. Divide the dough into 14 pieces and form into balls. With a rolling pin, flatten each ball into a 10-inch tortilla. In a 12-inch skillet or griddle, cook 1 minute on each side. Be sure not to overcook or the tortillas will become too brittle. As you remove them from the pan, wrap them in a large clean dish towel. *Yields 14 tortillas.*

PUREED PINTO BEANS

2 tablespoons olive oil
1 medium onion, diced
6 cloves garlic, crushed
1 can pinto beans, drained and rinsed, or 1 cup dry beans, soaked and cooked
1 teaspoon powdered cumin
A generous pinch salt
A handful chopped cilantro

In a skillet, heat 2 tablespoons olive oil and add the diced onion. Cook 10 minutes over very low heat, stirring frequently, until onion is golden brown. Add the crushed garlic and sauté a few more minutes. Add the beans and spices and cook another few minutes. Put in the blender and puree until very smooth. You might have to scrape down the blender once or twice. Sprinkle with cilantro and serve. *Serves 4.*

Legumes and Grains

LIMA BEANS WITH GOAT CHEESE AND SCALLIONS

(O, B)

1 package frozen baby limas or 1 cup dried or 2 cups fresh
1 tablespoon olive oil
2 scallions, finely sliced
2 cloves garlic, crushed
2 to 3 tablespoons dressing of choice
4 ounces goat cheese

Prepare the lima beans and place them into a serving bowl. In a skillet, heat the oil and sauté the scallions for a minute or two until fragrant. Add the crushed garlic, turning briefly until it just begins to color. Add scallions and garlic to limas. Pour 2 to 3 tablespoons of the chosen dressing over the beans and toss gently. Crumble the goat cheese over the top. Serve at room temperature. *Serves 4.*

BLACK-EYED PEAS, OKRA, AND LEEK MELANGE

(A)

½ small yellow onion
1 leek

⅛ teaspoon turmeric
½ teaspoon coriander
14 ounces frozen okra
16-ounce can of black-eyed peas
3 tablespoons wheat-free tamari

Chop the onion and sauté for 2 minutes. Add well-washed and sliced leek and dried spices. Immediately add the frozen okra. Cook on high until okra is warm and soft (about 5 minutes). Add the black-eyed peas and tamari and reduce the heat to medium. Cook until the peas are warm—about 5 minutes. Serve over rice.

BLACK-EYED PEAS WITH LEEKS

(O, A)

If you use canned beans, or if you think ahead to soak some the night before, this is an easy, delicious dish, served either hot or cold.

2 cups cooked black-eyed peas
1 tablespoon olive oil
1 small leek, thinly sliced
1 clove garlic, crushed
Pinch of salt
½ handful cilantro

Put the beans in a pot. In a skillet, heat the oil and add the leeks and garlic, turning well to coat with oil. Add ¼ cup of water, cover, and braise the leeks over low heat until soft. Add more water as needed, a tablespoon at a time. When the leeks are tender, add them to the beans and heat thoroughly.

LENTIL SALAD

(A, AB)

Bean salads taste great and are excellent backdrops to other, interesting ingredients. This is a slightly "sweet" salad that is perfect for lunch.

2 cup lentils
8 cups water
½ cup dried cherries
½ cup raisins
½ cup broken walnuts
2 tablespoons olive oil

Juice of ½ lemon
Pinch of salt

Cook the lentils in the water until done, 30 to 40 minutes. Start checking at 30 minutes because lentils can get overcooked very quickly. Drain and let cool. Add the cherries, raisins, and walnuts. Whisk together the olive oil, lemon, and salt and pour over the salad, mixing gently and thoroughly. *Serves 4 to 6.*

PUREED PINTO BEANS WITH GARLIC

(O, A, AB)

2 tablespoons olive oil
1 medium onion, diced
6 cloves garlic, crushed
1 can pinto beans, drained and rinsed, or 1 cup dry beans, soaked and cooked
1 teaspoon powdered cumin (or more to taste)
Generous pinch salt
Handful chopped cilantro (garnish)

In a skillet, heat the olive oil and add the diced onion. Cook 10 minutes over very low heat, stirring frequently, until onion is golden brown. Add the crushed garlic and sauté a few more minutes. Add the beans and spices and cook another few minutes. Put in the blender and puree until very smooth. You might have to scrape down the blender once or twice. Serve sprinkled with the cilantro. *Serves 4.*

FARO PILAF

(O, A, B, AB)

Faro, the Italian word for "spelt," makes a delectable change from rice in this pilaf.

1 cup faro
2 cups water
2 tablespoons olive oil
3 cloves garlic, crushed
2 small zucchini, cut into small dice
Salt
Pecorino Romano cheese

Place the faro and water in saucepan. Bring to a boil, reduce heat, cover, and steam until all the water is absorbed, about 20 minutes. Meanwhile, add olive oil to a heavy skillet. Heat the oil and add the garlic. Sauté a few moments over low-medium heat, then add the zucchini. Continue to stir until coated with oil. Cover and steam until soft, about 5 minutes. Remove from the heat and toss in the bowl with the faro. Add salt to taste. Grate on a little Pecorino Romano if you'd like. *Serves 3 to 4.*

WILD AND BASMATI RICE PILAF

(O, A, AB)

1 cup wild rice, cooked in 2 to 3 cups water
1 cup basmati rice, cooked in 2 cups water
3 green scallions, sliced
¼ cup olive oil
2 teaspoons salt

In two separate saucepans, cook the rices. When done, combine the two rices, toss with the scallions and olive oil, and season with salt.

MILLET TABBOULEH

(O, A, B, AB)

2 cups water (Vegetable Stock makes for more flavor; see page 354)
1 cup millet (lightly toasted in pan, no oil please)
3 scallions, sliced thinly
1 cucumber, peeled and seeded, small dice (Type O omit cucumber)
3 plum tomatoes, chopped (optional)
¼ cup chopped fresh mint
2 tablespoons olive oil
Juice of 1 lemon
Salt to taste

Bring 2 cups of water to a boil, add 1 cup of millet, stir, return to boil, reduce heat, and simmer 15 to 20 minutes, or until all the water is absorbed. Let sit off heat for 10 minutes. Remove to a bowl and let cool slightly. Add the scallions, cucumber, tomatoes, and mint. Mix well and dress with oil and lemon and add salt to taste.

MILLET COUSCOUS

(O, A, B, AB)

1 cup millet (lightly toasted, no oil, please)
2½ cups water or Vegetable Stock (page 354)
2 carrots, small dice
1 small red onion, small dice
¼ cup raisins, plumped (by soaking in hot water)
3 tablespoons sunflower seeds (Types O and A)
or 3 tablespoons chopped walnuts (Types O, B, and AB)
2 tablespoons olive oil
1 lemon, juiced
Salt to taste

Cook the millet (as directed in the Millet Tabbouleh recipe, page 348) and remove to a bowl. Add the carrots, red onion, raisins, and sunflower seeds or walnuts. In a small bowl, whisk together the olive oil and lemon juice and pour over
the millet. Add salt to taste. This is also delicious topped with silken tofu.

SPELTBERRY AND BASMATI RICE PILAF

(O, A, B, AB)

1 cup cooked speltberries
1 cup cooked basmati rice (more rice works well, too)
2 scallions, diced
2 tablespoons olive oil
Salt to taste

Combine all of the ingredients and let sit for at least 15 minutes. Serve at room
temperature.

SPELTBERRY AND RICE SALAD

(O, B, AB)

1 cup cooked speltberries
1 to 2 cups cooked rice (any kind)
1 yellow pepper, diced small

3 tablespoons chopped sweet basil
1 tablespoon finely diced jalapeños (not for Type AB)
3 tablespoons olive oil
Salt to taste

Combine all of the ingredients and serve at room temperature. This salad can be refrigerated for up to four days.

QUINOA RISOTTO

(O, A, B, AB)

2 tablespoons olive oil
1 onion, diced
2 cloves garlic, minced
1 red pepper, very small dice (optional)
3 tablespoons chopped sweet basil
2 cups quinoa
3¼ cups Vegetable Stock (page 354)
Salt and pepper to taste

Heat the oil in a medium saucepan and add the onion and garlic. Cook a few minutes on medium heat, being careful not to burn the garlic. Add the red pepper and chopped sweet basil and continue cooking for another minute. Rinse the quinoa before adding. Cook the quinoa for a few moments, then add the vegetable stock (water will do, although vegetable broth is so sweet and delicious). Bring to a boil, reduce to a simmer, and cover for 15 minutes. Season with salt and pepper. Serve immediately. This recipe is also delicious cold the following day for lunch. *Serves 4.*

BROWN RICE PILAF

(O, A, B, AB)

1 cup brown rice
2 cups water
2 tablespoons olive oil
4 cloves garlic, crushed
1 large carrot, diced
½ cup water

½ handful chopped coriander
Salt to taste

Place rice and 2 cups of water in a saucepan. Bring to a boil, reduce heat, cover, and steam for 40 minutes, or until all water has been absorbed. Always check your rice toward the end of the cooking time. Rices are particular and vary slightly. While the rice is cooking, heat 2 tablespoons of olive oil in a heavy skillet, add the crushed garlic cloves, and sauté gently for a few moments. Add the carrot, stir to coat with oil, and add the water. Reduce the heat, cover the pan, and simmer until the carrot is tender but not soft. Check carefully that there is always sufficient water to braise the carrot, adding water in small quantities if necessary. Add the chopped coriander for the last moments, letting it steam. When the rice is done, place the carrot and rice in a bowl and mix gently. Add salt to taste. *Serves 4.*

WILD RICE SALAD

(O, A, AB)

3 cups water
1 cup wild rice
1 cup walnuts
1 cup dried cherries
1 cup dried diced apricots
¼ cup olive oil
Juice of 1 lemon
1 tablespoon maple syrup
Salt

Boil 3 cups of water and add the wild rice. Cover, reduce heat, and simmer for about 45 minutes, or until tender. Drain any remaining water and reserve for stock. Toss the rice lightly with a fork. Plump unsulphured apricots over boiling water until soft. When the rice has cooled somewhat, add walnuts, cherries, and apricots, mixing well. Whisk together olive oil, lemon juice, maple syrup, and pinch of salt. Pour the dressing over the salad, turning well. Taste for seasoning. *Serves 3 to 4.*

SPELTBERRY SALAD

(O, A, B, AB)

4 cups water
1 cup speltberries

1 cucumber, peeled, if not organic, and diced
2 scallions, sliced finely
¼ cup finely chopped red onion
½ handful cilantro, chopped
2 tablespoons olive oil
Juice of 1 lemon
Salt to taste
Goat cheese

Cook spelt in 4 cups of water until tender and chewy, not mushy, about 45 minutes. Add the cucumber, scallions, red onion, and cilantro and mix gently to combine. Dress with olive oil, juice of 1 lemon, and salt to taste. Sprinkle with goat cheese. *Serves 4.*

BLACK-EYED PEAS AND BARLEY SALAD

(O, A)

1 cup cooked black-eyed peas (if canned, then rinse and drain)
1 cup cooked barley
½ red onion, diced small
2 tablespoons chopped cilantro
1 tablespoon salt
2 tablespoons olive oil
1 tablespoon diced jalapeño pepper (Type O)
½ cup cooked corn (Type A)

Combine all ingredients and let flavors mingle for at least 15 minutes before serving.

BARLEY BLACK BEAN SALAD

(O, A)

½ cup black beans
1 tablespoon ground cumin
½ cup barley
3 ears fresh corn (Type O omit)
Handful chopped coriander
½ red onion, diced small
¼ cup olive oil
Lemon juice to taste

Salt
1 jalapeño, diced (optional)

Soak the black beans overnight in water to cover. Drain. Cover with fresh water, add the cumin, and cook on low heat until tender, about 40 minutes. Drain, rinse well, and reserve in a bowl. Boil the barley until done, about 15 to 20 minutes. Drain, rinse, and add to the black beans in the bowl. Cut the corn off the cob, steam until tender, and add to the beans and barley. Mix in the coriander and red onion and cool all ingredients. Whisk the olive oil, lemon juice, and salt to taste and pour over the salad. Add the jalapeño if desired. Gently turn all ingredients to mix. This can be eaten at room temperature or cool. *Serves 4.*

ADZUKI BEAN AND SWEET BROWN RICE

(O, A)

2 to 3 cups cooked adzuki beans (leftover or canned is fine)
2 cups sweet brown rice
4 cups water or Vegetable Stock (page 354)
2 teaspoons salt
1 small red onion, diced small
¼ cup chopped fresh cilantro (always wash first)
2 ounces crumbled goat cheese

If the beans have not been cooked, then cook according to the directions on package. Adzuki are small and delicate and really do not have to be soaked overnight. If you start soaking them in the morning, they will be ready to cook by that afternoon.

Cook the rice by placing the rice, stock or water, and salt in a 2-quart saucepan. Bring to a boil, turn down the heat, and simmer, covered, until done (about 35 to 40 minutes).

Heat the beans if canned (rinse first) or leftover. In a large serving bowl, combine the hot rice, beans, onion, and cilantro. Mix well, but gently. Top with crumbled cheese and serve. *Serves 4 to 6.*

Soups and Stews

BASIC STOCK (CHICKEN OR TURKEY)

(O, A, B, AB)

It's always a good idea to have stocks on hand. They are basic to any sauce, soup, or stew. Making a stock really takes very little effort, but there are a couple of ways to approach it. The first is to roast a chicken or a turkey and use the carcass and neck and other organs packed inside the bird. The second is to buy necks and backs from the butcher and go from there. Either way is great, and since you are going through the effort, make a lot! Since turkey is neutral for Types O, A, B and highly beneficial for Type AB, it makes sense to make a stock from the ends of a roasted turkey.

The ingredients for stock should always be fresh. A stock can be enriched by the stems of mushrooms and herbs, the peels of onions, tops of leek, or leaves of celery. Everything should be washed well and free of dirt and grit. Do not add the sulfur vegetables like broccoli, cauliflower, or Brussels sprouts. They add a distinct and not so pleasant odor to the basic stock. This is the time to clean out your vegetable bin.

1 medium turkey carcass, picked fairly clean (reserve any meat for soup)
2 onions, roots removed, skins on, cut in quarters
3 large carrots, cut into chunks
3 ribs of celery, washed and cut into large pieces
¼ bunch fresh parsley, washed with stems
Fresh herbs like basil, bay leaf, mint, or tarragon

Fill a very large stock or lobster pot ¾ full with water. Add all the ingredients, bring to a boil, reduce heat, and simmer at least 2½ hours. The stock should reduce by ⅓. Let the stock cool to room temperature and skim any obvious scum or fat from the surface. It's not that critical to get all the fat because once strained and cold the fat will harden on the top. At the same time, the scum sinks to the bottom. Strain out the vegetables. Stock made with bones will gel when cold. The stock can be frozen.

VEGETABLE STOCK

(O, A, B, AB)

1 large yellow onion, cut into quarters
2 carrots, washed, with ends removed, cut into large pieces
2 celery ribs, washed and cut
Parsley stems
Garlic skins
Apple skins and cores
Mushroom stems
Parsnips
Leeks

Bring a large pot of water to a boil and add all the ingredients. Simmer for 40 minutes. Cool and strain. Refrigerate or freeze.

TURKEY SOUP

(O, A, B, AB)

8 cups Turkey Stock (page 353)
2 carrots, diced small
2 ribs of celery, diced small
1 scallion, sliced (optional)
1 cup turkey meat, torn into small pieces
1 cup noodles (rice or spelt)
1 tablespoon salt

In a 3-quart saucepan, bring the stock to a boil. Add the carrots and celery and simmer for about 20 minutes, or until the vegetables are done. Add the scallion, turkey, and noodles and cook another 10 minutes, or until the noodles are done. *Serves 4.*

BEEF STEW WITH GREEN BEANS AND CARROTS

(O, B)

2 pounds stew beef
¼ cup spelt flour (or less, for dredging meat)
3 tablespoons canola oil
1 teaspoon salt
1 tablespoon ground cumin
½ tablespoon ground kelp
1 tablespoon chili powder
Water
3 cups stock (chicken or vegetable) (page 353–354)
1 tablespoon Garlic-Shallot Mixture (page 409)
or 1 medium onion plus 2 cloves garlic (optional)
4 skinny carrots, peeled and sliced on the diagonal
1 pound green beans

Cut away any fat from the meat and cube into bite-sized pieces. Roll lightly in the flour and shake off any excess. Heat oil in a large pot and brown the beef in two batches. After the second one is almost done, replace the first batch of meat and add all the spices. Cook with the meat for 5 minutes on a low heat, then add water to deglaze. Add 2 cups of the stock and stir in the shallot mixture. If you are using onions and garlic add them at this point. Simmer, covered for 1 hour. Check to see if more liquid is needed and add it at this time. Add the carrots and cover again for another 30 minutes. Check for tenderness. Add the green beans and cook another 10 to 15 minutes.

MIXED ROOTS SOUP

(O, A, B, AB)

2 tablespoons olive oil
1 cup diced leeks or onions (Type O use onion)
6 cloves garlic, crushed
1 cup diced turnips and/or 1 cup diced rutabagas
1 cup diced carrots
1 cup diced parsnips
Boiling water to cover, about 8 cups
Salt
Bay leaf
Handful of basil, chopped

Cut all vegetables into a roughly uniform dice so that they will cook at the same rate. Heat olive oil in a heavy Dutch oven. Add your chosen onion and the garlic. Sauté in oil until fragrant, about 5 minutes. Add hardest vegetables first (turnips and rutabagas) and turn in oil a few minutes. Add carrots and parsnips, turning for several minutes more. Pour enough boiling water over all these vegetables to cover by an inch, add the salt and bay leaf, and simmer for 45 minutes, or until vegetables are tender. The soup can be coarsely mashed in its cooking pot using a potato masher or you may put it through a blender, food processor, or food mill. Garnish with chopped basil. *Serves 10 to 12.*

FRESH CHERRIES AND YOGURT SOUP

(A, B, AB)

1 pound pitted cherries
3 tablespoons sugar
3 2-inch slivers of orange peel
2 cloves
3 cups water

2 cups yogurt
Mint leaves

Combine the cherries, sugar, orange peel, and cloves with water in a pot and poach gently until fruit is tender, 8 to 10 minutes. Remove the cloves and coarsely mash the cherries in their own liquid. Let cool. Add yogurt, mix well, and garnish with mint leaves. *Serves 8.*

LENTIL SOUP

(A, AB)

6 cups water
1 package dried lentils
1 carrot, chopped
1 celery stalk, chopped
2 to 3 portabello mushrooms, chopped
½ onion, chopped
1 teaspoon sweet basil
2 Vegex cubes (vegetable boullion)
1 tablespoon salt

In a large pot, combine all the ingredients. Bring to a boil, then turn down heat and simmer for about 1 hour.

CARROT-TOFU SOUP WITH DILL

(O, A, AB)

2 cups water
1½ pounds carrots, peeled and sliced
1 small onion
1 teaspoon salt
2 cups vegetable broth
12 ounces soft silken tofu, regular or low-fat
1 tablespoon dill
1 teaspoon red miso, or to taste
White pepper (optional)

In a medium saucepan, combine carrots, onion, salt, and vegetable broth, and cook over medium heat until carrots are tender, about 15 minutes. Scoop carrots and onion out of cooking water; place in a blender or food processor. Add tofu, dill, miso, white pepper, and a small amount of the cooking water; puree. Return the puree to the cooking water, mix well and serve immediately. *Makes 4 to 6 servings.*

CREAM OF LIMA BEAN SOUP

(B)

1 small onion, minced
1 tablespoon butter
2 cups low-fat milk
2 cups fresh, 1 package frozen, or 1 can thoroughly drained limas
Salt
Parsley, chopped

Sauté the onion in butter until soft. Add the milk and beans, bring to a boil, reduce heat, and simmer gently until beans are tender. If using frozen, 5 to 7 minutes. If fresh, about the same, but please check often, since they will vary in size. When the beans are done, puree the milk and beans in a blender until smooth. Season with salt. Garnish with chopped parsley. *Serves 4 to 6.*

FARMER'S VEGETABLE SOUP

(O, A, B, AB)

3 medium leeks, trimmed and cut into 1-inch cubes (Type O use onion)
1 medium rutabaga, peeled and cut into 1-inch cubes
1 medium turnip, peeled and cut into 1-inch cubes
1 small parsnip, peeled and cut into 1-inch cubes
1 large carrot, peeled and sliced
1 large stalk of celery with leaves, sliced
½ cup or more of baby spinach leaves
2 5-inch sprigs rosemary
Salt to taste
Hot pepper sauce (optional)
6 cups water
6¾ cups beef or chicken broth

In a Dutch oven add the vegetables and seasonings to 6 cups of water, plus 6¾ cups of beef or chicken broth. Bring to a boil. Reduce the heat and simmer with the lid on for about 30 to 45 minutes. Note: Many different root vegetables will work in this versatile, homey soup. Fennel can be used in place of or in addition to one of the other root vegetables, for example. For a heartier meal, add diced cooked chicken or cooked rice to the bottom of the soup bowl before ladling soup into the bowl.

MISO SOUP

(O, A, AB)

1 piece (about 8 to 10 inches) of giant kelp, wiped quickly with a damp cloth
1 quart water
4 tablespoons miso
½ cake tofu, cut into ½-inch cubes
Additional vegetables according to taste (scallions, thinly sliced mushrooms,
delicate celery leaves, tender dandelion leaves, light green spinach leaves)

Place the kelp and water in a large bowl and let it stand overnight. In the morning, discard the kelp and pour the water into a pot. Bring the kelp stock to a simmer. Put the miso in a bowl and add a few tablespoons of kelp stock, stirring to soften and "melt" the miso. Add the softened miso to the pot and bring back to a low simmer. Add the tofu and any vegetables you would like. Let this simmer briefly and serve for breakfast with rice. A quicker, although more temperamental, version of the stock preparation follows: Place kelp and water in a pot and bring just to a boil, slowly. Do not let the water boil or the stock will be ruined. Pull out the kelp and if it is soft, the stock is ready. If the kelp is still too firm, return it to the pot and cook another minute or two. Again, do not boil, adding a few tablespoons of cold water over the brief cooking time. Proceed with the recipe as above.

JERUSALEM ARTICHOKE SOUP

(O, A)

1 pound of Jerusalem artichokes
Juice from ½ lemon
4 tablespoons butter (or oil)
2 leeks, the white part, sliced
2 carrots, sliced
3 cups Chicken Stock (page 353)
Salt
1 pound soft tofu

Scrub the Jerusalem artichokes well. (You don't need to peel them if they are well scrubbed.) Slice and toss with lemon juice. Melt the butter in a pan. Add the leeks, carrots, and Jerusalem artichokes. Cover and cook over low heat 20 to 25 minutes. Add 2½ cups stock and a pinch of salt, cover, and cook 30 minutes longer. Puree with the rest of the stock and the tofu. *Makes 4 servings.*

CUCUMBER-YOGURT SOUP

(A, B, AB)

1 cucumber
1 cup yogurt
Handful fresh dill
Squeeze of lemon
Pinch of salt
Dill leaves (garnish)

If the cucumber skin is not too tough, leave it on. Dice the cucumber and put it in the blender with the yogurt, dill, lemon, and salt. Blend until smooth. Pour into a bowl and garnish with some dill leaves.

ADZUKI BEAN AND PUMPKIN OR WINTER SQUASH SOUP

(A)

2 tablespoons olive oil
2 medium leeks, washed well and sliced thin
6 large cloves garlic, chopped
Water for cooking
1 small sugar pumpkin, 6 to 8 inches across, or
1 acorn or butternut squash, peeled and cut into ½-inch pieces
6 cups water
1 can adzuki beans, drained and rinsed well
Salt to taste

In a heavy pot, heat the oil and add the leeks and garlic. Turn to coat with oil and cook for a few minutes, until they begin to color. Add enough water to cover the vegetables, bring to a boil, reduce heat, and let simmer 10 minutes. Add the squash to the pot and cover vegetables with 6 cups of water. Bring to a boil, reduce heat, and simmer 15 to 20 minutes, depending on squash, or until tender. Add drained beans, let them heat through. Salt to taste. *Serves 4 to 6.*

WHITE BEAN AND WILTED GREENS SOUP

(O, A, B, AB)

1 can cooked cannellini beans, drained and rinsed
1 clove garlic, peeled and end trimmed
1½ to 2 cups stock (according to type and preference); water will also do, but the flavor
of the soup will not be so deep
2 handfuls (about 1 cup) Swiss chard, chopped
½ teaspoon salt
Black pepper to taste (optional)

In a 2-quart saucepan, bring the beans, garlic, and stock to a boil. Reduce the heat and simmer for 10 to 15 minutes. Carefully, with a slotted spoon, scoop out the beans with ½ cup of liquid into the bowl of a food processor or blender. Or, if you own a handheld household processor, leave the soup in the saucepan. (This piece of kitchen equipment is invaluable for just this.) Puree until smooth and return to the saucepan, stirring into the remaining stock. Add the greens, season with salt, and cook another 5 minutes. *Serves 2.*

MUSHROOM BARLEY SOUP WITH SPINACH

(A, B)

1 tablespoon olive oil
1 small onion, diced
½ cup barley (uncooked)
1 tablespoon water
1 portabello mushroom, halved then sliced
8 cups liquid, either Chicken, Turkey, or Vegetable
Stock, according to type (pages 353–354);
water is acceptable but the flavor will be less deep
1 tablespoon salt
1 large handful of fresh spinach, washed; stems cut or chopped

In a 3-quart saucepan, heat the oil and add the onion. Cook 2 minutes or until the onion is wilted. Add the uncooked barley, stirring well into the onion. Cook 2 minutes, and add the water and the mushroom, stirring again. Cover for 2 minutes and reduce heat. When the mushroom is softer, add the 8 cups of stock and bring to a boil. Reduce heat and simmer for 45 to 50 minutes. Season with salt and add the chopped spinach; it will "cook" in a few moments. *Serves 4.*

CUBAN BLACK BEAN SOUP

(O, A)

½ pound dried black beans
1 onion, peeled and chopped
4 cloves garlic, peeled and smashed
4 to 5 cups Chicken or Vegetable Stock (pages 353–354)
¼ cup fresh lemon juice
2 teaspoons salt (or to taste)
Lemon for garnish
Dollop plain yogurt (Type A only)

Wash and soak beans in three times the water to cover and refrigerate overnight or for at least 8 hours. Drain and rinse. Put the beans, onion, and garlic in a pot with the stock. Cook the beans slowly on a low heat until very tender, about 1 hour. Let cool slightly, then transfer to the bowl of a food processor and puree in batches, adding liquid from cooking to desired consistency. Stir in lemon juice and salt. Serve immediately with a slice of lemon on top, or chill and serve with a dollop of plain yogurt (Type A only).

INDIAN LAMB STEW WITH SPINACH

(B, AB)

3 tablespoons olive oil
1 large onion
2 tablespoons ground mustard seed
2 tablespoons ground cumin
2 tablespoons ground coriander
1 tablespoon ground chili powder
4 pound leg of lamb, cubed small
1 cup plain low-fat yogurt
Water as needed
4 to 5 cloves fresh garlic, peeled and diced
2 pounds fresh spinach, cleaned and chopped
Salt to taste

In a large stew pot or sauce pan, heat the oil and add the onion. Cook several minutes until translucent. Add all the spices and cook 2 to 3 minutes to release the flavors. Add the lamb, mixing well into the spices. Bit by bit, stir in the yogurt and add enough water to cover. Stir in the garlic. Simmer the meat, covered, until tender, about 1 hour and 15 minutes. Remove cover and simmer another 15 minutes, if necessary, to reduce liquid. Add the spinach in batches, stirring it down to incorporate it into the stew. It will cook in just a few minutes. Season with salt to taste.

SIMPLE FISH SOUP

(O, A, B, AB)

1 tablespoon olive oil
1 carrot, diced small
2 small ribs of celery, diced small
½ onion, diced small
4 cups water
¾ pound sole or monkfish, cut into 1-inch pieces
Salt and pepper to taste

Heat the olive oil and sauté the carrot, celery, and onion for several minutes. Add water and cook until the vegetables are soft, about 10 minutes. Add the sole or monkfish and cook a few minutes longer, until the fish is thoroughly done. Season with salt and pepper. *Serves 2.*

Salads

COLE SLAW

(B, AB)

White cabbage, ½ head
Red cabbage, ¼ head
Chinese cabbage, ½ head
2 carrots, grated
1 red onion, chopped
¾ to 1 cup Egg-Free Mayonnaise (page 406)
2 tablespoons horseradish
½ teaspoon celery salt
1 teaspoon caraway seeds
¾ to 1 cup broken walnuts

The leaves of all 3 cabbages should be finely shredded to make 6 to 8 cups. Mix in the grated carrots and chopped onion. Combine mayonnaise, horseradish, celery salt, and caraway seeds in a small bowl and pour over the cabbage leaves. Mix well and let marinate in refrigerator several hours to develop flavors. This can be served at room temperature. Add the walnuts just before serving. *Serves 6 to 8.*

MESCLUN SALAD

(A, B, AB)

Walnut Vinaigrette to taste (page 409)
1 pound fresh Mesclun mix
2 medium tomatoes, sliced (Types O, AB)
1 cucumber, sliced (Types A, B, AB)
¼ cup crumbled Roquefort (sheep's milk)
Fresh pepper to taste (optional)

In a large bowl, spoon in 2 tablespoons of the dressing. Add the Mesclun and toss with another tablespoon of the dressing so there is a light coating on the greens. Top with sliced tomato and/or cucumber (according to blood type) and crumbled cheese. Add fresh pepper to taste.

SUPER BROCCOLI SALAD

(O, A, B, AB)

⅓ to ½ cup mayonnaise
2 tablespoons sugar
2 tablespoons lemon juice
2 large heads of broccoli, broken up into small pieces
½ to 1 cup raisins
¼ to ½ cup imitation soy-based bacon bits (Types O, A, AB only)
or diced turkey bacon (all types)
½ cup sunflower seeds or almond slices

Combine the mayonnaise, sugar, and lemon juice, and allow it to sit. Combine the broccoli, raisins, and soy-based bacon bits or diced turkey bacon. Pour the dressing over the broccoli, raisins, and imitation bacon bits or diced turkey bacon. Stir to distribute dressing and let it sit overnight refrigerated. Dressing melds well as it sits. Just before serving, sprinkle with the seeds or nuts and toss. *Serves 4 to 6.*

"WATCHDOG SALAD"

(O)

Romaine lettuce, thinly sliced
¼ cup bean sprouts, rinsed
⅓ cup broken walnuts
1 green onion, sliced
1 grated carrot
⅛ cup raisins
4 to 8 ounces cooked roast beef, sliced thinly and cut into matchstick-sized-pieces

Combine the lettuce, sprouts, walnuts, onion, carrot, raisins, and roast beef in a salad bowl. Serve with Honey Mustard Dressing.

HONEY MUSTARD DRESSING

½ cup mayonnaise
1 tablespoon dry mustard
1 teaspoon minced onion
¼ cup honey
1 tablespoon minced sweet basil

In a small bowl, combine the mayonnaise, mustard, onion, honey, and sweet basil, and mix thoroughly. Pour the honey mustard dressing over the salad.

SPINACH SALAD

(O, A, B, AB)

1 pound fresh spinach
Olive Oil and Lemon Dressing (page 407)
1 hard-boiled egg, chopped
2 slices organic turkey bacon, cooked and chopped
2 tablespoons grated Romano cheese
Salt and pepper to taste

Wash the spinach several times to clean it of dirt and grit and then dry. Place it in a large salad bowl. Heat the dressing and pour it over the spinach. Toss well to mix. If not wilted enough, then put spinach and dressing into a pan for 1 minute only. Top with chopped egg, turkey bacon, and Romano cheese. Add salt and pepper to taste. *Serves 2.*

SARDINE SALAD

(O, A, B, AB)

1 large can water-packed sardines
3 to 4 cloves garlic, minced
2 tablespoons tahini
½ teaspoon salt
1 teaspoon cumin
2 medium onions, diced
1 pepper, diced
1 tablespoon olive oil
Juice of ½ lemon

Drain and mash the sardines well in a mixing bowl. Add the next four ingredients. In a 7-inch skillet, sauté the onions and pepper in oil until lightly browned. Add the sautéed mixture to the sardines while still hot. Mix well and add freshly squeezed lemon juice. Chill and serve.

GREEK SALAD

(A, B, AB)

1 head crisp Romaine, washed, dried, and torn into bite-sized pieces
½ cup Olive Oil and Lemon Dressing (see page 407)
2 cucumbers, washed, peeled, and sliced
1 green pepper, halved, seeded, and cut into bite-sized pieces (Types A and AB omit)
1 small red onion, sliced
¼ cup crumbled feta
Greek olives (for Type AB only)
1 teaspoon dried tarragon

In a large salad bowl, toss the Romaine with the dressing. Top with all other ingredients and mix well. *Serves 2 to 4.*

SALMON WITH WAKAME SEAWEED

(O, A, B, AB)

6-ounce can salmon with bones
1 organic yellow onion

1 cup wakame seaweed from your favorite health-food store
2 tablespoons cold-pressed olive oil
Garlic (as much as you like)
Salt

Drain the salmon. Mince or chop the onion. Soak the wakame seaweed for 5 minutes in a separate bowl, then drain. Combine the salmon, onion, and wakame in a bowl. Add the olive oil and garlic. Salt to taste.

MIXED MUSHROOM SALAD

(O, A, B, AB)

10 to 12 ounces mushrooms:
TYPE A *enoki and oyster*
TYPE O *enoki, oyster, and abalone*
TYPES B *and* **AB** *domestic, oyster, and enoki*
1 cup vinaigrette
2 tablespoons chopped parsley
2 tablespoons chopped chives
2 cups shredded lettuce

Choose a salad dressing appropriate to your blood type. For most, the Vidalia Onion Vinaigrette (page 407) or Olive Oil and Lemon Dressing (page 407) works nicely. Marinate the mushrooms in 1 cup of the dressing for 1 to 2 hours. Mix in the fresh herbs. Using a slotted spoon, serve on a bed of lettuce. *Serves 4.*

CARROT RAISIN SALAD

(O, A, B, AB)

2 pounds carrots, washed, ends removed and grated
½ cup raisins, plumped in hot water
3 tablespoons Egg-Free Mayonnaise (see recipe on page 406)
3 tablespoons chopped cilantro
1 scallion, sliced thin, or 1 tablespoon chopped chives

Place the carrots in a serving bowl. Drain the raisins and add them to the carrots. Mix in the rest of the ingredients and toss well. *Serves 4.*

CAESAR SALAD

(O, A, B, AB)

THE SALAD

1 head Romaine, washed and dried
4 anchovy fillets

Tear or cut the lettuce, place in a bowl, and set aside.

THE DRESSING

1 egg
2 lemons, juiced
1 cup extra virgin olive oil
2-ounce can anchovy filets or 2 tablespoons kelp powder
5 large cloves garlic
¼ cup grated Pecorino Romano cheese

Place the egg, lemon juice, and olive oil in a Cuisinart and blend thoroughly. Remove the mayonnaise to a mixing bowl. Without washing the Cuisinart, blend the anchovy, garlic, and cheese into a paste. If it gets lumpy and needs thinning, add 2 tablespoons of the mayonnaise and blend until smooth. Combine the two mixtures by hand for a truly pungent dressing.

THE CROUTONS

¼ cup olive or canola oil, or ⅛ cup olive oil and ⅛ cup canola oil
2 cloves garlic, through a press
1 tablespoon salt
2 cups cubed stale bread made from spelt flour (or cubed bread of any sort that is
appropriate to your blood type; large cubes make a nice change from the tiny packaged
ones we've all grown up with; it's also a lot easier to make)

Preheat the oven to 425 degrees. Whisk together the oil, garlic, and salt. Coat the cubed bread with the mixture and place on a cookie sheet with plenty of room between them for toasting. Bake 5 minutes, check, turn, and bake another 2 minutes or until golden brown. Remove from the oven and cool thoroughly. Croutons can be stored in an airtight container for several days.

TO ASSEMBLE THE SALAD

Toss the lettuce with the dressing. Top with the croutons and the anchovy fillets. Serve chilled.

GRILLED SWEET POTATO SALAD

(O, B, AB)

2 pounds sweet potatoes, sliced and grilled
3 tablespoons olive oil
1 scallion, sliced
2 tablespoons chopped cilantro
1 lime, juiced
Salt and pepper to taste

Cube the sweet potatoes after they've cooled. Add the remaining ingredients, toss well, and serve. *Serves 4 to 6.*

SMOKED MACKEREL SALAD

(O, A, B, AB)

4 smoked mackerel fillets, skinned and boned
½ red onion, diced small
⅓ to ½ cup Egg-Free Mayonnaise (see recipe, page 406)
Juice of 1 lemon

Chop fillets by hand, add onion, mayonnaise, and lemon juice. Mix well and serve with crackers. *Yields approximately 2 cups.*

GRILLED CHICKEN SALAD

(O, A)

1 to 2 cups cooked diced chicken
3 tablespoons homemade mayonnaise
1 lime, juiced
3 tablespoons chopped cilantro
2 scallions, sliced thin
1 red pepper, either roasted or grilled, with the skin removed, or fresh,
cut in half, then sliced (Type O only)
Salt and pepper to taste

Put the chicken in a bowl. Thin the mayonnaise with the lime juice and add that to the chicken. Add all other ingredients, toss well, and serve with crackers, on Ezekiel bread, or rolled in a Romaine lettuce leaf. *Serves 2 to 4.*

GREEN BEAN SALAD WITH WALNUTS AND GOAT CHEESE

(O, A, B, AB)

2 pounds green beans, stems removed
¼ cup walnut pieces and halves
2 tablespoons crumbled goat cheese
2 tablespoons extra virgin olive oil
Salt and pepper to taste
Squeeze of lemon

Quickly blanch the green beans by throwing them in a pot of boiling water, counting to 30, then removing them to an ice bath. Drain well and dry. On a serving plate, layer the beans, walnuts, and crumbled goat cheese. Dress with good olive oil, salt and pepper to taste, and a squeeze of the lemon. *Serves 4 to 6.*

Vegetables

GLAZED TURNIPS AND ONIONS

(O, A, B, AB)

2 tablespoons butter
2 tablespoons olive oil
1 yellow onion, quartered
4 turnips, cut into wedges
4 cloves garlic, crushed
¾ to 1 cup Chicken Stock (page 353) or water
Salt
½ handful parsley, chopped

In a heavy skillet, melt the butter in the oil over low heat and add the onion, turning to coat with butter and oil. Cook gently over very low heat until soft and very golden, about 20 minutes. Add the turnips and garlic, turning well. Add the chicken stock or water and a little salt, bring to a boil, reduce heat, and cover. Simmer until done, about 20 minutes. Check to be sure there is always liquid in the skillet. Add a few tablespoons at a time as needed. There should be very little liquid left. Take the lid off and allow the last of the liquid to evaporate. Continue to turn the vegetables. Serve at once, spooning the "syrup" over them. Salt to taste and sprinkle with parsley. *Serves 4.*

EGGPLANT CASSEROLE

(B, AB)

1 medium to large eggplant, sliced thin
4 zucchini, sliced
1 8-ounce package of sliced mushrooms
1 cup Pesto (page 409)
1 cup shredded mozzarella cheese
Sea salt to taste

Divide all ingredients in half. Layer everything in a large Pyrex baking dish. Start with half the eggplant slices, then half the zucchini and mushrooms, dot with half the Pesto, and then sprinkle half the mozzarella. Salt to taste. Repeat all layers. Cover with foil and bake at 300 degrees for 1 hour and 20 minutes.

CARROTS AND PARSNIPS WITH GARLIC AND CILANTRO

(O, A, B, AB)

2 carrots
2 parsnips
1 to 2 tablespoons olive oil
6 cloves garlic, peeled and crushed
½ cup water (or more if needed)
½ handful coriander, chopped
Salt to taste

Slice carrots and parsnips on the diagonal. Heat 1 to 2 tablespoons of olive oil in a heavy skillet, add sliced vegetables, and turn in oil a few moments until coated. Add garlic, stirring in oil another moment. Add ½ cup of water, bring to boil, reduce heat, cover, and braise 15 to 20 minutes or until carrots and parsnips are tender. Be sure that there is always a little water in the skillet, adding a tablespoon or two as needed. By the end of the cooking time, the water should be absorbed. For the last moments of cooking, add the chopped coriander and salt.

GRILLED PEPPER MEDLEY

(O, B)

3 peppers, mixed (sweet red, green, yellow, or orange)
1 large onion
2 cloves garlic
2 tablespoons olive oil
Salt

Core and seed the peppers, then slice thinly. Chop the onion into small pieces. Crush the garlic. Heat the oil in a heavy cast-iron skillet over medium heat. Add the garlic and onions and sauté gently until translucent. Add the peppers and toss to coat with the oil. Sauté the mixture until peppers are soft. Add salt to taste. *Serves 4.*

SWEET POTATO PANCAKES

(O, B, AB)

1 large sweet potato or 4 cups grated
¼ red onion, grated
2 tablespoons chopped fresh cilantro
1 large egg
¼ cup spelt flour
¼ teaspoon salt
¼ cup canola oil for cooking

Wash and rinse the sweet potato. Do not peel. Grate over a large plate. Add the onion and cilantro. Mix in the egg and flour until all is well incorporated and add the salt. The mixture will be loose, yet easy to form patties. Heat oil and carefully panfry each pancake 4 to 5 minutes on each side. At this point, the pancakes can be held in the oven for an hour or so. *Yields 6 large dinner-sized pancakes or 15 appetizer-sized pancakes.*

CAULIFLOWER WITH GARLIC AND PARSLEY

(A, B, AB)

1 head cauliflower
2 tablespoons olive oil
4 to 6 cloves garlic, crushed

1 cup water
Salt to taste

Cut the cauliflower into reasonably uniform "flowers." In a large, heavy skillet, heat 2 tablespoons olive oil and add garlic, sautéing until fragrant. Add the flowers and turn in oil. Then add about 1 cup of water, bring to a low boil, and cover. The cauliflower will steam in this. When the cauliflower is soft but firm, the water should be almost absorbed. If not, remove the lid and allow the rest to boil away, leaving a rich garlic/oil residue. With the back of a wooden spoon, roughly mash the cauliflower and add the salt. This is a delicious pasta sauce or serve as a vegetable with pan-roasted chicken. *Serves 4 to 6.*

MASHED PLANTAINS

(B, AB)

2 ripe plantains
Water
2 to 3 tablespoons butter
Salt

Peel the plantains. They do not peel as bananas do; you will probably have to cut them into smaller pieces first. Once peeled, cut them into 1- to 2-inch lengths and place them in a pot. Cover completely with water, bring to a boil, and cook until they are fully tender, 20 to 30 minutes, but check because riper ones will cook more quickly. Do not overcook. Drain, reserving a little of the broth. Mash well and add 2 to 3 tablespoons of butter and salt to taste. You may also use the cooking water, a tablespoon at a time, in the mashing process.

VEGETABLE FRITTERS

(O, A, B, AB)

3 cups grated vegetables (choose vegetables such as peppers, mushrooms,
cauliflower, broccoli, eggplant, and zucchini)
1 tablespoon finely minced onion
2 eggs
Olive oil
Salt to taste

Mix the grated vegetables, used either alone or in combination, with the onion and eggs. In a large, heavy skillet, heat the olive oil. Lightly shape a handful of the batter for each fritter and gently drop into the oil, being careful not to splatter yourself. Flatten with a spatula. Let them fry over medium heat until the bottoms begin to color. Carefully turn over and fry several more minutes. Drain on paper towels, sprinkle with salt, and serve.

STEAMED ARTICHOKE

(O, A)

1 stalk of lemongrass, peeled and cut into pieces (large is okay)
1 teaspoon olive oil
4 cloves garlic, peeled and smashed
1 artichoke per person
Squeeze of lemon

Place all ingredients in the steamer. With or without trimming, the stem long or short, the bottoms up or tips down, an artichoke usually takes between 45 and 55 minutes to cook. Keep plenty of water in the bottom of the pan, and the pot mostly covered. Serve with a squeeze of lemon. *Allow one artichoke per person.*

SWISS CHARD WITH SARDINES

(O, A, B, AB)

2 pounds Swiss chard
2 tablespoons olive oil
3 cloves garlic, minced
1 small onion, sliced thin
6 sardines, chopped
1 tomato (Types O and AB only)
Salt to taste

Wash the chard well, slice into 1-inch strips, and quickly steam. Remove them from the pan and set aside. In a large skillet, heat the oil and add the garlic and onion and cook until slightly browned and soft. Add the sardines and tomato (Types O and AB only). Salt to taste. Add the greens and toss lightly. *Serves 4.*

SESAME BROCCOLI

(O, A, B, AB)

1 cup water
1 head of broccoli, cut into bite-sized flowerettes; reserve stems for another purpose
Juice of ½ lemon
1 teaspoon black sesame seeds

Bring the water to a boil (you can use your kettle). Put all the broccoli in a steamer or a large skillet. Make sure there is a top to cover. When the water is boiling, pour evenly over the broccoli, cover, and put heat on high. Cook for only 3 to 4 minutes. Remove to a plate, squeeze the lemon generously, and sprinkle on the seeds. *Serves 4.*

BRAISED COLLARDS

(O, A, B, AB)

3 tablespoons of olive oil
1 large Vidalia onion, peeled and sliced thin
1 bunch of fresh collard greens, washed well and tips of stems removed
(the stems themselves are quite delicious)
2 tablespoons tamari

Heat the oil in a very large skillet or saucepan. Cook the onion for 5 minutes. Meanwhile, slice the collards by rolling them in one large bunch and cutting across the leaves in 1-inch intervals. Add all the collards at once and cover. Turn the heat down and, after 5 minutes, with a pair of tongs, turn the collards so the wilted greens are on top. Add the tamari sauce and cover again. From time to time, over 40 minutes, turn the collards so as to cook them evenly. Unlike other greens, these are much more tasty if they are allowed to cook longer. *Serves 4.*

GRILLED PORTABELLO MUSHROOMS

(O, A, B, AB)

4 large portabello mushrooms, stems removed and saved for soups or stews
4 teaspoons Garlic-Shallot Mixture (page 409)

Salt to taste
Chopped parsley or basil

Brush the mushrooms with plenty of the Garlic-Shallot Mixture. Grill over medium heat for 5 to 8 minutes. Turn over. If making cheeseburgers, place cheese on top. Whether you use cheese or not, grill another 5 to 8 minutes. Season with salt and serve on a bun, or plate together with grilled meats or tempeh. Top with parsley or basil.

Sandwiches, Eggs, Tarts, and Frittata

Sandwiches

Try these sandwich fillings on bread that is right for your type:

Grilled peppers (yellow, red, green, orange), goat cheese	(O, B)
Grilled eggplant, feta	(B, AB)
Sliced tomatoes, fresh mozzarella, and basil	(O, AB)
Braised red peppers and onions with feta	(O, B)
Grilled eggplant, braised shiitake mushrooms, goat cheese	(B)
Almond butter and sliced bananas	(O, B)
Ricotta, chopped walnuts, raisins, honey drizzle	(O, A, B, AB)
Peanut butter, raisins, honey	(A, AB)
Tofu, avocado, Lemon Vinaigrette	(A)
Tofu, sliced tomato, chopped Spanish olives, Lemon Vinaigrette	(AB)
Mashed sardines, minced clove garlic	(O, A, B, AB)
Soft goat cheese and your best preserves	(O, A, B, AB)
Sunflower butter and plum preserves	(O, A)
Sliced lamb with homemade mango (O, B) or peach (AB) chutney	(O, B, AB)
Fresh mozzarella, sautéed zucchini, and garlic	(O, A, B, AB)

GRILLED OR ROASTED PEPPERS ON RYE CRACKERS WITH CHÈVRE

(O, B)

2 red or yellow peppers, grilled or roasted with some olive oil
4 Rye-Krisp crackers
2 ounces crumbled goat cheese

Slice the peppers to the size and shape of the crackers. Crumble goat cheese on top. This makes a great snack or light lunch.

GRILLED GOAT CHEDDAR ON EZEKIEL OR SPELT

(O, A, B, AB)

2 slices Ezekiel or spelt bread
3 to 4 slices goat cheddar
2 tablespoons butter or margarine

Mix all ingredients together and serve on Ezekiel bread or rice crackers.

CURRIED EGG SALAD

(O)

4 eggs, hard-boiled, peeled, and mashed
2 tablespoons mayonnaise
1 tablespoon salt, or to taste
1 teaspoon good curry powder

Mix all ingredients together and serve on Ezekiel bread or rice crackers.

Eggs

ONE-EGG OMELET

(O, A)

1 tablespoon plus 1 teaspoon olive oil
1 small green zucchini, washed and grated
1 large organic egg
1 tablespoon water
2 basil leaves

1 tablespoon grated Romano cheese
Salt and pepper to taste

In a medium frying pan, heat 1 tablespoon of olive oil and quickly cook the zucchini for 2 to 3 minutes, then set aside on plate. Briskly beat the egg, add 1 tablespoon of water, and beat again. The idea is to get the egg as fluffy as possible. Add 1 teaspoon of olive oil to grease the pan and pour in the egg. Let the egg run around the whole bottom of the pan. Since there's only one egg, it's bound to be thin. Quickly add the zucchini, basil, and Romano cheese. With a spatula, lift the edges of the omelet and carefully fold over the filling to make a half moon. "Roll" onto plate. Add salt and pepper to taste.

OTHER FILLINGS

Any leftover vegetables from last night's dinner
Braised collards
Steamed carrots
Freshly grated carrot with crumbled goat cheese and fresh dill
Tomato and basil
Tofu and scallion with hoisin sauce
Wild rice tempeh with basmati
Fresh spinach and feta
Feta cheese and chopped parsley
Mozzarella cheese and broccoli
Zucchini and grated carrots with crumbled goat cheese

Make sure to warm any leftovers before filling the omelet.

Tarts

ARTICHOKE AND VIDALIA ONION TART

(A)

1½ cups white spelt flour
½ cup whole spelt flour
½ teaspoon salt
1 stick unsalted butter, cold, cut into small pieces (Type A substitute
3 tablespoons soy oil margarine)
4 to 5 tablespoons cold water

In a large mixing bowl, combine both flours and the salt. Cut in the cold butter or margarine. Work the flour into the butter using your fingertips. When mix resembles coarse meal, add water 1 tablespoon at a time; it may not take all the water. The dough should be formed into a ball, but not be too wet. Wrap in plastic and chill in the refrigerator for at least 2 hours. At this point, it will last for 5 days.

When ready to use, remove the dough from the refrigerator and let sit for 45 minutes. Slice into two pieces and roll out on a floured board. Roll to ⅛-inch thick, cut in a circle shape, and brush with olive oil. Pierce with fork at intervals over the surface.

Bake on a cookie sheet in a 350-degree oven for 5 to 8 minutes. Let cool. At this point, you can store the baked crust in an airtight container in the refrigerator for a couple of days.

FILLING

1 Vidalia onion, sliced thin
1 tablespoon olive oil
2 cooked artichoke hearts, sliced
2 tablespoons crumbled goat cheese
Salt and pepper to taste

Sauté the onion in the oil until lightly caramelized. Cool. Top the crust with onion, artichoke, and goat cheese. Add salt and pepper to taste.

Frittatas

ZUCCHINI AND MUSHROOM FRITTATA

(O, A, B, AB)

3 tablespoons olive oil
2 shallots or ½ small onion, chopped
2 medium zucchini, cut lengthwise, then on the diagonal
1 portabello mushroom, sliced
5 eggs
1 tablespoon water
¼ cup grated Romano cheese
Salt to taste

Preheat the oven to 350 degrees. In a large, heavy skillet, heat 1 tablespoon of oil and gently cook the shallots. Add the zucchini and sliced mushroom and cook until soft. Meanwhile, beat the eggs with a tablespoon of water. Add the cheese and the vegetables to the egg mixture. Mix well. Add 2 more tablespoons of oil to the skillet. When the oil is hot, add the egg mixture. Cook on low heat until halfway done, then finish in the oven. The frittata will puff up nicely. Salt to taste.

SPINACH FRITTATA

(O, A, B, AB)

5 eggs
1 teaspoon water
1 package spinach, washed, dried, and chopped fine
2 tablespoons olive oil
1 tablespoon Garlic-Shallot Mixture (page 409)
¼ cup grated Pecorino Romano cheese
Salt and pepper to taste

Preheat the broiler. Beat the eggs with a teaspoon of water and add the spinach. In a large skillet, heat the oil and cook the Garlic-Shallot Mixture for 2 minutes. Add the spinach-egg mixture all at once and cook on medium heat until almost done. While the top is still a bit runny, sprinkle with cheese and run under the broiler until done, about 2 minutes. Season with salt and pepper and serve.

Breads, Muffins, Pancakes, and Batters

Breads

Type O can use all spelt flour.

BANANA PLUM BREAD

(O, B)

1 cup spelt flour
¾ cup oat flour
2½ teaspoons baking powder
½ teaspoon salt
5 tablespoons softened butter
⅔ cup sugar
1 to 2 teaspoons lemon rind
1 to 2 eggs, beaten
1 cup mashed banana

3 ripe plums, diced
½ to 1 cup broken walnuts

Preheat oven to 350 degrees. Sift flours, baking powder, and salt. Blend the butter, sugar, and lemon rind until creamy. Beat in the eggs and mashed banana. Add dry ingredients to butter mixture in 3 parts, beating well after each addition. Fold in plums and walnuts. Pour into 2 small, well-buttered loaf pans. Bake about 40 minutes or until a straw comes out clean. Cool.

PUMPKIN-ALMOND BREAD

(O, A, AB)

1 cup white spelt flour
¾ cup ground almonds
½ teaspoon baking powder
1 teaspoon baking soda
½ teaspoon salt
⅛ teaspoon cloves
¼ teaspoon mace
¾ cup sugar
¼ cup butter, at room temperature
2 eggs
1 cup pumpkin
⅓ cup soy milk
½ cup raisins or chopped figs
Butter or oil for pan

Preheat oven to 350 degrees. Prepare a 9- by 13-inch glass pan. In a large bowl, mix thoroughly the flour, ground almonds, baking powder, baking soda, salt, cloves, and mace. In a separate bowl, beat the sugar, butter, and eggs until very light. Add the pumpkin and beat again. Swiftly add the dry ingredients alternately with the soy milk in two additions. Stir in the raisins or figs. Pour into pan and bake about 30 minutes or until a straw comes out clean.

SPELT BREAD
(for Bread Machine)

(O, A, B, AB)

1½ cups water
1½ teaspoons yeast
2 tablespoons soy powder

2 tablespoons canola oil (Type B substitute light olive oil)
2 tablespoons honey
2 tablespoons molasses
1½ teaspoons salt
3⅓ cups whole spelt flour

Measure the ingredients in the baking pan in the order listed. Insert into the baking chamber and close the lid. Select a whole-grain setting, and bake according to the machine. Let cool before slicing. For a lighter loaf, substitute 1 cup white spelt for 1 cup whole-grain spelt.

Muffins

QUINOA ALMOND MUFFINS

(O, A, B, AB)

1 cup quinoa flour
1 cup white spelt flour
⅓ cup Sugar in the Raw
2½ teaspoons baking powder
¼ teaspoon salt
1 egg
1 cup almond milk
½ cup canola oil (Type B use butter)

Preheat oven to 400 degrees and prepare muffin tins using butter, oil, or paper liners. Combine all dry ingredients. Beat egg. Add almond milk and oil. Fold quickly into dry ingredients. Fill tins to almost full. Add water to remaining empty tins and bake 15 to 20 minutes.

BANANA WALNUT BREAD OR MUFFINS

(O, B)

Butter for pans
2 cups white spelt flour
1 teaspoon salt
2 teaspoons baking soda
⅔ cup canola oil (Type B use butter)
1 cup sugar in the raw
1½ cups banana, ripe and cut into chunks (about 2 large bananas)

3 eggs, beaten
½ cup chopped walnuts

Preheat the oven to 350 degrees. Prepare pans: If nonstick, they do not need buttering; otherwise butter and flour the pan(s), or if you're making muffins, you can use paper liners. Mix the flour, baking soda, and oil in one bowl and all the sugar, bananas, and eggs in another. Blend together and add the walnuts for the last few turns with the spoon. Be careful not to overmix the batter. Fill the pans ¾ full, and bake 25 to 30 minutes for muffins and 30 to 35 minutes for breads, or until a cake tester comes out clean. Let cool on a rack. For whole-wheat banana bread, substitute 1 cup whole spelt flour for 1 cup white spelt flour.

BLUEBERRY BUCKWHEAT MUFFINS

(A, AB)

1 cup buckwheat flour
1 cup white spelt flour
2½ teaspoons baking powder
½ teaspoon salt
⅓ cup sugar
2 tablespoons honey
1 cup soy milk
¼ cup canola oil
1 egg, beaten
½ cup blueberries
Oil or margarine for tins

Preheat the oven to 350 degrees. In a large bowl, mix the dry ingredients together. In another bowl, stir together the honey, soy milk, oil, and egg. Lightly combine the dry and wet ingredients. Fold in the blueberries. Grease the muffin tins or use paper liners and fill each muffin cup to the top. Bake for 20 minutes or until a toothpick comes out clean.

CORNBREAD

(A)

¾ cup white spelt flour
¾ cup stone-ground cornmeal
½ cup buckwheat flour
2 tablespoons brown sugar
2½ teaspoons baking powder
Pinch salt
2 eggs

4 tablespoons melted butter
1 cup soy milk

Butter a 9-inch square pan or cast iron skillet and preheat it in a 425-degree oven. Mix together the spelt flour, cornmeal, buckwheat flour, brown sugar, baking powder, and salt. In another bowl, beat the eggs very well and add the melted butter and soy milk. Add the liquid ingredients to the dry, stirring quickly until just thoroughly mixed. Do not overbeat. Pour into the hot pan or skillet and bake for 20 to 25 minutes. Serve hot.

BANANA SPELT BREAD OR MUFFINS

(O)

This recipe can make either 12 large muffins or 3 small loaves.

Butter for pans
2 cups white spelt flour
1 teaspoon salt
2 teaspoons baking soda
⅔ cup canola oil (Type B use butter)
1 cup Sugar in the Raw
1½ cups banana, ripe and cut into chunks (about 2 large bananas)
3 eggs, beaten
½ cup chopped walnuts

Preheat oven to 350 degrees. Prepare pans: If nonstick, they do not need buttering; otherwise butter and flour the pan(s), or if you're making muffins, you can use paper liners. Mix all dry ingredients in one bowl and all wet ingredients in another. Blend together and add walnuts for the last few turns with the spoon. Be careful not to overmix the batter. Fill pans ¾ full, and bake 25 to 30 minutes for muffins and 30 to 35 minutes for breads, or until a cake tester comes out clean. Let cool on rack.

Pancakes and Batters

BARLEY-SPELT PANCAKES

(O, A)

1 cup barley flour
1 cup spelt flour

2 teaspoons baking powder
Pinch salt
2 eggs
1½ cups soy milk
Water as needed
Butter, margarine, or oil for skillet

Combine the two flours, the baking powder, and the salt in a large bowl. In a separate bowl, beat the eggs very well and stir in the soy milk. Pour the liquid into the dry ingredients and stir until blended. The addition of water here depends on whether you prefer thick or thin pancakes. Heat butter, margarine, or oil in a heavy skillet and when hot, ladle in the batter. Cook on low heat until bubbles fully cover the surface of the pancakes. Turn once and cook until beautifully colored. Serve with maple syrup, honey, or your favorite preserve. *Makes 15 to 20 pancakes.*

MILLET-SPELT-SOY PANCAKES

(O, A, AB)

1 cup millet flour
½ cup spelt flour
½ cup soy flour
1 tablespoon baking powder
Pinch salt
2 eggs
1½ cups soy milk
Water as needed
Butter, margarine, or oil for skillet

Combine flours, baking powder, and salt and stir well. In a separate bowl, beat eggs and add soy milk, mixing well. Pour liquid into dry ingredients and blend thoroughly. Melt butter, margarine, or oil in a heavy skillet and when hot ladle in the batter. Cook over low heat until bubbles cover the surface of the pancakes. Flip over and cook until lightly colored on the underside. Serve with maple syrup, honey, or your favorite preserve. *Makes 15 to 20 pancakes.*

AMARANTH PANCAKES

(O, A, AB)

1 cup amaranth flour
1 cup white spelt flour

> *1 teaspoon sugar*
> *½ teaspoon salt*
> *1 teaspoon baking powder*
> *2 eggs, beaten*
> *1 cup ricotta cheese*
> *1 cup filtered water*
> *½ teaspoon almond extract*
> *Butter, margarine, or oil for skillet*

In a medium bowl, mix together both flours, sugar, salt, and baking powder. In another bowl, blend the eggs, ricotta, water, and almond extract. Combine the two mixtures without overmixing. The batter may seem a bit thin, but after sitting 5 minutes it thickens. Melt butter, margarine, or oil in a heavy skillet. Spoon the batter into the skillet and cook until bubbles form on the surface. Turn over, and cook until lightly colored.

BROWN RICE–SPELT PANCAKES

(O, A, B, AB)

> *1 cup brown rice flour*
> *1 cup whole spelt flour*
> *1 teaspoon baking powder*
> *2 eggs*
> *1½ cups rice milk*
> *Butter, margarine, or oil for skillet*

Combine the two flours and the baking powder, mixing well. Beat in the eggs and the rice milk and stir thoroughly. Melt the butter in a hot skillet, ladle in the batter, and flip over when bubbles appear on the surface. Serve with maple syrup. *Makes 15 to 20 pancakes.*

WHEAT-FREE WAFFLE BATTER

(O, A, B, AB)

> *1 cup brown rice flour*
> *1 cup millet flour*
> *1 tablespoon rice bran*
> *½ teaspoon salt*
> *1½ teaspoons corn-free baking powder*
> *1 egg*

1½ cups low-fat soy milk (Type B use 1% cow's milk)
¼ cup canola oil

Mix all the ingredients to the proper consistency. You may need a little more flour or milk. Bake in a waffle iron 3 minutes or according to the directions of your waffle maker. Serve with sugar-free applesauce or banana slices. The batter keeps in the refrigerator for at least a week.

Snacks

TRAIL MIX OR GORP

Combine all ingredients and store in a glass container.

TYPE O
1 cup broken walnuts
½ cup halved filberts
½ cup quartered dried apricots
½ cup dried cherries
½ cup chocolate or carob chips
or
1 cup pumpkin seeds
½ cup sunflower seeds
½ cup chopped dried pears
½ cup chopped dried pineapple

TYPE A
1 cup peanuts
½ cup quartered dried apricots
½ cup raisins
or
1 cup pumpkin seeds
½ cup sunflower seeds
½ cup broken walnuts
1 cup chopped dried pineapple

TYPE B
1 cup chopped Brazil nuts
½ cup sliced dried bananas

½ cup quartered dried apricots
or
1 cup halved macadamia nuts
1 cup chopped dried pineapple
1 cup dried cranberries

TYPE AB
1½ cups peanuts
1 cup walnuts
½ cup raisins
½ cup quartered dried apricots
or
½ cup cashews
½ cup pignoli
½ cup dried cranberries

RAISIN PEANUT BALLS

(A, AB)

1 cup shelled peanuts
1 cup seeded raisins
Molasses or honey
Finely chopped peanuts

Put peanuts and raisins into a food processor or grinder and grind. Moisten slightly with molasses or honey to hold together. Make into little balls and roll in finely chopped peanuts.

TAMARI TOASTED SUNFLOWER SEEDS

(O, A)

4 ounces raw shelled sunflower seeds
1 tablespoon tamari sauce
Handful of raisins

In a large skillet, heat seeds until almost popping. Flip around to toast evenly, then add the tamari. Toss only for a few more seconds so they are well coated but the tamari doesn't burn. Mix with raisins for a sweet and savory snack.

TOASTED TAMARI PUMPKIN SEEDS

(O, A, B, AB)

4 ounces raw pumpkin seeds
1 tablespoon tamari sauce

In a large skillet, heat the pumpkin seeds until almost popping. They behave a lot like popcorn. Shake the pan so the bottom seeds don't burn. Toss over a few times and add the tamari. Toss again and let cook a few more seconds. Remove from the pan and cool.

Desserts

WALNUT COOKIES

(O, A, B)

¼ pound butter, room temperature
¼ cup sugar
1 cup walnuts
1 cup spelt flour

Preheat the oven to 350 degrees. Cream the butter and sugar. Finely chop the walnuts with a heavy kitchen knife. Add the nuts and flour to the butter/sugar mixture. Drop teaspoonful-sized mounds on to buttered baking sheets, about 2 inches apart. Bake about 25 minutes, watching carefully that the cookies not get darker than golden. Remove at once from pans and cool on a wire rack. Sprinkle lightly with sugar. *Makes 20 to 30 cookies.*

CARROT RAISIN CAKE

(O, A, AB)

Butter, margarine, or oil for pans
2 cups whole spelt flour
2 teaspoons baking soda
2 teaspoons baking powder
1 teaspoon salt
1⅓ cups canola oil
1½ cups light brown sugar
4 eggs, slightly beaten

3 cups grated carrots
½ cup raisins
1 cup chopped walnuts

Preheat the oven to 325 degrees, and grease and flour two 8-inch round cake pans. Mix together the flour, baking soda, baking powder, and salt. In a separate bowl combine the oil, sugar, eggs, and carrots. Add them to the dry ingredients with a minimum of strokes, then stir in the raisins and walnuts. Do not overmix. Fill the pans almost to the top. Bake 55 minutes, or until a cake tester comes out clean. Let cool and remove from pan.

WILD OR BASMATI RICE PUDDING

(B, AB)

8 eggs
3 cups milk
10 tablespoons sugar
4 tablespoons melted butter
2 teaspoons vanilla
Pinch salt
Grated rind of 1 orange
2 tablespoons orange juice
4 handfuls of raisins
4 cups cooked wild or Basmati rice

Preheat the oven to 325 degrees. Beat the eggs with a whisk until light. Add milk, sugar, melted butter, vanilla, and salt. Beat again until well combined. Add grated orange rind and orange juice. Add raisins to the rice and blend well. Place rice and raisins in a buttered 9- by 13- by 2-inch glass baking dish. Pour in the milk and egg mixture and stir lightly. Bake for 45 minutes or until set. Delicious hot or cold.

CRANBERRY BISCOTTI

(O, A, B, AB)

3 eggs
¼ cup sugar
3 tablespoons butter or margarine, melted and cooled
1 teaspoon vanilla
1 tablespoon pineapple or orange juice

Zest of 1 lemon or orange
1⅔ cups spelt flour
1 teaspoon baking powder
¼ teaspoon salt
¼ teaspoon mace
½ cup chopped fresh cranberries

Preheat the oven to 350 degrees. In a mixer, beat the eggs until foamy, then slowly add the sugar and, on high speed, beat until light. Add butter, vanilla, pineapple or orange juice, and the zest. In a separate bowl, mix the flour, baking powder, salt, and mace. On low speed, add the dry ingredients to the egg mixture and blend well. Stir in the cranberries. The dough will be soft. Divide the dough in half and, on a greased cookie sheet, mold each half into a long thin loaf (about 8 by 3 inches). Bake for 25 minutes. Remove from the oven, and reduce heat to 325 degrees. Let the loaves cool for 10 minutes. Put the loaves on a cutting board and slice on the diagonal into ½-inch pieces. Return the cookies to the baking sheet and toast on one side for 5 minutes, then turn each cookie and toast on the other side for another 10 minutes. Remove from oven when golden brown. Cool completely.

RICE CRISPY CAKES

(O, A, B, AB)

2 tablespoons butter or canola margarine (depending on type)
¼ cup honey, maple syrup, or brown rice syrup
2 tablespoons brown sugar
¼ teaspoon salt
3 cups crispy rice cereal (brown rice is always preferable)

In a 3-quart saucepan, melt the butter or margarine, then add the honey (or other liquid sweetener), sugar, and salt. Add the rice cereal all at once. Stir to incorporate thoroughly. Immediately press into a flat, rectangular plastic or glass container. A 5- by 8-inch dish works well. The cakes should be about 1-inch high by 2-inches square. Unlike the ones made with marshmallows, these must be refrigerated to hold together.

OATMEAL COOKIES

(A, B, AB)

1¼ cups butter (Types A and AB use margarine)
½ cup brown sugar
½ cup raw sugar
1 egg
1 teaspoon vanilla
1½ cups white spelt flour
1 teaspoon baking soda
1 teaspoon salt
3 cups rolled oats
1 tablespoon water (for moistening hands)

In a mixing bowl or with electric beater, cream together the butter (or margarine), the two sugars, the egg, and vanilla. In a separate bowl, mix the dry ingredients. Slowly add the dry ingredients to the wet ingredients and combine well. Chill the dough for at least half an hour. Preheat oven to 375 degrees and grease a couple of cookie sheets. Remove the dough from the refrigerator and scoop out a tablespoon at a time and place on a cookie sheet. Flatten each scoop a bit with the palm of your hand. If the dough is too sticky, moisten your hand with water. Bake at 375 degrees for 15 minutes. Note: Cookies can be made either small or large. If large, bake 2 extra minutes.

PEANUT BUTTER COOKIES

(A, AB)

½ cup butter
½ cup brown sugar
¼ cup white sugar
2 eggs
1¼ cups chunky, unsalted peanut butter
1 teaspoon vanilla
½ teaspoon baking soda
Generous pinch of salt
1 cup spelt flour
½ cup oat flour

Preheat the oven to 350 degrees. Beat the butter until soft, then add the sugars, beating until creamy. Beat in the eggs, peanut butter, vanilla, baking soda, and salt, fully incorporating all the peanut butter. Stir in both flours and mix well.

Roll between your palms into 1-inch balls and place on buttered cookie sheet or unbuttered parchment paper. Flatten to about ¼ inch with the tines of a fork. Bake for about 7 to 10 minutes, or until the cookies are beginning to color. Cool on wire racks. *Makes about 40 cookies.*

RICE PUDDING WITH SOY MILK

(O, A, B, AB)

Butter for baking dish
2 cups Basmati rice, cooked
4 eggs
2 cups soy milk
½ cup sugar
2 tablespoons melted butter
Grated rind of 1 lemon
Juice of ½ lemon
½ cup raisins

Preheat the oven to 350 degrees. Butter a baking dish and add the rice. In a large mixing bowl, beat the eggs with a whisk until frothy. Add the rest of ingredients and mix thoroughly. Pour these ingredients over the rice, combining well with a fork. Bake the pudding until set, about 40 to 50 minutes. *Serves 6 to 8.*

TOFU BANANA PUDDING

(O, B)

1 cake tofu
2 ripe bananas

Place both ingredients in a blender and puree for a few moments. Pour into individual little bowls and chill. *Serves 2 to 4.*

TOFU PUMPKIN PUDDING

(O, A, AB)

1 cake tofu
1 cup canned pumpkin
Honey as needed (start with 1 to 2 tablespoons)

Puree the ingredients in a blender, pour into bowls, and chill.

SAUTÉED PEARS OR APPLES

(O, A, B, AB)

2 pears or apples
2 tablespoons butter (Types A and AB can use soy or canola margarine)

Peel and thinly slice the pears or apples. Melt the butter in a heavy skillet and add the fruit, turning gently to coat with butter. Turn heat very low and cover the pan, stewing the fruit in the butter and whatever water the fruit expresses. If there doesn't seem to be enough liquid, add 1 tablespoon of water at a time. Cook 7 to 10 minutes or until the fruit is soft. There should be a little syrup. Types A and AB can sprinkle the fruit with cinnamon or nutmeg. Type B can sprinkle nutmeg.

SAUTÉED BANANAS

(O, B)

2 ripe bananas
2 tablespoons butter
1 tablespoon lemon juice, optional
1 grated lemon rind

Cut bananas in half, then slice them lengthwise. The bananas should be quartered. Melt the butter in a heavy skillet, lower the heat, and add the bananas, turning carefully in the butter. They will brown and get softer. They will be done in just a few minutes. Sprinkle on the lemon juice and rind and serve. *Serves 2.*

FRESH FIG SALAD

(O, A, B, AB)

Fresh figs
Goat cheese

Slice figs lengthwise. Fan out on a plate and top with bits of broken goat cheese.

RICOTTA ORANGE CREAM

(B)

1 cup ricotta
1 tablespoon orange blossom water
1 grated orange rind

Whip ingredients in blender and refrigerate.

CITRUS SALAD

(O, A, B, AB)

Grapefruit, orange, and tangerine make sparkling salads either on their own or mixed together for interesting combinations. Serve topped with a little of the Ricotta Orange Cream (Type B) or any other dressing of your type. One grapefruit, two oranges, and two tangerines. *Serves 4.*

Grapefruit (O, A, B, AB)
Orange (B)
Tangerine (B, AB)
Whole mint leaves

Peel and section fruits over the serving bowl in order to catch the juices. Cut grapefruit wedges into halves or thirds and halve the orange and tangerine wedges. Toss to mix well (if using more than one fruit) and pour dressing over the top of the fruits. Garnish with some small, whole mint leaves.

TROPICAL SALAD

(O, A, B, AB)

Combine these lovely, fragrant fruits according to your taste and type. A generous squeeze of lemon or lime keeps the colors intact and is dressing enough for many people. If you prefer, swirl Ricotta Orange Cream (see recipe above) over the top of each portion for a richer version.

Papaya (O, B, AB)
Mango (O, B)
Kiwi (O, A, B, AB)
Pineapple (O, A, B, AB)
Carambola (O, A)
Banana (O, B)

Guava (O, A, B)
Juice of 1 lemon
Juice of 1 lime

Peel, seed, and cut the papaya and mango, so that they are of uniform size. Peel the kiwi and either cut into slices or wedges. Cut the pineapple into small chunks. Slice the carambola so that each piece is a little star. Slice the banana. Peel and slice the guava. This salad can be layered in a glass bowl, each individual fruit in its own layer, or very gently turned to mix the fruits. Sprinkle each layer with lemon or lime juice or pour the squeezed juice over the salad before turning.

POACHED FRUIT

(O, A, B, AB)

1 cup water
¾ cup sugar
1 lemon, juiced, rind peeled and cut into strips
3 cloves
Apples
Pears
Peaches
Plums
Apricots
Grapes
Nectarines
Cherries
Handful torn mint leaves

Make a poaching syrup: Bring to a boil the water, sugar, lemon juice, strips of lemon rind, and cloves. Prepare the fruits: If you prefer, you do not have to peel them. In general, just remove all seeds and pits, slice larger fruits, and halve the smaller ones like apricots and plums. If you have a cherry pitter, leave the cherries whole; if not, halve them, too. Leave the grapes whole. Add any combination of fruits to the boiling syrup, allowing one large and several smaller fruits per person. Poach, uncovered, for about 10 to 15 minutes. Lift the fruit carefully from the syrup with a slotted spoon and place it in a serving bowl. Reduce the syrup another 8 to 10 minutes, remove the cloves, and pour over the fruits. Cool in the refrigerator. Sprinkle with mint leaves if desired.

BAKED APPLES

(O, A, B, AB)

4 Rome apples
½ cup chopped walnuts
½ cup mixed dried figs and apricots
½ lemon, juiced
Grated rind of ½ lemon
2 tablespoons maple syrup
Pat of butter
1 cup boiling water

Core the apples, being careful not to pierce the bottoms. Mix the walnuts, dried fruit, lemon juice, and rind together. Pour enough maple syrup over this to moisten well, about 2 tablespoons. Fill the apples with this, but don't pack the filling in too tightly. If the filling mounds at the top of the apple, that's okay. Put a generous pat of butter on top of the filling, place apples in a glass baking dish, and pour 1 cup boiling water into the dish, around the apples. Bake at 350 degrees for 20 to 30 minutes, or until the apples are tender. During the baking time, you can baste the apples with the pan juices. When the apples are done, remove to a serving dish, transfer the liquid to a small skillet, and reduce. Spoon over the apples before serving. *One apple per serving.*

Beverages

Super Baby Smoothies

These blood type–specific protein smoothies provide an excellent nutritional boost. For the protein base use either *Proteus ABO*, our specially formulated product, or a commercial protein powder suitable for your blood type.

SUPER BABY SMOOTHIE—TYPE O

2 tablespoons Protein Blend 4 Types protein powder for Type O
or egg albumin–based commercial protein powder
1 cup blueberries
1 banana
½ cup pineapple juice

Blend well and serve.

SUPER BABY SMOOTHIE—TYPE A

2 tablespoons Protein Blend 4 Types for Type A
or soy-based commercial protein powder
1 cup blueberries
½ cup blackberries
½ cup pineapple juice

Blend well and serve.

SUPER BABY SMOOTHIE—TYPE B

2 tablespoons Protein Blend 4 Types for Type B
or whey–based commercial protein powder
1 banana
1 papaya, peeled and sliced
½ cup pineapple juice

Blend well and serve.

SUPER BABY SMOOTHIE—TYPE AB

2 tablespoons Protein Blend 4 Types for Type AB
or whey–based commercial protein powder
1 kiwi, peeled and sliced
½ cup pitted cherries
½ cup pineapple juice

Blend well and serve.

Yogurt Drinks

PINEAPPLE

(A, B, AB)

1 cup yogurt
1 cup chopped pineapple
½ cup pineapple juice
Mint leaves

Put the yogurt, pineapple, and pineapple juice in a blender and blend well. Pour into a tall glass and garnish with mint leaves. *Serves 1 or 2.*

APRICOT

(A, B, AB)

1 cup yogurt
1 cup fresh apricots
½ cup apricot juice

Put the ingredients into a blender and blend well. *Serves 1 or 2.*

BANANA

(O, B)

1 cup yogurt
1 large, ripe banana
½ cup pineapple juice

Put ingredients into a blender and blend well. *Serves 1 or 2.*

MINT

(A, B, AB)

1 cup yogurt
½ handful fresh mint leaves
1 cup water
½ teaspoon ground, roasted cumin seeds
Sprinkle of salt

Puree all ingredients in a blender. Drink ice cold. *Serves 1.*

ROSE WATER LASSI

(A, B, AB)

Types A and AB can use low-fat yogurt.

1 cup whole milk yogurt
2 teaspoons rose water
3 tablespoons sugar

Blend all ingredients. *Serves 1.*

STRAWBERRY-BANANA SMOOTHIE

(B)

1 cup low-fat vanilla yogurt
1 cup low-fat milk
1 cup frozen unsweetened strawberries
2 ripe bananas
1 teaspoon honey

Place all ingredients in a blender and mix for about 1 minute. *Makes 2 servings.*

Soy Drinks

TOFU CAROB PROTEIN DRINK

(O, A, AB)

8 ounces extra-soft tofu
3 cups Rice Dream
¼ teaspoon Stevia
1 tablespoon carob powder

Blend and chill. *Makes 1 quart.*

PINEAPPLE PROTEIN SHAKE

(A)

¾ cup egg substitute
¾ cup vanilla soy milk
6 ounces pineapple juice
4 ice cubes

Combine ingredients in blender. Mix on high for 30 seconds.

SASSY SMOOTHIE

(O, A)

1 cup of 100% pineapple or black cherry juice
3 to 4 tablespoons of 100% almond butter
2 medium-sized ripe bananas
1 cup of frozen blueberries or cherries

Blend all ingredients until smooth and creamy. *Serves 1 or 2.*

MANGO-LIME SMOOTHIE

(O, B)

1 cup soy milk
1 ripe mango, peeled, pitted, and cut into chunks
½ cup pineapple juice
Juice of ½ lime

Blend all ingredients until smooth and serve very cold. *Serves 1 or 2.*

PAPAYA-KIWI DRINK

(O, B, AB)

1 cup soy milk
½ small papaya, peeled, seeded, cut into chunks
1 kiwi, peeled, cut into chunks
½ cup papaya juice

Blend all ingredients until smooth and serve very cold. *Serves 1.*

CHERRY-PEACH SMOOTHIE

(O, A, B, AB)

1 cup soy milk
½ cup pitted black cherries
2 ripe peaches, pitted and cut into chunks
1 cup cherry juice

Blend well and serve ice cold. *Serves 2.*

BANANA-PAPAYA SMOOTHIE

(O, B)

1 cup soy milk
1 ripe banana
½ ripe papaya
½ cup pineapple juice

Blend well and drink well chilled. *Serves 2.*

DATE-PRUNE SMOOTHIE

(O, A, B, AB)

1 cup soy milk
4 pitted prunes
2 to 3 pitted dates
1 cup prune juice

Blend very well and enjoy ice cold. *Serves 2.*

GRAPE-PEACH SMOOTHIE

(O, A, B, AB)

½ cup soy milk
½ cup apple juice
1 small peach, pitted
Handful of seedless grapes (green or red)
½ lime, juiced

Blend thoroughly. *Serves 1.*

PINEAPPLE-APRICOT SILKEN SMOOTHIE

(O, A, AB)

Instead of using soy milk, this recipe calls for the softest tofu: silken.

1 cup fresh pineapple chunks
3 ounces silken tofu
½ cup pineapple juice

1 fresh apricot
4 ice cubes

Combine all ingredients in a blender and mix for 2 minutes or until smooth. Drink immediately.

HEIDI'S EARLY MORNING SHAKE

(O, A, AB)

1 cup soy milk or carob soy milk or 2 to 3 tablespoons carob powder
(if not using carob soy milk)
1 teaspoon raw honey
1½ frozen bananas or 1 cup frozen blueberries
1 teaspoon flaxseeds

In a blender, combine the milk and honey. Add all other ingredients and blend.

Rice/Almond Milk

HIGH-ENERGY PROTEIN SHAKE

(O, A, B, AB)

8 to 12 ounces almond milk (rice milk or soy can be used)
3 heaping tablespoons rice protein powder (health-food store)
½ cut-up banana (or desired fruit)
1 tablespoon flaxseed oil (must be kept refrigerated)
½ tablespoon honey
(Note: For a lower carbohydrate/sugar shake, use half almond milk, half water, and substitute stevia to taste for the honey.)

Combine all ingredients and blend until smooth.

CARROT-CUCUMBER-APPLE SMOOTHIE

(O, A, B)

4 carrots
1 cucumber
1 apple

½ cup of rice milk
Honey to taste
2 ice cube trays or use crushed ice

Cut ends off carrots. Peel the cucumber. Cut the apple, removing the seeds and keeping the skin. Place in a blender with rice milk. Add honey and ice. Blend.

Fruit and Vegetable Juices

CARROT-CELERY

(O, A, B, AB)

4 washed carrots, ends removed
2 washed stalks celery, leaves on

Combine ingredients in a juicer and juice until smooth.

CARROT-ROMAINE-BROCCOLI

(O, A, B, AB)

4 carrots
2 Romaine leaves, or more
1 stalk of broccoli, peeled

Combine ingredients in a juicer and juice until smooth.

CARROT-CUCUMBER

(A, B, AB)

4 carrots
1 cucumber, peeled if not organic

Combine ingredients in a juicer and juice until smooth.

CARROT-APPLE

(O, A, B, AB)

4 carrots
1 apple, peeled if not organic

Place ingredients in a juicer and juice until smooth.

APPLE-GRAPE

(O, A, B, AB)

3 apples
1 cluster of grapes

Place ingredients in a juicer and juice until smooth.

Dressings and Relishes

TAHINI DRESSING

(O, A)

½ cup tahini
1 tablespoon honey
1 to 2 tablespoons water (or more as needed)

Combine well in small bowl and drizzle over fruit.

TOFU MISO DRESSING

(O, A, AB)

½ cake tofu
1 tablespoon miso
2 to 3 tablespoons Vegetable Stock (page 354)
2 tablespoons sesame seeds

Place all ingredients in a blender and puree until smooth.

EGG-FREE MAYONNAISE

(O, A, B, AB)

Pour into blender:

¼ cup egg substitute
½ teaspoon dry mustard
½ teaspoon salt
1½ tablespoons lemon juice

Blend on low, and pour in slowly:

½ cup cold-pressed, extra virgin olive oil
2 teaspoons very hot water to emulsify the mayonnaise

Then, pouring in slowly again:

½ cup of olive oil

Follow with:

1 teaspoon of very hot water

This mayonnaise may be stored in the refrigerator for three weeks.

LEMON-HONEY DRESSING

(O, A, B, AB)

2 lemons, juiced
¼ cup olive oil
1 to 2 tablespoons honey
1 to 2 teaspoons tamari sauce

Put all the ingredients into a jar and shake well.

SEAWEED DRESSING

(O, A, B, AB)

1 cup dulse flakes, wakame, or nori
½ cup olive oil
¼ cup sesame seeds

1 tablespoon sesame oil
1 teaspoon rice vinegar
1 teaspoon soy sauce
¼ cup water (approximately)

Place all ingredients in a blender to mix. Thin with water to desired consistency.

OLIVE OIL AND LEMON DRESSING

(O, A, B, AB)

½ cup extra virgin olive oil
2 lemons, juiced
½ teaspoon dry mustard
½ teaspoon salt
¼ teaspoon honey

Whisk all the ingredients together and serve on any salad.

VIDALIA ONION VINAIGRETTE

(O, A, B, AB)

½ small Vidalia onion
Juice of 2 lemons
1 tablespoon chopped basil
1 teaspoon salt
½ teaspoon sugar
1½ cups olive oil

Grate or finely chop the onion. Add all the other ingredients except the oil and allow to marinate for 1 hour. Drizzle the oil on to the onion-lemon mixture and whisk briskly. When the vinaigrette separates, shake or whisk again.

BALSAMIC MUSTARD VINAIGRETTE

(B)

2 tablespoons honey
2 tablespoons Dijon mustard

½ cup balsamic vinegar
1 cup olive oil

In the bowl of a food processor, mix the first three ingredients. Slowly drizzle the oil, so it incorporates completely. This can last in the refrigerator indefinitely.

CUCUMBER YOGURT SAUCE

(A, AB)

2 cups plain yogurt
½ red onion, diced small
1 tablespoon chopped fresh mint
1 tablespoon chopped cilantro
1 small cucumber
2 teaspoons ground cumin
Squeeze of lemon

Combine all the ingredients in a blender until smooth.

FRESH MINT SAUCE

(O, A, B, AB)

1 cup fresh mint leaves, cleaned and dried
1½-inch piece fresh ginger, peeled and cut into quarters
1 scallion
3 stalks lemongrass, bottom quarter cut and peeled to the soft layer;
reserve tough outer leaves for broth
1 tablespoon brown rice vinegar
Juice of 1 lime
½ teaspoon sugar
¼ cup olive oil

In a blender or food processor, puree the first seven ingredients. Slowly drizzle the oil into the bowl of the machine and blend 10 more seconds. Chill and serve.

GARLIC-SHALLOT MIXTURE

(O, A, B, AB)

10 cloves garlic, peeled
10 shallots, peeled
Olive oil to cover

In a food processor or blender, finely chop the garlic and shallots by pulsing the blade and scraping down the sides. Put the mixture in an airtight container and cover with oil. This mixture will last refrigerated for 10 days or so.

CHUTNEY YOGURT MAYONNAISE

(A)

½ cup plain yogurt
⅓ cup homemade canola or olive oil mayonnaise
3 tablespoons mango-ginger or pineapple chutney
1 teaspoon ground cumin

Stir all the ingredients together.

WALNUT VINAIGRETTE

(O, A, B, AB)

½ cup olive oil
¼ cup walnut oil
2 tablespoons fresh lemon juice
½ teaspoon dry mustard
¼ teaspoon salt
¼ cup broken walnuts
2 tablespoons chopped basil

Combine all the ingredients in a blender and mix for 1 to 2 minutes.

PESTO

(O, A, B, AB)

1 teaspoon coarse salt
2 handfuls basil

½ handful parsley
2 to 3 cloves garlic
½ cup broken walnuts
Olive oil

Place the salt in a mortar and begin adding basil and parsley leaves while crushing with a pestle. Add some garlic, continuing to work in each new addition. Add broken nuts, more leaves, then garlic, until mixture is well ground but not necessarily smooth. Add the oil slowly, stirring until desired consistency is achieved.

PLUM BARBECUE SAUCE

(O, A, B, AB)

6 ounces plum jam
2 ounces pineapple juice
3 tablespoons tamari sauce
2 cloves garlic, through a press
2 scallions, sliced thin

Combine all the ingredients and brush lightly over any fish, especially tuna. It also works very well for chicken.

APPLE ONION CONFIT

(O, A, B, AB)

1 stick butter (Types O, B) or margarine (Types A, AB)
1 very large yellow onion
6 apples

Melt the butter or margarine in heavy, lidded pot. Peel and halve the onion, slice it very thin, and add to melted butter, turning well. Peel and core the apples; slice into thin wedges and add to pot, incorporating into the onion. Let simmer over very low heat until tender. The apples will "melt" and the onion will be in long, thin pieces. Serve warm or at room temperature.

RAW ENZYME RELISH

(A, B, AB)

1 pound fresh (cleaned/spun dry) cranberries
2 cups raw pumpkin seeds

1 large Fuji apple (tart/crisp)
½ cup diced raw pineapple
½ cup thinly sliced celery
¼ cup plain yogurt
¼ cup blackstrap molasses (or maple syrup)
¾ cup raw cane sugar
3 tablespoons lemon juice
Poppy seeds
Allspice
Salt

In a food processor, coarsely chop cranberries and pumpkin seeds. In a large bowl, combine cranberry/seed mixture with Fuji apple, raw pineapple, celery, yogurt, blackstrap molases, raw cane sugar, and lemon juice. Sprinkle with poppy seeds, allspice, and a pinch of salt.

For Baby

Contents

Vegetables
Fruits
Biscuits and Cereals
Rice
Meats

Vegetables

VEGETABLE PUREES

(O, A, B, AB)

Cut vegetables (according to blood type) into small pieces and steam them in a vegetable steamer over 1 or 2 inches of water in a tightly covered pot. Use this water as a thinner when pureeing vegetables. The approximate ratio of vegetables to liquid is 2 cups of fresh vegetables to between ⅓ to ½ cup of liquid. Place steamed vegetables and a little of the steaming water in a food processor or baby-food grinder and puree to a soft consistency. To add flavor and protein, try adding an equal amount of baked or steamed potato to the steamed vegetables and puree together. Thin the mixture with infant formula or breast milk to desired consistency. Freeze unused portions immediately.

PUREED BLACK-EYED PEAS

(O, A)

Carefully rinse and pick over 1 cup of black-eyed peas. Soak in water overnight or bring to a boil for 2 minutes, cover, and then allow to sit for 2 hours. Drain off the soaking water or the cooking water, then add 3 cups fresh water and bring the beans to a boil. Reduce the heat and simmer, covered, until the beans are tender. Skim the surface often as beans are simmering. Puree with ¾ cup soy or breast milk.

BAKED SWEET POTATOES

(O, B, AB)

Scrub the sweet potatoes thoroughly and prick several times with a fork. Bake at 350 degrees until soft and tender. Scoop the meat of the sweet potato out of the skin and mash it with a fork. Cool to warm and serve.

PUREED GREEN BEANS

(O, A, B, AB)

1 cup green beans
2 tablespoons water or breast milk

Steam the beans until tender. Add water or breast milk and puree to a smooth texture.

CRUSTLESS SWEET POTATO AND CARROT PIE

(B, AB)

1 sweet potato
1 carrot, finely grated
¼ cup plain yogurt
1 egg

In a microwave oven, cook the sweet potato at 100 percent for 5 minutes, or longer if it is very big. Prick the skin before cooking. Carefully remove the meat of the potato. In a bowl, mix in the carrot and yogurt, then the egg; blend until smooth. If the mixture appears dry, add another tablespoon of yogurt. Cook at 100 percent, uncovered, for 2 minutes. Stir, cook 1½ minutes more. Let rest 2 to 3 minutes. This tastes best if served as soon as it cools. Serve with a dollop of cold yogurt. *Yield: 2 cups.*

Fruits

BLUEBERRY BANANA YOGURT

(B, AB)

1 cup blueberries
1 whole banana
1 cup plain yogurt

Microwave the blueberries just until the juices start to run, about 30 seconds. Place the banana, yogurt, and blueberries in a blender and puree until smooth.

STRAWBERRIES AND BANANA

(O)

Mash ½ a banana and mix with 1 tablespoon of pureed strawberries. Serve immediately.

STRAWBERRY YOGURT

(A, B)

Mix ¼ cup of plain whole yogurt with 1 tablespoon pureed strawberries and serve.

STRAWBERRY-TOFU PARFAIT

(O, A)

Puree 3 tablespoons of silken tofu until real smooth and add 1 tablespoon of pureed strawberries. Blend well.

APPLESAUCE

(O, A, B, AB)

Wash, quarter, and core 5 apples just before cooking. Place apple quarters in a steamer basket in a pot filled with a low level of boiling water. Cover the pot tightly and steam the apples for 10 minutes or until they are tender. You may have to add more water. The apples should pierce easily when they're ready. Cool the apples, then strain them in a food mill or food processor. Add 1 tablespoon of the cooking liquid per apple to the puree.

BABY'S FIRST PEARS

(O, A, B, AB)

Peel, core, and slice pears thickly. Steam 5 to 10 minutes, until tender. Blend or puree to a smooth consistency. Cool and serve.

PLUMS

(O, A, B, AB)

Simmer 2 pounds of plums in a covered saucepan with a ¼ cup of water for 10 minutes, until tender. *Two pounds yields 3 cups.*

Biscuits and Cereals

Biscuits

TEETHING BISCUIT NO. 1

(O, A, B, AB)

1 egg
¼ teaspoon salt
1 tablespoon soy flour
1 cup spelt flour
1 tablespoon breast milk or formula

Preheat the oven to 350 degrees. Beat the egg in a mixing bowl. Add the remaining ingredients and mix thoroughly. Roll onto a flour-dusted surface until about 1 inch thick and cut into the size you want. (Use cookie cutters, if you prefer.) Place on a greased baking sheet and cook for 7 minutes. Flip over and cook for 4 minutes.

TEETHING BISCUIT NO. 2

(B, AB)

½ cup brown rice flour
½ cup whole barley flour
½ teaspoon blackstrap molasses
Water for consistency

Combine the flours and molasses and stir in water until the dough is a pasty consistency. Place approximately ¼-inch-thick rounds on a cookie sheet. Bake at 250 degrees for 90 minutes.

Cereals

BABY CEREAL

(A, B, AB)

1 tablespoon rolled oats
2 tablespoons organic plain yogurt
4 tablespoons breast milk or formula

Mix together the oats and yogurt. Bring the milk to a boil and pour over the oat-yogurt mix, stirring constantly. Cool to taste and serve.

Rice

RICE-VEGETABLE PUREE

(O, A, B, AB)

2 tablespoons brown rice
4 carrots, chopped into small pieces
1⅓ cups water

Place the rice and carrots in a saucepan with water. Cover and simmer until the water is absorbed—about 30 minutes. Cool to warm temperature and blend in the food processor until smooth.

RICE WITH MUSHROOMS

(O, A, B, AB)

2 tablespoons long-grain rice
6 to 8 small mushrooms, cleaned and chopped
1 tablespoon breast milk or formula
Water

Place rice, mushrooms, and milk in a pan and cover with water. Bring to a boil and simmer for 15 minutes or until rice is tender. Drain and puree. Add the milk as needed for consistency.

Meats

PUREED MEATS

(O, A, B, AB)

Cut meat (according to blood type) into ½-inch cubes. Trim off all fat. Add 1 cup of stock (either meat or vegetable) to 1 cup of meat. Simmer until meat is tender—45 minutes to an hour. Drain stock, reserving the liquid. When you puree, use ½ cup of cooking liquid for each cup of meat. Freeze extra portions immediately.

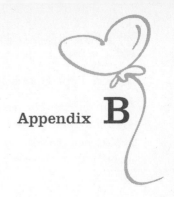

Appendix **B**

Resources and Products

General

DR. PETER D'ADAMO

The D'Adamo Naturopathic Center in Stamford, Connecticut, blends time-honored natural healing techniques with state-of-the-art diagnostics. The clinic staff is comprised of naturopathic physicians (ND) working with medical doctors (MD), nurses (RN), and other licensed health professionals, all under the precepts and guidance of Dr. Peter D'Adamo. To find out more or to schedule an appointment, please contact:

> The D'Adamo Clinic
> 2009 Summer Street
> Stamford, CT 06905
> 203-348-4800

www.dadamo.com

The World Wide Web has proven to be a valuable venue for exploring and applying the tenets of the Blood Type Diet and Lifestyle. Since January 1997, hundreds of thousands have visited the site to participate in the ABO chat groups, to peruse the scientific archives, to share experiences and recipes, and to learn more about the science of blood type.

Blood Type Specialty Products and Supplements

North American Pharmacal, Inc., is the official distributor of Blood Type Specialty Products. The product line includes supplements, books, tapes, teas, meal-replacement bars, cosmetics, and support material that make eating and living right for your type easier.

> North American Pharmacal, Inc.
> 12 High Street
> Norwalk, CT 06851
> Tel: 203-866-7664
> Fax: 203-838-4066
> Toll-free: 877-ABO-TYPE (877-226-8973)
> www.4yourtype.com

Home Blood Typing Kits

North American Pharmacal, Inc., is the official distributor of Home Blood Type Testing Kits. Each kit costs $9.95 (plus shipping and handling) and is a single-use, disposable, educational device capable of determining one individual's ABO and Rhesus (Rh) blood type. Results are obtained within about 4 to 5 minutes. If you have several friends or family members who need to learn their blood type, you will need to order a separate home blood typing kit for each individual.

The Blood Type Library

The following books are available in bookstores, health-food stores, selected grocery and specialty stores, on the Web, and through North American Pharmacal.

Eat Right 4 Your Type: The Individualized Diet Solution to Staying Healthy, Living Longer, and Achieving Your Ideal Weight
By Dr. Peter J. D'Adamo, with Catherine Whitney
G. P. Putnam's Sons, 1996
   The original blood type diet book, with more than two million copies sold in more than fifty languages.

Cook Right 4 Your Type: The Practical Kitchen Companion to Eat Right 4 Your Type
By Dr. Peter J. D'Adamo, with Catherine Whitney
G. P. Putnam's Sons, 1999 (Berkley Trade Paperback, 2000)
   Includes more than two hundred original recipes, thirty-day meal plans, and guidelines for each blood type.

Live Right 4 Your Type: The Individualized Prescription for Maximizing Health, Metabolism, and Vitality in Every Stage of Your Life
By Dr. Peter J. D'Adamo, with Catherine Whitney
G. P. Putnam's Sons, 2001

A total health and lifestyle plan based on the individual variations observed for each blood type. Includes new research on the mind-body connection and the importance of blood type secretor status.

Eat Right 4 Your Type Complete Blood Type Encyclopedia
By Dr. Peter J. D'Adamo, with Catherine Whitney
Riverhead Books, 2002

The A to Z reference guide for the blood type connection to symptoms, diseases, conditions, medications, vitamins, supplements, herbs, and food.

4 Your Type Pocket Guides: Blood Type, Food, Beverage, and Supplement Lists
By Peter J. D'Adamo, with Catherine Whitney
Berkley Books, 2002

The Eat Right 4 Your Type Portable and Personal Blood Type Guides are pocket-sized and user-friendly. They serve as a handy reference tool while shopping, cooking, and eating out. Each book contains the food, beverage, and supplement list for each blood type, plus handy tips and ideas for incorporating the blood type diet into your daily life.

Eat Right 4 Your Baby: The Individualized Guide to Fertility and Maximum Health During Pregnancy, Nursing, and Your Baby's First Year
By Dr. Peter J. D'Adamo, with Catherine Whitney
G. P. Putnam's Sons, 2003 (Berkley Trade Paperback, 2004)

An invaluable guide for couples looking to combine the best of naturopathic and blood type science to maximize the health of mother and baby—with practical blood type–specific guidelines for achieving a healthy state before pregnancy, eating and living right during pregnancy, and how to continue in good health during baby's first year.

Dr. Peter J. D'Adamo's Eat Right 4 Your Type Health Library

Cancer: Fight It with the Blood Type Diet
Diabetes: Fight It with the Blood Type Diet

Resources for Pregnancy, Labor, and Delivery

Association of Labor Assistants and Childbirth Educators (ALACE)
www.alace.org

Doulas of North America (DONA)
P.O. Box 626
Jasper, IN 47547
888-788-DONA
www.dona.org

Birthworks
P.O. Box 2045
Medford, NJ 08055
888-TO-BIRTH
www.birthworks.net

Birth Balance: A Resource for Waterbirth, Doulas,
Labor, and Pregnancy
www.birthbalance.com

Midwives Alliance of North America (MANA)
www.mana.org

Pregnancy and Childbirth Therapy Sources

Chico Water Cure Spa
6670 Chico Way, NW
Bremerton, WA 98312
360-692-5554
crogers5@aol.com

Cathy Rogers, N.D., the naturopath/midwife whose advice appears in this book, practices her healing principles at her Chico Water Cure Spa in Washington State. Cathy also produces a line of healing products, which can be ordered direct. They include: Seaweed Rubedo Herbal Seaweed Washbag, a reusable blend of lavender, rose, and rich seaweed gel in a healing washbag; Seaweed Rubedo Sea Salt Bathing Crystals; and Lavender Cleanse Sea Salt Bathing Crystals. These products can be used in showers and baths for relief of arthritis, fibromyalgia, allergies, chronic pain, and skin conditions.

American Massage Therapy Association
820 Davis Street
Suite 100
Evanston, IL 60201
847-864-0123
www.amtamassage.org
    Information and resources on massage, massage therapists, and use of massage to relieve pain.

Reflexology Association of America
4012 Rainbow Suite K-PMB #585
Las Vegas, NV 89103
www.reflexology-usa.net
    Information and resources on the practice of reflexology and its uses for pain and stress relief.

American Academy of Medical Acupuncture
4929 Wilshire Boulevard
Suite 428
Los Angeles, CA 90010
323-937-5514
www.medicalacupuncture.org
    Information and resources on acupuncture, its uses, and practitioners.

LABOR TUBS:
    Labor Tubs Northwest
    888-217-2229 (toll-free)
    www.labortubs.com

    AquaDoula Tubs to Go
    3101 111th Street SW, Bay A
    Everett, WA 98204
    waterbirth@aquadoula.com

    Birth Balance: A Resource for Waterbirth, Doulas, Labor, and Pregnancy
    www.birthbalance.com

    Waterbirth Resources
    3204 Elliot Ave. S.
    Minneapolis, MN 55407
    612-622-3263

Tender Loving Childbirth
www.watermama.com

Dolphin Circle Waterbirth Tub Kits
505-294-4359
www.tubsntea.com

Organic Baby Foods

Each of the following companies offers a line of high-quality organic baby food that can be ordered over the Web.

Baby Organic
800-259-9774
www.babyorganic.com

Diamond Organics
www.diamondorganics.com

Earth's Best
www.earthsbest.com

Abortion, Rh sensitization and, 12
A Type baby, 303–7; colds and congestion,
    303–4; colic, 304; diaper rash, 304–5; diar-
    rhea, 304; diet, 305–7; ear infections, 303;
    restlessness/sleep problems, 305; skin
    rashes, 304
A Type blood, anti-B antibodies, 6
A Type mother, 275–79; breast-feeding power
    foods, 292
A Type pregnancy, 95–152; appetite, 127; blood
    flow, 135; blood pressure, 135–36; blood
    sugar, 127–28; detoxification, 112; diet,
    95–143; digestive enzymes, 117; emotional
    health, 114–15; exercise, 115–16, 143–48;
    fatigue, 118, 136; food cravings and aver-
    sions, 118; immunity, 127; labor and deliv-
    ery, 151–52; mood swings, 118; mucus
    production, 128; stress, 136; supplements,
    112–14; weight control, 111
AB Type baby, 315–19; colds and congestion,
    315; diaper rash, 316; diarrhea, 316; diet,
    316–19; ear infections, 315
AB Type mother, 282–85; breast-feeding power
    foods, 293
AB Type pregnancy, 213–319; appetite, 243–44;
    blood flow, 253; blood pressure, 253; blood
    sugar, 244; detoxification, 229–30; diet,
    213–61; digestive enzymes, 234; emotional
    health, 232; exercise, 232–33, 261–64;
    fatigue, 235; food aversions and cravings,
    236; immunity, 245; labor and delivery, 268;
    mood balance, 234–35; mucus production,
    245; supplements, 231–32, 264–68; urinary
    tract infections, 244; weight control, 228–29
Acupressure in pain control, 35
Adzuki Bean; and Pumpkin or Winter Squash
    Soup, 360; and Sweet Brown Rice, 353
Allergies, 26; B Type baby, 310; O Type baby,
    297; O Type pregnancy, 69–70
Amaranth Pancakes, 385–86
Amniocentesis, 7
Anise, milk production and, 289
Anxiety, relieving, 22
Appetite; A Type pregnancy, 126; AB Type
    pregnancy, 243–44; B Type pregnancy,
    184–85; lack of, 30; O Type pregnancy, 69

Apples; Applesauce, 413–14; Baked, 397; -Grape
    Juice, 405; Onion Confit, 410; Sautéed, 394
Apricot Yogurt Drink, 399
Arginine, fertility and, 19
Artichokes; Jerusalem, Soup, 359–60; Steamed,
    374; and Vidalia Onion Tart, 378–79

Babies, recipes, 411–16
Baby Cereal, 415
Baby's First Pears, 414
Baked Apples, 397
Baked Sweet Potatoes, 412
Balsamic Mustard Vinaigrette, 407–8
Bananas; -Papaya Smoothie, 402; Plum Bread,
    380–81; Sautéed, 394; Spelt Bread or
    Muffins, 384; Walnut Bread or Muffins,
    382–83; Yogurt Drink, 399
Barley Black Bean Salad, 352–53
Barley-Spelt Pancakes, 384–85
Basic Stock, 353–54
Beans and legumes; A Type baby, 306, 307;
    A Type pregnancy, 102–3; AB Type baby, 317,
    318; AB Type pregnancy, 220–21; Adzuki
    Bean and Pumpkin or Winter Squash Soup,
    360; Adzuki Bean and Sweet Brown Rice,
    353; Barley Black Bean Salad, 352–53;
    Black-Eyed Peas, Okra, and Leek Melange,
    345–46; Black-Eyed Peas and Barley Salad,
    352; Black-Eyed Peas with Leeks, 346;
    Brown Rice Pilaf, 350–51; B Type baby, 311,
    312–13; B Type pregnancy, 160; Cream of
    Lima Bean Soup, 358; Cuban Black Bean
    Soup, 362; Faro Pilaf, 347–48; Lentil Salad,
    346–47; Lentil Soup, 357; Lima Beans with
    Goat Cheese and Scallions, 345; Millet
    Couscous, 349; Millet Tabbouleh, 348;
    O Type baby, 301–2; O Type pregnancy,
    44; Pureed Pinto Beans with Garlic, 347;
    Quinoa Flour Tortillas with Pureed Pinto
    Beans, 344–45; Quinoa Risotto, 350; Spelt-
    berry and Basmati Rice Pilaf, 349; Spelt-
    berry and Rice Salad, 349–50; Speltberry
    Salad, 351–52; Tofu and Black Bean Chili,
    334; White Bean and Wilted Greens Soup,
    361; Wild and Basmati Rice Pilaf, 348; Wild
    Rice Salad, 351

Beef. *See also* Meats and poultry; Cellophane Noodles with Grilled Sirloin and Green Vegetables, 341–42; Flank Steak, 327; Great Meatloaf, 326; Old-Fashioned Yankee Pot Roast, 325; Pan-Fried Liver and Onions, 326–27; Stew with Green Beans and Carrots, 355–56

Beverages; A Type pregnancy, 109–10; AB Type pregnancy, 227–28; B Type pregnancy, 166–68; Fruit and Vegetable Juices, 404–5; O Type pregnancy, 51–52; Rice/Almond Milk, 403–4; Soy Drinks, 400–403; Super Baby Smoothies, 397–98

Black-Eyed Peas; and Barley Salad, 352; with Leeks, 346; Okra, and Leek Melange, 345–46

Bleeding gums, 26; O Type pregnancy, 71

Blood-clotting ability in O Type pregnancy, 71

Blood flow; A Type pregnancy, 136; AB Type pregnancy, 253

Blood pressure; A Type pregnancy, 136; AB Type pregnancy, 253; B Type pregnancy, 195–96; O Type pregnancy, 78

Blood sugar, 27; A Type pregnancy, 127; AB Type pregnancy, 244; B Type pregnancy, 185; O Type pregnancy, 69

Blood type; fertility and, 5–13; genetics and, 10–11

Blueberr(ies); Banana Yogurt, 413; Buckwheat Muffins, 383

Boiled Lamb Chops, 323

Borage, milk production and, 289

Braised Collards, 375

Braised Rabbit, 322

Breads. *See also* Grains, breads, rice, and pasta; Banana Plum Bread, 380–81; Banana Spelt Bread or Muffins, 384; Banana Walnut Bread or Muffins, 382–83; Blueberry Buckwheat Muffins, 383; Cornbread, 383–84; Pumpkin-Almond Bread, 381; Quinoa Almond Muffins, 382; Spelt Bread, 381–82

Breast-feeding, 287–93

Breath, shortness of, 30

Broccoli; Carrot-Romaine-, Juice, 404; Sesame, 375; Super, Salad, 364

Broiled Salmon Steaks, 329

Broiled Salmon with Lemongrass, 328

Bromelain in B Type pregnancy, 172

Brown Rice Pilaf, 350–51

Brown Rice-Spelt Pancakes, 386

B Type baby, 309–13; diaper rash, 310; diarrhea, 310; diet, 310–13; food allergies, 310; respiratory/ear infections, 309; restlessness/hyperactivity, 310

B Type blood, anti-B antibodies, 6

B Type mother, 279–82; breast-feeding power foods, 293

B Type pregnancy, 153–212; appetite, 184–85; blood building needs, 211; blood pressure,

195–96; blood sugar, 185; detoxification, 170–71; diet, 153–203; emotional health, 173; exercise, 173–74, 203–7; food cravings and aversions, 177; food intolerances, 186–87; herbal remedies, 208–9, 210; infection resistance, 186, 196; labor and delivery, 211–12; supplements, 172–73, 207–11; swelling and edema, 194–95; urinary tract infections, 185; weight control, 169–70

Butternut Squash and Tofu with Mixed Vegetables, 333

Caesar Salad, 368–69

Calcium in O Type pregnancy, 57

Candida infections in O Type pregnancy, 70–71

Carbohydrate cravings, 274

Carnitine, fertility and, 19

Carrots; -Apple Juice, 405; Beef Stew with Green Beans and, 355–56; -Celery Juice, 404; -Cucumber-Apple Smoothie, 403–4; -Cucumber Juice, 404; and Parsnips with Garlic and Cilantro, 371; Raisin Salad, 367; -Romaine-Broccoli Juice, 404; -Tofu Soup with Dill, 357–58

Catecholamines, 57

Cauliflower with Garlic and Parsley, 372–73

Cellophane Noodles with Grilled Sirloin and Green Vegetables, 341–42

Cereals, baby, 300, 301, 305, 307, 311, 312, 316, 318, 415–16

Chamomile in A Type pregnancy, 113

Cherries; Fresh, and Yogurt Soup, 356–57; -Peach Smoothie, 401

Chicken. *See also* Meats and poultry; Basic Stock, 353–54; Grilled, Salad, 369–70; Kung Pao Tofu and, 334–35; Peanut, 323; Roast, with Garlic and Herbs, 328; Sesame, 322–23

Chutney; -Yogurt Mayonnaise, 409; -Yogurt Sauce, 323

Coenzyme Q_{10}, fertility and, 19

Cold Buckwheat Noodles with Peanut Sauce, 343

Colds and congestion; A Type baby, 303–4; AB Type baby, 315

Cole Slaw, 363–64

Colic; A Type baby, 304; O Type baby, 298

Collards, Braised, 375

Condiments; A Type pregnancy, 108–9; AB Type pregnancy, 226; B Type pregnancy, 166; O Type pregnancy, 50–51

Constipation, 21, 30; B Type pregnancy, 175; O Type pregnancy, 61

Cornbread, 383–84

Cream of Lima Bean Soup, 358

Creative visualization, 152, 212

Crustless Sweet Potato and Carrot Pie, 412

Cuban Black Bean Soup, 362

Cucumber; Yogurt Sauce, 408; -Yogurt Soup, 360

Curried Egg Salad, 377

Dairy. *See* Eggs and dairy

D'Amado, Peter J., 37, 96, 153, 214

Dandelion; A Type pregnancy, 113; AB Type pregnancy, 232; B Type pregnancy, 172; O Type pregnancy, 57

Date-Prune Smoothie, 402

Deep breathing in A Type pregnancy, 146–47

Desserts; Baked Apples, 397; Carrot Raisin Cake, 389–90; Citrus Salad, 395; Cranberry Biscotti, 390–91; Fresh Fig Salad, 394; Oatmeal Cookies, 392; Peanut Butter Cookies, 392–93; Poached Fruit, 396; Rice Crispy Cakes, 391; Rice Pudding with Soy Milk, 393; Ricotta Orange Cream, 395; Sautéed Bananas, 394; Sautéed Pears or Apples, 394; Tofu Banana Pudding, 393; Tofu Pumpkin Pudding, 393; Tropical Salad, 395–96; Walnut Cookies, 389; Wild or Basmati Rice Pudding, 390

Detoxification, 17–18; A Type pregnancy, 112; AB Type pregnancy, 229–30; B Type pregnancy, 170–71; O Type pregnancy, 55

DHA supplementation, 23–24

Diaper rash; A Type baby, 304–5; AB Type baby, 316; B Type baby, 310; O Type baby, 299

Diarrhea; A Type baby, 304; AB Type baby, 316; B Type baby, 310; O Type baby, 298

Diet; A Type baby, 305–7; A Type mother, 277, 278; A Type pregnancy, 95–110; AB Type baby, 316–19; AB Type mother, 283–85; AB Type pregnancy, 213–61; B Type baby, 310–13; B Type mother, 281; B Type pregnancy, 153–203; fertility and, 9–10; O Type baby, 299–302; O Type mother, 274; O Type pregnancy, 37–85

Digestive discomforts; B Type pregnancy, 175–76; O Type baby, 297–98; O Type pregnancy, 60–61

Digestive enzymes; A Type pregnancy, 117; AB Type pregnancy, 234

Doula, 32–33, 35

Down's syndrome, 7

Dressings; Balsamic Mustard Vinaigrette, 407–8; Chutney-Yogurt Mayonnaise, 409; Egg-Free Mayonnaise, 406; Honey Mustard, 365; Lemon-Honey Dressing, 406; Olive Oil and Lemon Dressing, 407; Seaweed Dressing, 406–7; Tahini Dressing, 405; Tofu Miso Dressing, 405; Vidalia Onion Vinaigrette, 407; Walnut Vinaigrette, 409

Dry skin brushing, 171, 230–31

Ear infections; A Type baby, 303; AB Type baby, 315; B Type baby, 309; O Type baby, 298

Ectopic pregnancy, Rh sensitization and, 12

Edema, 30; B Type pregnancy, 194–95; O Type pregnancy, 77

Egg-Free Mayonnaise, 406

Eggplant Casserole, 371

Eggs and dairy; A Type baby, 306, 307; A Type pregnancy, 99–100; AB Type baby, 317–18; AB Type pregnancy, 218–19; B Type baby, 312, 313; B Type pregnancy, 157–58; Curried Egg Salad, 377; One-Egg Omelet, 377–78; O Type baby, 302; O Type pregnancy, 42

Emotional health; A Type pregnancy, 114–15; AB Type pregnancy, 232; B Type pregnancy, 173; O Type pregnancy, 57–58

Escargot, Peter's, 329

Exercise; A Type pregnancy, 115–16, 143–48; AB Type pregnancy, 232–33, 261–64; B Type pregnancy, 173–74, 203–7; during first trimester, 25–26, 85–86, 143–44, 203–4, 261–62; kegel, 28; in O Type pregnancy, 58–59, 85–89; postpartum; A Type mother, 276–79; AB Type mother, 283–85; B Type mother, 280–82; O Type mother, 272–75; during second trimester, 27–28, 87–88, 144–46, 204–5, 262–63; during third trimester, 31, 88–89, 146–47, 206–7, 263–64

Farmer's Vegetable Soup, 358–59

Faro Pilaf, 347–48

Fatigue, 22, 30; A Type pregnancy, 118, 136; AB Type pregnancy, 235; B Type pregnancy, 176

Fats. *See* Oils and fats

Fertility; blood type and, 5–13; diet and, 9–10; impediments to, 15, 16

Fettuccine with Grilled Lamb Sausages and Vegetables, 342–43

Figs, Fresh, Salad, 394

First trimester, 20; common conditions, 20–23; diet and meal plans, 59–68, 116–26, 174–84, 233–34; exercise, 25–26, 85–86, 143–44, 203–4, 261–62

Flank Steak, 327

Food aversions, cravings, intolerances, 22–23; A Type pregnancy, 118; AB Type pregnancy, 236; B Type pregnancy, 177, 186–87; O Type pregnancy, 62–63

Fresh Cherries and Yogurt Soup, 356–57

Fresh Mint Sauce, 408

Fried Monkfish, 329–30

Frittatas; Spinach, 380; Zucchini and Mushroom, 379–80

Fruits; A Type baby, 306, 307; A Type pregnancy, 106–7; AB Type baby, 317, 318; AB Type pregnancy, 223–24; Applesauce, 413–14; Baby's First Pears, 414; Blueberry Banana Yogurt, 413; B Type baby, 311, 312; B Type pregnancy, 163–64; Fruit Silken Scramble, 336; Juices, 404–5; O Type baby, 300, 301; O Type pregnancy, 47–48; Plums, 414; Poached, 396; Strawberries and Banana, 413; Strawberry-Tofu Parfait, 413; Strawberry Yogurt, 413

Gelsemium, 35
Genetics, blood type and, 10–11
Ginger rhizome, miscarriage and, 61
Glazed Turnips and Onions, 370–71
Grains, breads, rice, and pasta. *See also* Pasta and noodles; A Type baby, 306, 307; A Type pregnancy, 103, AB Type baby, 317, 318; AB Type pregnancy, 221–22; B Type baby, 312, 313; B Type pregnancy, 160–61; O Type baby, 301, 302; O Type pregnancy, 44–46
Grape-Peach Smoothie, 402
Great Meatloaf, 326
Greek Salad, 366
Green Beans; Beef Stew with, and Carrots, 355–56; Salad with Walnuts and Goat Cheese, 370
Green Leafy Pasta, 340
Green tea; A Type pregnancy, 113; AB Type pregnancy, 232; B Type pregnancy, 173; O Type pregnancy, 57
Grilled Chicken Salad, 369–70
Grilled Curried Leg of Lamb, 325
Grilled Goat Cheddar on Ezekiel or Spelt, 377
Grilled Loin of Lamb Chops, 324–25
Grilled or Roasted Peppers on Rye Crackers with Chèvre, 377
Grilled Pepper Medley, 372
Grilled Portabello Mushrooms, 375–76
Grilled Sweet Potato Salad, 369
Grilled Wild Rice Tempeh, 337

Hasidic Jews, fertility and, 8
Hatha yoga, in AB Type pregnancy, 232–33
Heartburn, 30; B Type pregnancy, 175; O Type pregnancy, 60–61
Heidi's Early Morning Shake, 403
Hemorrhoids, 27; in O Type pregnancy, 70
Herbs and herbal remedies; A Type pregnancy, 109–10, 114, 149, 150, 151; AB Type pregnancy, 226–27, 232, 265–67; avoiding during pregnancy, 24; B Type pregnancy, 166–67, 172–73, 208–9, 210; milk production and, 289; O Type pregnancy, 51–52, 57, 90, 91, 92
High blood pressure, 30. *See also* Blood pressure
High-Energy Protein Shake, 403
Holy basil in A Type pregnancy, 113
Homeopathy, 35
Honey Mustard Dressing, 365
Hops, milk production and, 289
Hydrotherapy, 35

Immunity; A Type pregnancy, 127; AB Type pregnancy, 245
Indian Lamb Stew with Spinach, 362–63
Infection resistance in B Type pregnancy, 186, 196
Ingestion, 30
Iron in A Type pregnancy, 113

Jerusalem Artichoke Soup, 359–60

Kegel exercise, 28
Kung Pao Tofu and Chicken, 334–35

Labor and delivery, 32–36; A Type pregnancy, 151–52; AB Type pregnancy, 268; B Type pregnancy, 211–12; O Type pregnancy, 93–94
Lamb. *See also* Meats and poultry; Broiled, Chops, 323; Fettuccine with Grilled, Sausages and Vegetables, 342–43; Grilled Curried Leg of, 325; Grilled Loin of, Chops, 324–25; Indian, Stew with Spinach, 362–63
Landsteiner, Karl, 12
Lasagna with Portabello Mushrooms and Pesto, 340–41
Legumes. *See* Beans and legumes
Lemon-Honey Dressing, 406
Lentil Salad, 346–47
Lentil Soup, 357
Licorice (DGL); B Type pregnancy, 173; miscarriage and, 61; O Type pregnancy, 57
Live Right 4 Your Type (D'Adamo), 37, 96, 153, 214

Magnesium in B Type pregnancy, 172
Mango-Lime Smoothie, 401
Marinades. *See also* Sauces; Spicy Curry, 337–38; Tamari-Mustard, 324–25
Mashed Plantains, 373
Massage in pain control, 35
Meats and poultry. *See also* Beef; Chicken; Lamb; Turkey; A Type baby, 306, 307; A Type pregnancy, 97–98; AB Type baby, 318, 319; AB Type pregnancy, 216; B Type baby, 312, 313; B Type pregnancy, 155–56; O Type baby, 301, 302; O Type pregnancy, 39–40; Pureed Meats, 416
Medications, avoiding during pregnancy, 24
Meditation; A Type pregnancy, 146–47; B Type pregnancy, 206–7
Membrane fluidizer cocktail, 176, 235–36
Menu plans; A Type pregnancy, 128–35, 136–43; AB Type pregnancy, 236–43, 245–53, 254–61; B Type pregnancy, 177–84, 187–94, 196–203; O Type pregnancy, 63–68, 71–77, 78–85
Mesclun Salad, 364
Millet; Couscous, 349; -Spelt-Soy Pancakes, 385; Tabbouleh, 348
Minerals. *See* Supplements
Mint Yogurt Drink, 399
Miscarriages; blood type and, 6–7; Rh sensitization and, 12
Miso. *See also* Tofu; Miso Dressing, 405; Miso Soup, 359
Mixed Mushroom Salad, 367
Mixed Roots Soup, 356

Mood swings, 21; A Type pregnancy, 118; AB
  Type pregnancy, 234–35; B Type pregnancy,
  176; O Type pregnancy, 62
Morning sickness, 20; B Type pregnancy,
  175–76; O Type pregnancy, 61
Mothers, recipes, 321–411
Motherwort, milk production and, 289
Movement in pain control, 35
Mucus production; A Type pregnancy, 128;
  AB Type pregnancy, 245
Mushrooms; Barley Soup with Spinach, 361;
  Grilled Portabello, 375–76; Lasagna with
  Portabello, and Pesto, 340–41; Mixed, Salad,
  367; Zucchini and, Frittata, 379–80

Nausea, 20
Nosebleeds, 26
Nuts and seeds; A Type pregnancy, 101–2; AB
  Type pregnancy, 219–20; B Type pregnancy,
  159; O Type pregnancy, 43–44

Oils and fats; A Type pregnancy, 101; AB Type
  pregnancy, 219; B Type pregnancy, 158–59;
  O Type pregnancy, 43
Old-Fashioned Yankee Pot Roast, 325
Olive Oil and Lemon Dressing, 407
One-Egg Omelet, 377–78
Onions; Artichoke and Vidalia, Tart, 378–79;
  Vidalia, Vinaigrette, 407
O Type baby, 297–302; colic, 298; diaper rash,
  299; diarrhea, 298; diet, 299–302; ear infections, 299; food allergies, 297; gastric distress, 297–98; restlessness/hyperactivity, 299
O Type blood, anti-A and anti-B antibodies, 6
O Type mother, 271–75; breast-feeding power
  foods, 292
O Type pregnancy, 37–94; allergic reactions,
  69–70; appetite, 69; blood-building needs,
  93; blood-clotting ability, 71; blood pressure,
  78; blood sugar, 69; Candida infections,
  70–71; detoxification, 55; diet, 37–85;
  emotional health, 57–58; exercise, 58–59;
  85–89; food cravings and aversions, 62–63;
  hemorrhoids, 70; herbal remedies, 90, 91,
  92; labor and delivery, 93–94; mood swings,
  62; supplements, 56–57, 89–92; swelling and
  edema, 77; thyroid activity, 54–55; varicose
  veins, 70; weight control, 53–54

Pain control in labor and delivery, 35–36
Pancakes; Amaranth, 385–86; Barley-Spelt,
  384–85; Brown Rice-Spelt, 386; Millet-Spelt-
  Soy, 385; Wheat-free Waffle Batter, 386–87
Pan-Fried Liver and Onions, 326–27
Papaya-Kiwi Drink, 401
Pasta and noodles. See also Grains, breads, rice,
  and pasta; Cellophane Noodles with Grilled
  Sirloin and Green Vegetables, 341–42; Cold
  Buckwheat Noodles with Peanut Sauce,
  343; Fettuccine with Grilled Lamb
  Sausages and Vegetables, 342–43; Green
  Leafy Pasta, 340; Lasagna with Portabello
  Mushrooms and Pesto, 340–41; Pasta (Rice
  or Spelt) with Rappini, 343–44; Quinoa
  Flour Tortillas with Pureed Pinto Beans,
  344–45; Soba Noodles with Pumpkin and
  Tofu, 339; Stuffed Shells with Pesto,
  339–40
Peanut Chicken, 323
Peanut Sauce, 343
Pears; Baby's First, 414; Sautéed, 394
Perineal massage, 31
Pesto, 409–10
Peter's Escargot, 329
Pineapple; -Apricot Silken Smoothie, 402–3;
  Protein Shake, 400; Yogurt Drink, 398–99
Plantains, Mashed, 373
Plums, 414; Barbecue Sauce, 410
Postpartum period, 269–71; A Type mother,
  275–79; AB Type mother, 282–85; B Type
  mother, 279–82; O Type mother, 271–75
Poultry. See Chicken; Meats and poultry; Turkey
Pregnancy; herbs to avoid during, 24; medica-
  tions to avoid during, 24
Prenatal supplements, 23
Pre-pregnancy checklist, 16–17
Pumpkin-Almond Bread, 381
Pureed Black-Eyed Peas, 412
Pureed Green Beans, 412
Pureed Meats, 416
Pureed Pinto Beans, 345
Pureed Pinto Beans with Garlic, 347

Quinoa; Almond Muffins, 382; Flour Tortillas
  with Pureed Pinto Beans, 344–45; Risotto,
  350

Rabbit, Braised, 322
Raisin Peanut Balls, 388
Rashes in A Type baby, 304
Raw Enzyme Relish, 410–11
Recipes. See Specific recipes
Relaxation techniques, in pain control, 35
Respiratory infection, in B Type baby, 309
Restlessness; A Type baby, 305; B Type baby,
  310; O Type baby, 299
Rh factor, 11–12
Rice. See also Grains, breads, rice, and pasta;
  Adzuki Bean and Sweet Brown, 353;
  /Almond Milk, 403–4; Brown, Pilaf, 350–51;
  Brown, -Spelt Pancakes, 386; Grilled Wild,
  Tempeh, 337; with Mushrooms (cereal),
  416; Speltberry and, Salad, 349–50; Spelt-
  berry and Basmati, Pilaf, 349; Sticks and
  Tofu with Vegetables, 332; -Vegetable
  Puree, 415; Wild, Salad, 351; Wild and
  Basmati, Pilaf, 348; Wild or Basmati,
  Pudding, 390

Roast Chicken with Garlic and Herbs, 328
Roast Turkey, 327–28
Rose Water Lassi, 399–400

Salads; Barley Black Bean, 352–53; Black-Eyed Peas and Barley, 352; Caesar, 368–69; Carrot Raisin, 367; Citrus, 395; Cole Slaw, 363–64; Fresh Fig, 394; Greek, 366; Green Bean, with Walnuts and Goat Cheese, 370; Grilled Chicken, 369–70; Grilled Sweet Potato, 369; Lentil, 346–47; Mesclun, 364; Mixed Mushroom, 367; Salmon with Wakame Seaweed, 366–67; Sardine, 366; Smoked Mackerel, 369; Speltberry, 351–52; Spelt-berry and Rice, 349–50; Spinach, 365; Super Broccoli, 364; Tropical, 395–96; Watchdog, 365; Wild Rice, 351
Salmon with Wakame Seaweed, 366–67
Sandwiches, 376–77
Sardines; Salad, 366; Swiss Chard with, 374
Sassy Smoothie, 401
Sauces. See also Marinades; Apple Onion Confit, 410; Chutney-Yogurt, 323; Cucumber Yogurt, 408; Fresh Mint, 408; Peanut, 343; Pesto, 409–10; Plum Barbecue, 410; Tamari Dipping, 342
Seafood; A Type pregnancy, 98–99; AB Type pregnancy, 216–18; Broiled Salmon Steaks, 329; Broiled Salmon with Lemongrass, 328; B Type pregnancy, 156–57; Fried Monkfish, 329–30; O Type pregnancy, 40–41; Peter's Escargot, 329; Salmon with Wakame Sea-weed, 366–67; Shrimp Kabobs, 330; Simple Fish Soup, 363; Smoked Mackerel Salad, 369; Steamed Whole Red Snapper, 330–31
Seaweed Dressing, 406–7
Second trimester, 26; common conditions, 26–27; diet and meal plans, 68–77, 126–35, 184–94, 243–53; exercise, 27–28, 87–88, 144–46, 204–5, 262–63
Seeds. See also Nuts and seeds; Tamari Toasted Sunflower, 388; Toasted Tamari Pumpkin, 389
Sesame Broccoli, 375
Sesame Chicken, 322–23
Shrimp Kabobs, 330
Silica in O Type Pregnancy, 57
Silken Scramble, 336
Simple Fish Soup, 363
Sitz baths for postpartum discomfort, 270
Smoked Mackerel Salad, 369
Snacks; Raisin Peanut Balls, 388; Tamari Toasted Sunflower Seeds, 388; Toasted Tamari Pumpkin Seeds, 389; Trail Mix or Gorp, 387–88
Soba Noodles with Pumpkin and Tofu, 339
Solid foods, 294–95
Soups and stews; Adzuki Bean and Pumpkin or Winter Squash Soup, 360; Basic Stock, 353–54; Beef Stew with Green Beans and Carrots, 355–56; Carrot-Tofu Soup with Dill, 357–58; Cream of Lima Bean Soup, 358; Cuban Black Bean Soup, 362; Cucum-ber-Yogurt Soup, 360; Farmer's Vegetable Soup, 358–59; Fresh Cherries and Yogurt Soup, 356–57; Indian Lamb Stew with Spinach, 362–63; Jerusalem Artichoke Soup, 359–60; Lentil Soup, 357; Miso Soup, 359; Mixed Roots Soup, 356; Mushroom Barley Soup with Spinach, 361; Simple Fish Soup, 363; Turkey Soup, 355; Vegetable Stock, 354–55; White Bean and Wilted Greens Soup, 361
Soy Drinks, 400–403
Speltberry; and Basmati Rice Pilaf, 349; and Rice Salad, 349–50; Salad, 351–52
Spelt Bread, 381–82
Spices and Sweeteners; A Type pregnancy, 107–8; AB Type pregnancy, 224–26; B Type pregnancy, 164–66; O Type pregnancy, 49–50
Spicy Stir-Fried Tofu with Apricots and Al-monds, 337–38
Spinach; Frittata, 380; Indian Lamb Stew with, 362–63; Mushroom Barley Soup with, 361; Salad, 365
Squash; Adzuki Bean and Pumpkin or Winter, Soup, 360; Butternut, and Tofu with Mixed Vegetables, 333
Steamed Artichoke, 374
Steamed Whole Red Snapper, 330–31
Strawberries; and Banana, 413; -Banana Smoothie, 400; -Tofu Parfait, 413; Yogurt, 413
Stress; A Type pregnancy, 136; weight gain and, 31
Stuffed Shells with Pesto, 339–40
Super Baby Smoothie, 397–98
Super Broccoli Salad, 364
Supplements; A Type pregnancy, 112–14, 148–51; AB Type pregnancy, 231–32, 264–68; B Type pregnancy, 172–73, 207–11; O Type pregnancy, 56–57, 89–92
Sweeteners. See Spices and Sweeteners
Sweet Potatoes; Grilled, Salad, 369; Pancakes, 372
Swelling; B Type pregnancy, 194–95; O Type pregnancy, 77
Swiss Chard with Sardines, 374

Tahini Dressing, 405
Tamari; Dipping Sauce, 342; -Mustard Marinade, 324–25; Toasted Sunflower Seeds, 388
Tarts, Artichoke and Vidalia Onion Tart, 378–79
Tasty Tofu-Pumpkin Stir-Fry, 338
Teething Biscuits, 414–15
Tempeh. See also Tofu; Grilled Wild Rice, 337; Kabobs, 332–33

Teriyaki Tofu Steak, 338–39

Third trimester, 28–30; common conditions, 30–31; diet and meal plans, 77–85, 135–43, 194–203, 253–61; exercise, 31, 88–89, 146–47, 206–7, 263–64

Thyroid activity in O Type pregnancy, 54–55

Toasted Tamari Pumpkin Seeds, 389

Tofu. See also Miso; Tempeh; Banana Pudding, 393; and Black Bean Chili, 334; Butternut Squash and, with Mixed Vegetables, 333; Carob Protein Drink, 400; Carrot-, Soup with Dill, 357–58; Fruit Silken Scramble, 336; Jerusalem Artichoke Soup, 359–60; Kung Pao, and Chicken, 334–35; Miso Dressing, 405; Pumpkin Pudding, 393; Rice Sticks and, with Vegetables, 332; -Sesame Fry, 335–36; Silken Scramble, 336; Spicy Stir-Fried, with Apricots and Almonds, 337–38; Tasty, -Pumpkin Stir-Fry, 338; Teriyaki, Steak, 338–39; Vegetable Stir-Fry, 331

Trail Mix or Gorp, 387–88

Turkey; Basic Stock, 353–54; Burgers, 324; Cutlets, 326; Great Meatloaf, 326; Roast, 327–28; Soup, 355

Urinary tract infections, 31; AB Type pregnancy, 244; B Type pregnancy, 185

Varicose veins, 27; O Type pregnancy, 70

Vegetables; A Type baby, 305–6, 307; A Type pregnancy, 104–5; AB Type baby, 317, 318; AB Type pregnancy, 222–23; Baked Sweet Potatoes, 412; Braised Collards, 375; B Type baby, 311, 312; B Type pregnancy, 161–63; Carrots and Parsnips with Garlic and Cilantro, 371; Cauliflower with Garlic and Parsley, 372–73; Crustless Sweet Potato and Carrot Pie, 412; Eggplant Casserole, 371; Farmer's, Soup, 358–59; Fritters, 373–74; Glazed Turnips and Onions, 370–71; Grilled Pepper Medley, 372; Grilled Portabello Mushrooms, 375–76; Juices, 404–5; Mashed Plantains, 373; O Type baby, 300, 301; O Type pregnancy, 46–47; Pureed Black-Eyed Peas, 412; Pureed Green Beans, 412; Purees, 411; Sesame Broccoli, 375; Steamed Artichoke, 374; Stock, 354–55; Sweet Potato Pancakes, 372; Swiss Chard with Sardines, 374; Vegetable Purees, 411

Vitamin B; A Type pregnancy, 113; O Type pregnancy, 56

Vitamin B_{12}, fertility and, 19

Vitamin C; A Type pregnancy, 113; fertility and, 19

Vitamin E; A Type pregnancy, 113; fertility and, 19

Vitamin K in O Type pregnancy, 56

Vitamins. See Supplements

Walnut Vinaigrette, 409

Watchdog Salad, 365

Weight control; A Type pregnancy, 111; AB Type pregnancy, 228–29; B Type pregnancy, 169–70; O Type pregnancy, 53–54; stress and, 31

Weight lifting for O Type mother, 275

Wheat-Free Waffle Batter, 386–87

White Bean and Wilted Greens Soup, 361

Wild and Basmati Rice Pilaf, 348

Wild Rice Salad, 351

Yogurt; Chutney-, Sauce, 323; Cucumber-, Soup, 360; Drinks, 398–400; Fresh Cherries and, Soup, 356–57

Zinc; A Type pregnancy, 113; AB Type pregnancy, 232; fertility and, 19

Zucchini and Mushroom Frittata, 379–80

A FINAL NOTE

Dear Reader,

Eat Right 4 (for) Your Baby represents the next stage in a publishing success story that began seven years ago with *Eat Right 4 (for) Your Type*. With more than two million copies in print, in more than fifty languages, *Eat Right 4 (for) Your Type* has demonstrated that the blood type diet works to address the most pressing issues of health and well-being for people of all ages. *Cook Right 4 (for) Your Type*, the companion cookbook, available in hardcover and paperback, has enabled followers of the blood type diet to easily incorporate it into their daily lives.

The publication of *Live Right 4 (for) Your Type* in January 2001 took the blood type science to a deeper level, utilizing the ever-expanding body of scientific research to provide practical strategies for living fully according to your blood type. Each blood type life prescription shows how to adapt your lifestyle, achieve emotional balance, maximize your health, deal with stress, and fight the effects of aging and disease.

Live Right 4 (for) Your Type was so well received that in 2002 we added a further tool—*The Eat Right 4 (for) Your Type Complete Blood Type Encyclopedia*. This comprehensive reference guide introduces revolutionary blood type–specific protocols for more than three hundred medical conditions.

The study of blood type is at its heart the study of human individuality. The science of blood type tells us the ways in which people are unique. My goal has been to provide you with the tools you need to make the most of the special genetic blueprint provided by your blood type. I am delighted to offer the benefits of blood type living to a whole new generation, with the publication of *Eat Right 4 (for) Your Baby*.

I invite you to join me in reaping the benefits of living right for your blood type.

SINCERELY,
DR. PETER J. D'ADAMO

The Essential Companion to
Eat Right 4 (for) Your Baby

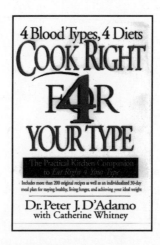

Cook Right 4 (for) Your Type
By Peter J. D'Adamo, with Catherine Whitney

This practical kitchen companion to *Eat Right 4 (for) Your Type*
includes more than 200 original recipes as well as an individualized
30-day meal plan for staying healthy, living longer, and achieving
your ideal weight. Now available in trade paperback.